# 100 CASE STUDIES
# IN PATHOPHYSIOLOGY

**Harold J. Bruyere, Jr., Ph.D.**

PROFESSOR EMERITUS
UNIVERSITY OF WYOMING
LARAMIE, WYOMING

Wolters Kluwer | Lippincott Williams & Wilkins
Health

Philadelphia • Baltimore • New York • London
Buenos Aires • Hong Kong • Sydney • Tokyo

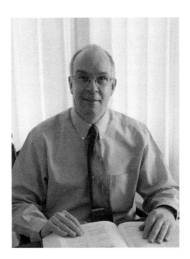

Professor Bruyere has 30 years of experience teaching students in human medicine, pharmacy, nursing, and the allied health professions. He has been a member of the faculty at the University of Wisconsin, the University of Wyoming, and the University of Washington.

T he primary purpose of *100 Case Studies in Pathophysiology* is to provide students beginning their formal education in the health sciences with a resource they can use to begin to develop their clinical problem-solving and critical thinking skills. This workbook, which provides a strong link between theory and practice, was designed for use by medical, pharmacy, nursing, and allied health educators and their students. The basic concept that underlies this workbook is that clinical manifestations of an illness are directly associated with the pathophysiology of human disease.

This workbook provides a straightforward approach to integrating basic pathophysiology, risk factors, physical examination findings, and clinical laboratory data for 100 significant health problems in the United States today. Some of the case studies were written from comprehensive interviews with patients, some are composites of case studies reported in the medical literature, and others are drawn from my personal experiences. Review summaries of selected major health problems allow students to develop effective methods of clinical assessment and disease management. In addition, the principles and concepts of underlying disease processes presented here will further prepare students for the study of basic pharmacology.

## Goals of This Workbook

The three major goals of this workbook are:

* To provide a basic, straightforward, and current resource tool for medical, pharmacy, nursing, and allied health students who have minimal experience interpreting a medical case study or a patient's medical record;
* To provide students in the health sciences with an opportunity to develop their clinical problem-solving skills by identifying clinical manifestations, abnormal clinical laboratory data, and risk factors for a variety of significant health disorders;
* To provide an opportunity for students in the health sciences to develop their clinical critical thinking skills by selecting appropriate disease management options through a case study approach.

## The Audience

This workbook is unique in that it was designed for students in human medicine, pharmacy, nursing, and the allied health sciences to support early courses in basic pathophysiology or general pathology. I made the assumption that students who would use this workbook had not completed courses in pharmacology and were novices regarding drug treatment. I also assumed that students would be learning for the first time how to problem solve and think critically with a medical case study before them.

The use of case studies in this workbook does not require extensive knowledge and experience in human medicine, pharmacy, or nursing. Case studies are basic, concise, and introduce the student to new medical terms and medical abbreviations that are commonly used by health professionals. Each patient case also incorporates important clinical signs, symptoms, and laboratory data that are consistent with a specific health problem. The student will use tables of clinical laboratory reference values (e.g., normal white blood cell count, normal serum sodium or potassium concentrations) to recognize data collected from case study patients that are abnormal and suggestive of specific disease states.

The workbook can be used to complement a variety of basic pathophysiology or pathology textbooks. *100 Case Studies in Pathophysiology* also can be used by itself as a concise and effective review of concepts previously learned.

## ■■ Organizational Philosophy

This book uses the organ systems approach to categorize human diseases and other health conditions. This approach allows the instructor to cover conditions in a logical and efficient manner (e.g., cardiovascular disorders, gastrointestinal disorders, or respiratory disorders). However, instructors must ensure that an anatomic and physiologic review of the appropriate organ system has been completed before students begin each of the case studies. Success in working through each case presentation presupposes fundamental knowledge of the normal anatomy and physiology of the appropriate organ system. For example, a complete review of the anatomy and physiology of the heart is essential before completing the case studies in Part 1, Cardiovascular Disorders, such as "Acute Myocardial Infarction" and "Congestive Heart Failure."

This workbook contains a wide range of pertinent clinical information so that students may better interpret and assess each case study patient. Seven appendices are included for patient assessment purposes:

- Appendix A: Table of Clinical Reference Values
- Appendix B: Table of Normal Height and Weight in Children
- Appendix C: Table of Blood Pressure in Children
- Appendix D: Table of Karnovsky Performance Status
- Appendix E: Table of Common Medical Abbreviations
- Appendix F: Table of APGAR Scoring for Newborns
- Appendix G: Questionnaire of Quality of Life in Epilepsy (QOLIE-31)

## ■■ Case Study Structure

The organization of *100 Case Studies in Pathophysiology* provides health science instructors and students with a logical and efficient method for integrating the pathophysiology of health conditions with appropriate clinical information. Each case study is divided into a Patient Case of a specific health condition and the supporting Disease Summary (found on the accompanying CD-ROM).

### Patient Cases

Patient Cases are found in the printed workbook. Although the structure of each case is similar, it is not identical. This variability is intentional so that students will understand that patient medical records vary significantly by individual healthcare providers. The cases present detailed information that simulates real-life patients. I have included questions that assess understanding in each Patient Case. The basic structure of the Patient Case in this workbook includes the following components:

- **Patient's Chief Complaints**
- **History of Present Illness**
- **Past Medical History**
- **Family History**
- **Social History**
- **Medications**
- **Allergies**
- **Review of Systems**
- **Physical Examination Findings** (including vital signs)
- **Laboratory Blood Test Results**
- **Specialized Test Results** (e.g., urinalysis, chest x-ray, or electrocardiogram)

### Disease Summaries

There is one Disease Summary on the CD-ROM to accompany each Patient Case in the workbook. Questions within many of the Disease Summaries assess the student's understanding or require the student to conduct more extensive research of the medical literature. Boldface is used to draw students' attention to especially important key concepts, and many key terms are italicized and defined. Each Disease Summary is presented in the following order:

- **Definition** of the medical condition
- **Prevalence** of the medical condition in the United States with a focus on age, gender, and racial/ethnic group predispositions
- **Significance** of the medical condition with emphasis on bothersome symptoms, mortality rates, and national economic implications
- **Causes and Risk Factors** of the medical condition
- **Pathophysiology** of the medical condition based on established research findings
- **Diagnosis:** (based on) **Clinical Manifestations and Laboratory Tests**
- **Appropriate Therapy** with a focus on the primary goals of treatment and common non-pharmacologic, pharmacologic, and surgical approaches
- **Serious Complications and Prognosis** (i.e., the consequences of failure to treat the condition appropriately)

# Learning Objectives

The major objective of this case studies book is to provide a current and close correlation between basic principles of human disease and clinical practice. It is important for students to thoroughly understand the underlying pathophysiologic processes that are present in the patients they will serve. Additionally, understanding basic pathophysiologic mechanisms of human disease ultimately promotes better decision-making efforts by healthcare providers and a better quality of life for their patients.

By working through the case studies in this workbook, students will:

- Strengthen their vocabulary in human medicine, pharmacy, and nursing;
- Develop an ability to recognize clinical signs and symptoms that are consistent with a large group of common human health conditions;
- Develop an ability to identify abnormal clinical laboratory test results that are consistent with a variety of human health disorders;
- Develop clinical problem-solving and critical thinking skills;
- Gain insights for specific treatments and methods of clinical assessment.

# Student and Instructor Resources

## Student Resources

The CD-ROM included with this book and the Student Resource Center at http://thePoint. lww.com/bruyere includes the following materials:

- The Disease Summary for each case study, including definition, prevalence, significance, causes and risk factors, pathophysiology, diagnosis, appropriate treatment, and serious complications and prognosis.
- An Image Bank that contains more than 150 color photographs and illustrations from the text to enhance the student's understanding of a wide range of medical conditions presented in the workbook. These figures will help students master the concepts and principles of pathophysiology. The tables from the book are also included.

## Instructor Resources

We understand the demand on an instructor's time, so to help make your job easier, you will have access to Instructor Resources upon adoption of *100 Case Studies in Pathophysiology*. In addition to the student resources just listed, an Instructor's Resource Center at http://thePoint.lww.com/bruyere includes the following:

- Answers to the questions found in the Disease Summary and Patient Case sections of this product

## ■■ Suggestions for Future Editions

I made every effort to ensure that all information presented in *100 Case Studies in Pathophysiology* is current and accurate. However, I encourage readers to contact me by email at hbruyere@uwyo.edu with corrections and suggestions that will make the next edition of this workbook better than the first.

## ■■ Acknowledgments

This workbook is a direct result of my 30-year career of teaching pathology and pathophysiology to students in human medicine, pharmacy, nursing, and the allied health sciences. The workbook also is the product of an extensive medical literature search that spanned four years, numerous drafts of the manuscript, and a rigorous review process. However, a workbook such as *100 Case Studies in Pathophysiology* cannot be developed without the personal contributions of numerous individuals. I am indebted to them all and pleased to have the opportunity to provide some recognition to them.

Initially, I would like to extend my deepest appreciation to my beloved wife, Kathy, and my amazing children, Travis and Kimberly, for their strong support, encouragement, and understanding during this lengthy project.

Two professional colleagues to whom I owe so very much are Enid Gilbert-Barness, MD, PhD (my major professor at the University of Wisconsin—Madison) and H. John Baldwin, PhD (former Dean at the University of Wyoming School of Pharmacy). There is no one on this earth who has taught me as much pathology and as much about effectively teaching pathology as Dr. Gilbert-Barness. She has been a role model and friend whom I have respected and admired for more than 35 years. Furthermore, this workbook would never have been contemplated had it not been for the profound influence that Dr. Gilbert-Barness has had in my life.

Dr. H. John Baldwin recognized qualities and abilities in me that I apparently overlooked in myself. He hired me for my first tenure-track faculty appointment at the University of Wyoming in 1987. More importantly, he also provided me with strong leadership and support that allowed me to develop as a teacher and researcher and be promoted to full professor in 1999. I will always be grateful for his contributions to the success of my career.

Four of my former colleagues and friends at the University of Wisconsin—Madison were very instrumental in my decision to pursue a teaching and research career in pathology— Chirane Viseskul, MD; Sunita Arya, MD; Ken Gilchrist, MD; and Tom Warner, MD. I will not forget the encouragement and guidance that they afforded me during those early years of my career.

I would also like to thank all of those individuals who, with openness and honesty, have shared their medical histories with me during the last four years, but especially Mary Lee, Kathy Bruyere, and the late Merrill Buckley.

*100 Case Studies in Pathophysiology* is also a reflection of the talents of all those who participated in the development and review processes. These include eight expert reviewers and the staff at Lippincott Williams & Wilkins, coordinated by Meredith Brittain—my patient, understanding, and competent managing editor.

Finally, I would like to acknowledge the numerous medical, pharmacy, nursing, and allied health students at the University of Wisconsin—Madison and the University of Wyoming with whom I have worked closely in the classroom during the past 30 years. They have made significant contributions with their insights, stories, and questions and have helped to ensure that this case studies workbook was developed with both clarity and quality.

# REVIEWERS

**Yvonne Alles, MBA, RMT**

*Department Coordinator, Allied Health*
*School of Health Professions*
*Davenport University*
*Grand Rapids, Michigan*

**Kathy Bode, RN, MS**

*Professor, Division of Health*
*Flint Hills Technical College*
*Emporia, Kansas*

**Dana Marie Grzybicki, MD, PhD**

*Assistant Professor of Biomedical Informatics*
 *and Pathology*
*College of Medicine*
*University of Pittsburgh*
*Pittsburgh, Pennsylvania*

**Jeff Kushner, PhD**

*Associate Professor of ISAT*
*College of Integrated Science and Technology*
*James Madison University*
*Harrisonburg, Virginia*

**Treena Lemay, BScN**

*Professor, Health and Community*
 *Studies*
*Algonquin College of Applied Arts*
 *and Technology*
*Pembroke, Ontario, Canada*

**Ruth Martin-Misener, MN, PhD**

*Coordinator, NP Programs*
*Dalhousie University*
*Halifax, Nova Scotia, Canada*

**John P. McNamara, MS, DC**

*Associate Professor*
*Biomedical Sciences Department*
*Jefferson College of Health Sciences*
*A Carilion Clinic Affiliate*
*Roanoke, Virginia*

**M. Margaret Rayman Stinner, RN, MS**

*Instructor*
*Mount Carmel College of Nursing*
*Columbus, Ohio*

# CONTENTS

# PART

# 1

# CARDIOVASCULAR DISORDERS

# ACUTE MYOCARDIAL INFARCTION

 *For the Disease Summary for this case study, see the CD-ROM.*

# PATIENT CASE

## ■ Patient's Chief Complaints

"I'm having pain in my chest and it goes up into my left shoulder and down the inside of my left arm. I'm also having a hard time catching my breath and I feel somewhat sick to my stomach."

## ■ History of Present Illness

Mr. W.G. is a 53-year-old white man who began to experience chest discomfort while playing tennis with a friend. At first he attributed his discomfort to the heat and having had a large breakfast. Gradually, however, discomfort intensified to a crushing sensation in the sternal area and the pain seemed to spread upward into his neck and lower jaw. The nature of the pain did not seem to change with deep breathing. When Mr. G. complained of feeling nauseated and began rubbing his chest, his tennis partner was concerned that his friend was having a heart attack and called 911 on his cell phone. The patient was transported to the ED of the nearest hospital and arrived within 30 minutes of the onset of chest pain. En route to the hospital, the patient was placed on nasal cannulae and an IV D$_5$W was started. Mr. G. received aspirin (325 mg po) and 2 mg/IV morphine. He is allergic to meperidine (rash). His pain has eased slightly in the last 15 minutes but is still significant; was 9/10 in severity; now 7/10. In the ED, chest pain was not relieved by 3 SL NTG tablets. He denies chills.

## ■ Past Medical History

- Ulcerative colitis × 22 years
- HTN × 12 years (poorly controlled due to poor patient compliance)
- Type 2 DM × 5 years
- S/P AMI 5 years ago that was treated with cardiac catheterization and PTCA; chronic stable angina for the past 4 years
- BPH × 2 years
- Hypertriglyceridemia
- Adenomatous colonic polyps

## Family History

- Father died from myocardial infarction at age 55, had DM
- Mother died from breast cancer at age 79
- Patient has one sister, age 52, who is alive and well and one brother, age 44, with HTN
- Grandparents "may have had heart disease"

## Social History

- 40 pack-year history of cigarette smoking
- Married and lives with wife of 29 years
- Has two grown children with no known medical problems
- Full-time postal worker for 20 years, before that a baker for 8 years
- Occasional alcohol use, average of 2 beers/week
- Has never used street drugs

## Review of Systems

Positive for some chest pain with physical activity "on and off for a month or so," but the pain always subsided with rest

## Allergies

- Meperidine (rash)
- Trimethoprim-sulfamethoxazole (bright red rash and fever)

## Medications

- Amlodipine 5 mg po Q AM
- Glyburide 10 mg po Q AM, 5 mg po Q PM
- EC ASA 325 mg po QD
- Gemfibrozil 600 mg po BID
- Sulfasalazine 1.5 g po BID
- Terazosin 1 mg po HS

## Physical Examination and Laboratory Tests

### General Appearance

The patient is an alert and oriented white male who appears to be his stated age. He is anxious and appears to be in severe acute distress.

### Vital Signs

See Patient Case Table 1.1

| Patient Case Table 1.1 Vital Signs | | | | | | |
|---|---|---|---|---|---|---|
| BP | 160/98 right arm sitting | RR | 18 | HT | 5'10½" |
| P | 105 with occasional premature beat | T | 98.2°F | WT | 184 lbs |

## Skin

Cool, diaphoretic, and pale without cyanosis

## Neck

Supple without thyromegaly, adenopathy, bruits, or jugular venous distension

## Head, Eyes, Ears, Nose, and Throat

- Pupils equal at 3 mm, round, responsive to light and accommodation
- Extra-ocular muscles intact
- Fundi benign
- Tympanic membranes intact
- Pharynx clear

## Chest and Lungs

- No tenderness with palpation of chest wall
- No dullness with percussion
- Slight bibasilar inspiratory crackles with auscultation
- No wheezes or friction rubs

## Cardiac

- Tachycardia with occasional premature beat
- Normal $S_1$ and $S_2$
- No $S_3$, soft $S_4$
- No murmurs or rubs

## Abdomen

- Soft and non-tender
- Negative for bruits and organomegaly
- Bowel sounds heard throughout

## Musculoskeletal/Extremities

- Normal range of motion throughout
- Muscle strength on right 5/5 UE/LE; on left 4/5 UE, 5/5 LE
- Pulses 2+
- Distinct bruit over left femoral artery
- No pedal edema

## Neurological

- Cranial nerves II–XII intact
- Cognition, sensation, gait, and deep tendon reflexes within normal limits
- Negative for Babinski sign

## Laboratory Blood Test Results (3½ hours post-AMI)

See Patient Case Table 1.2

| Patient Case Table 1.2 Laboratory Blood Test Results | | | | | |
|---|---|---|---|---|---|
| Na | 133 meq/L | Mg | 1.9 mg/dL | CK-MB | 6.3 IU/L |
| K | 4.3 meq/L | $PO_4$ | 2.3 mg/dL | Troponin I | 0.3 ng/mL |
| Cl | 101 meq/L | Chol | 213 mg/dL | Hb | 13.9 g/dL |
| $HCO_3$ | 22 meq/L | Trig | 174 mg/dL | Hct | 43% |
| BUN | 14 mg/dL | LDL | 143 mg/dL | WBC | 4,900/mm$^3$ |
| Cr | 0.9 mg/dL | HDL | 34 mg/dL | Plt | 267,000/mm$^3$ |
| Glu, fasting | 264 mg/dL | CPK | 99 IU/L | $HbA_{1c}$ | 8.7% |

## Arterial Blood Gases

- pH 7.42
- $PaO_2$ 90 mm
- $PaCO_2$ 34 mm
- $SaO_2$ 96.5%

## Electrocardiogram

4 mm ST segment elevation in leads $V_2$–$V_6$

## Chest X-Ray

Bilateral mild pulmonary edema (<10% of lung fields) without pleural disease or widening of the mediastinum

## Clinical Course

Patient history showed no contraindications to thrombolysis. The patient received IV reteplase, IV heparin, metoprolol, and lisinopril. Approximately 90 minutes after initiation of reteplase therapy, the patient's chest pain and ST segment elevations had resolved and both heart rate and blood pressure had normalized. The patient was stable until two days after admission when he began to experience chest pain again. Emergency angiography revealed a 95% obstruction in the left anterior descending coronary artery. No additional myocardium was at risk—consistent with single-vessel coronary artery disease and completed AMI. Percutaneous transluminal coronary angioplasty of the vessel was successfully performed, followed by placement of a coronary artery stent. After the stent was placed, the patient received abciximab infusion. Ejection fraction by echocardiogram three days post-AMI was 50% and the patient's temperature was 99.5°F. The remainder of the patient's hospital stay was unremarkable. He was gradually ambulated, physical activity was slowly increased, and he was discharged eight days post-AMI.

*Patient Case Question 1.* Cite *six* risk factors that predisposed this patient to acute myocardial infarction.

*Patient Case Question 2.* In which Killip class is this patient's acute myocardial infarction?

*Patient Case Question 3.* For which condition is this patient taking amlodipine?

*Patient Case Question 4.* For which condition is this patient taking glyburide?

*Patient Case Question 5.* For which condition is this patient taking gemfibrozil?

*Patient Case Question 6.* For which condition is this patient taking sulfasalazine?

*Patient Case Question 7.* For which condition is this patient taking terazosin?

*Patient Case Question 8.* Are there any indications that this patient needed oxygen supplementation during his hospital stay?

***Patient Case Question 9.*** Cite *four* clinical signs that suggest that acute myocardial infarction has occurred in the left ventricle and not in the right ventricle.

***Patient Case Question 10.*** Which single laboratory test provides the clearest evidence that the patient has suffered acute myocardial infarction?

***Patient Case Question 11.*** Based on the patient's laboratory tests, what type of treatment approach may be necessary to prevent another acute myocardial infarction?

***Patient Case Question 12.*** What is suggested by the "distinct bruit over the left femoral artery"?

***Patient Case Question 13.*** What is the pathophysiologic mechanism for elevated temperature that occurred several days after the onset of acute myocardial infarction?

***Patient Case Question 14.*** Does this patient satisfy the clinical criteria for *metabolic syndrome*?

# 2 ANEURYSM OF THE ABDOMINAL AORTA

 *For the Disease Summary for this case study, see the CD-ROM.*

# PATIENT CASE

## ■ History of Present Illness

J.A. is an 83-year-old male who presents to his PCP complaining of a "strange rhythmic, throbbing sensation in the middle of his abdomen." He has sensed this feeling for the past three days. For the past several weeks he has also experienced deep pain in his lower back that "feels like it is boring into my spine." He describes the pain as persistent but may be relieved by changing position. "I think that I hurt my back lifting some firewood," he explains. The patient has never smoked.

*Patient Case Question 1.* Given the diagnosis, what is probably causing this patient's lower back pain?

## ■ Past Medical History

- Triple coronary artery bypass surgery at age 73
- History of cluster headache
- History of PUD
- History of OA
- History of psoriasis
- Recent history of hypercholesterolemia

## ■ Medications

- Celecoxib 200 mg po QD
- Aspirin 81 mg po QD
- Clopidogrel 75 mg po QD
- Simvastatin 20 mg po HS
- Multivitamin tablet QD

***Patient Case Question 2.*** For which health condition is the patient taking celecoxib, and what is the basic pharmacologic mechanism of action for this medication?

***Patient Case Question 3.*** For which health condition is the patient taking simvastatin, and what is the basic pharmacologic mechanism of action for this medication?

***Patient Case Question 4.*** For which health condition is the patient taking clopidogrel, and what is the basic pharmacologic mechanism of action for this medication?

# ▬ Physical Examination and Laboratory Tests

Auscultation of the abdomen revealed a significant bruit over the aorta. Palpation of the abdomen revealed an abnormally wide pulsation of the abdominal aorta with some tenderness. When questioned, the patient denied nausea, vomiting, urinary problems, loss of appetite, heart failure, drug allergies, and a history of family members who had been diagnosed with an aortic aneurysm.

***Patient Case Question 5.*** What is a bruit?

The patient's vital signs were as follows: BP 150/95; HR 83; RR 14; T 98.8°F; WT 158 lbs; HT 5′9″

***Patient Case Question 6.*** Based on the patient's vital signs, which type of medication is indicated?

A CBC was ordered and the results of the CBC are shown in Patient Case Table 2.1

| Patient Case Table 2.1 Complete Blood Count | | | |
|---|---|---|---|
| Hb | 13.9 g/dL | **WBC Differential** | |
| Hct | 43% | Neutrophils | 59% |
| WBC | 5,100/mm³ | Lymphocytes | 32% |
| RBC | 6.0 million/mm³ | Monocytes/Macrophages | 5% |
| Plt | 315,000/mm³ | Eosinophils | 3% |
| ESR | 6 mm/hr | Basophils | 1% |

***Patient Case Question 7.*** What important information can be gleaned from the patient's CBC?

Laboratory blood tests were ordered and the results are shown in Patient Case Table 2.2

| Patient Case Table 2.2 Laboratory Blood Test Results | | | | | |
|---|---|---|---|---|---|
| $Na^+$ | 145 meq/L | Glu, fasting | 112 mg/dL | AST | 15 IU/L |
| $K^+$ | 4.9 meq/L | Uric acid | 2.9 mg/dL | ALT | 37 IU/L |
| $Cl^-$ | 104 meq/L | BUN | 9 mg/dL | Total bilirubin | 1.0 mg/dL |
| $Ca^{+2}$ | 8.7 mg/dL | Cr | 0.7 mg/dL | Cholesterol | 202 mg/dL |
| $Mg^{+2}$ | 2.3 mg/dL | Alk Phos | 79 IU/L | HDL | 50 mg/dL |
| $PO_4^{-3}$ | 3.0 mg/dL | PSA | 11.6 ng/mL | LDL | 103 mg/dL |
| $HCO_3^-$ | 27 meq/L | Alb | 3.5 g/dL | Trig | 119 mg/dL |

***Patient Case Question 8.*** Which single abnormal laboratory value has to be of most concern?

An abdominal x-ray was performed, a localized dilation of the abdominal aorta was visualized, and calcium deposits were seen within the aortic aneurysm.

***Patient Case Question 9.*** What has caused the calcium deposits in the aorta?

***Patient Case Question 10.*** What type of imaging test is now most appropriate in this patient?

An abdominal aortic aneurysm of 6.5 cm in diameter was located at the level of the renal arteries and extended downward into the iliac arteries.

***Patient Case Question 11.*** Would a "wait-and-see" approach be appropriate or should surgery be advised for this patient?

***Patient Case Question 12.*** Would surgical excision and graft placement or endovascular stent placement be more appropriate treatment for this patient?

# CONGESTIVE HEART FAILURE

 *For the Disease Summary for this case study, see the CD-ROM.*

## PATIENT CASE

### ■ History of Present Illness

H.J. presented to the ER late one evening complaining of a "racing heartbeat." She is an over-weight, 69-year-old white female, who has been experiencing increasing shortness of breath during the past two months and marked swelling of the ankles and feet during the past three weeks. She feels very weak and tired most of the time and has recently been waking up in the middle of the night with severe breathing problems. She has been sleeping with several pillows to keep herself propped up. Five years ago, she suffered a transmural (i.e., through the entire thickness of the ventricular wall), anterior wall (i.e., left ventricle) myocardial infarction. She received two-vessel coronary artery bypass surgery 4½ years ago for obstructions in the left anterior descending and left circumflex coronary arteries. Her family history is positive for atherosclerosis as her father died from a heart attack and her mother had several CVAs. She had been a three pack per day smoker for 30 years but quit smoking after her heart attack. She uses alcohol infrequently. She has a nine-year history of hypercholesterolemia. She is allergic to nuts, shellfish, strawberries, and hydralazine. Her medical history also includes diagnoses of osteoarthritis and gout. Her current medications include celecoxib, allopurinol, atorvastatin, and daily aspirin and clopidogrel. The patient is admitted to the hospital for a thorough examination.

*Patient Case Question 1.* Based on the limited amount of information given above, do you suspect that this patient has developed *left-sided CHF*, *right-sided CHF*, or *total CHF*?

*Patient Case Question 2.* How did you arrive at your answer to Question 1?

*Patient Case Question 3.* What is a likely cause for this patient's heart failure?

*Patient Case Question 4.* From the information given above, identify *three* risk factors that probably contributed to the patient's heart attack five years ago.

*Patient Case Question 5.* Why is this patient taking allopurinol?

*Patient Case Question 6.* Why is this patient taking atorvastatin?

*Patient Case Question 7.* Why is this patient taking celecoxib?

*Patient Case Question 8.* Why is this patient taking aspirin and clopidogrel?

## ■■■ Physical Examination and Laboratory Tests

### Vital Signs

BP = 125/80 (left arm, sitting); P = 125 and regular; RR = 28 and labored; T = 98.5°F oral; Weight = 215 lb; Height = 5'8"; patient is appropriately anxious

### Head, Eyes, Ears, Nose, and Throat

- Funduscopic examination normal
- Pharynx and nares clear
- Tympanic membranes intact

### Skin

- Pale with cool extremities
- Slightly diaphoretic

### Neck

- Neck supple with no bruits over carotid arteries
- No thyromegaly or adenopathy
- Positive JVD
- Positive HJR

*Patient Case Question 9.* What can you say about this patient's blood pressure?

*Patient Case Question 10.* Why might this patient be tachycardic?

*Patient Case Question 11.* Why might this patient be tachypneic?

*Patient Case Question 12.* Is this patient technically *underweight, overweight, obese,* or is her weight *healthy?*

*Patient Case Question 13.* Explain the pathophysiology of the abnormal skin manifestations.

*Patient Case Question 14.* Do abnormal findings in the neck (JVD and HJR) suggest *left heart failure, right heart failure,* or *total CHF?*

### Lungs

- Bibasilar rales with auscultation
- Percussion was resonant throughout

### Heart

- PMI displaced laterally
- Normal $S_1$ and $S_2$ with distinct $S_3$ at apex
- No friction rubs or murmurs

### Abdomen

- Soft to palpation with no bruits or masses
- Significant hepatomegaly and tenderness observed with deep palpation

## Extremities

- 2+ pitting edema in feet and ankles extending bilaterally to mid-calf region
- Cool, sweaty skin
- Radial, dorsal pedis and posterior tibial pulses present and moderate in intensity

## Neurological

- Alert and oriented × 3 (to place, person, and time)
- Cranial and sensory nerves intact
- DTRs 2+ and symmetric
- Strength is 3/5 throughout

## Chest X-Ray

- Prominent cardiomegaly
- Perihilar shadows consistent with pulmonary edema

## ECG

- Sinus tachycardia with waveform abnormalities consistent with LVH
- Pronounced Q waves consistent with previous myocardial infarction

## ECHO

Cardiomegaly with poor left ventricular wall movement

## Radionuclide Imaging

EF = 39%

*Patient Case Question 15.* Which abnormal cardiac exam and chest x-ray findings closely complement one another?

*Patient Case Question 16.* Which abnormal cardiac exam and ECG findings closely complement one another?

## Laboratory Blood Test Results

See Patient Case Table 3.1

| Patient Case Table 3.1 Laboratory Blood Test Results | | | |
|---|---|---|---|
| $Na^+$ | 153 meq/L | $PaCO_2$ | 53 mm Hg |
| $K^+$ | 3.2 meq/L | $PaO_2$ | 65 mm Hg (room air) |
| BUN | 50 mg/dL | WBC | 5,100/mm$^3$ |
| Cr | 2.3 mg/dL | Hct | 41% |
| Glu, fasting | 131 mg/dL | Hb | 13.7 g/dL |
| $Ca^{+2}$ | 9.3 mg/dL | Plt | 220,000/mm$^3$ |
| $Mg^{+2}$ | 1.9 mg/dL | Alb | 3.5 g/dL |
| Alk phos | 81 IU/L | TSH | 1.9 µU/mL |
| AST | 45 IU/L | $T_4$ | 9.1 µg/dL |
| pH | 7.35 | | |

*Patient Case Question 17.* What might the abnormal serum $Na^+$ and $K^+$ levels suggest?

*Patient Case Question 18.* Explain the abnormal BUN and serum Cr concentrations.

*Patient Case Question 19.* What might be causing the elevated serum glucose concentration?

*Patient Case Question 20.* Explain the abnormal serum AST level.

*Patient Case Question 21.* Explain the abnormal arterial blood gas findings.

*Patient Case Question 22.* Which of the hematologic findings, if any, are abnormal?

*Patient Case Question 23.* What do the TSH and $T_4$ data suggest?

*Patient Case Question 24.* Identify four drugs that might be immediately helpful to this patient.

*Patient Case Question 25.* Ejection fraction is an important cardiac function parameter that is used to determine the contractile status of the heart and is measured with specialized testing procedures. If a patient has an SV = 100 and an EDV = 200, is EF abnormally *high, low,* or *normal?*

# ■■■ Clinical Course

After administration of low doses of the diuretics hydrochlorothiazide (which blocks sodium reabsorption) and triamterene (which reduces potassium excretion), the patient voided 4,500 mL clear, yellow urine during the first 24 hours and another 3,500 mL during the second day post-admission. Bibasilar "crackles" and dependent edema also subsided. The patient lost three pounds in total body weight.

Vital signs were as follows: BP = 115/80 (right arm, sitting); P = 88 and regular; RR = 16 and unlabored; $PaO_2$ (room air) = 90; $PaCO_2$ = 44. H.J. was discharged on day 4 with prescription medicines and orders to pursue a follow-up with a cardiologist as soon as possible.

# 4 DEEP VENOUS THROMBOSIS

 *For the Disease Summary for this case study, see the CD-ROM.*

## PATIENT CASE

### ■ History of Present Illness

J.B. is an overweight, 58-year-old man who has had swelling in his left foot and ankle and pain in his left calf for six days. The pain has been getting worse for the past 24 hours. The patient ranks the pain as 8/10. He has made an appointment today with his PCP.

### ■ Past Medical History

- Previous episode of DVT at age 54; treated with warfarin for 1 year
- Diagnosed with diabetes mellitus type 2, 5 years ago

A preliminary diagnosis of DVT is made and the patient is admitted to the hospital for a thorough clinical workup.

### ■ Family History

- Father died at age 63 from myocardial infarction
- Mother alive at age 80 with diabetes mellitus type 2
- Brother, age 56, alive and healthy
- No family history of venous thromboembolic disease reported

### ■ Social History

- Patient is single and lives alone
- Works as dean of pharmacy school, 11 years
- 28 pack-year smoking history, currently smokes 1 pack per day
- Drinks 3–4 beers/day during the week and a 6-pack/day on weekends
- No history of illicit drug use

# ■■ Medications

- Glyburide 5 mg po QD × 3 years
- Denies taking any over-the-counter or herbal products

---

**Patient Case Question 1.** For what condition is this patient taking glyburide?

**Patient Case Question 2.** What is the basic pharmacologic mechanism of action for glyburide?

---

# ■■ Allergies

- Penicillin causes a rash
- Cat dander causes watery eyes and sneezing

# ■■ Physical Examination and Laboratory Tests

## General

J.B. is a pleasant, overweight, white male in moderate acute distress from leg pain.

## Vital Signs

BP = 130/80; P = 110; RR = 16; T = 99.8°F; Ht = 5′10″; Wt = 245 lb; $SaO_2$ = 98% on room air

---

**Patient Case Question 3.** Which two of J.B.'s vital signs are abnormal and why are these abnormal vital signs consistent with a diagnosis of DVT?

**Patient Case Question 4.** Is J.B. considered *underweight, overweight,* or *obese* or is his weight technically considered *normal and healthy?*

---

## Head, Eyes, Ears, Nose, and Throat

- Atraumatic
- Pupils equal, round, and reactive to light and accommodation
- Extra-ocular movements intact
- Fundi normal
- Normal sclera
- Ears and nose clear
- Tympanic membranes intact
- Oral mucous membranes pink and moist

## Neck

- Supple
- No cervical adenopathy
- Thyroid non-palpable

- No carotid bruits
- No jugular venous distension

## Chest

- Bilateral wheezing
- No crackles

## Heart

- Regular rate and rhythm
- Distinct $S_1$ and $S_2$
- No $S_3$ or $S_4$
- No murmurs, rubs, or gallops

## Abdomen

- Soft, non-tender, and non-distended
- No masses, guarding, rebound, or rigidity
- No organomegaly
- Normal bowel sounds

## Genitalia

- Normal penis and testes

## Rectal

- No masses
- Heme-negative brown stool

## Extremities

- No clubbing or cyanosis
- Left foot and ankle swollen
- Left calf swollen to twice normal size
- No tenderness, pain, swelling, or redness, right lower extremity

## Neurological

- Alert and oriented × 3
- No neurologic deficits noted

## Laboratory Blood Test Results

See Patient Case Table 4.1

| Patient Case Table 4.1 Laboratory Blood Test Results | | | | | | | |
|---|---|---|---|---|---|---|---|
| $Na^+$ | 145 meq/L | Cr | 0.9 mg/dL | RBC | 5.2 million/mm³ | HDL | 30 mg/dL |
| $K^+$ | 4.9 meq/L | Glu, fasting | 160 mg/dL | AST | 17 IU/L | LDL | 152 mg/dL |
| $Cl^-$ | 112 meq/L | Hb | 15.1 g/dL | ALT | 8 IU/L | Trig | 160 mg/dL |
| $HCO_3^-$ | 23 meq/L | Hct | 42% | Alk phos | 100 IU/L | ESR | 23 mm/hr |
| $Ca^{+2}$ | 9.7 mg/dL | WBC | 12,200/mm³ | PT | 12.9 sec | | |
| BUN | 10 mg/dL | Plt | 270,000/mm³ | Cholesterol | 280 mg/dL | | |

## Specialized Serum Laboratory Testing

Homocys, 91 μmol/L

## Hypercoagulability Profile

- (−) factor V Leiden mutation
- (−) prothrombin 20210A mutation
- (+) protein C deficiency
- (−) protein S deficiency
- (−) antithrombin III deficiency

*Patient Case Question 5.* Identify *two* risk factors for DVT from the laboratory data directly above.

*Patient Case Question 6.* Identify *two* other abnormal laboratory findings consistent with a diagnosis of DVT.

*Patient Case Question 7.* Identify *three* other abnormalities from the laboratory data above that may be unrelated to DVT but nevertheless should be addressed by the patient's PCP.

## Doppler Ultrasound

- Left lower extremity shows no flow of the left posterior tibial vein
- Normal flow demonstrated within the left common femoral and iliac veins
- Right lower extremity shows normal flow of the deep venous system from the level of the common femoral to posterior tibial vein

## ▬ Diagnosis

Deep vein thrombosis of the left posterior tibial vein

*Patient Case Question 8.* Prior to warfarin therapy, list two drugs that may serve as *initial* treatment for this patient.

*Patient Case Question 9.* For how long should this patient be treated with warfarin?

# CASE STUDY

# 5

## HYPERTENSION

 *For the Disease Summary for this case study, see the CD-ROM.*

## PATIENT CASE

### ■ HPI

E.W. is a 40-year-old African American male, who has had difficulty controlling his HTN lately. He is visiting his primary care provider for a thorough physical examination and to renew a prescription to continue his blood pressure medication.

### ■ PMH

- Chronic sinus infections
- Hypertension for approximately 11 years
- Pneumonia 6 years ago that resolved with antibiotic therapy
- One major episode of major depressive illness caused by the suicide of his wife of 15 years, 5 years ago
- No surgeries

### ■ FH

- Father died at age 49 from AMI; had HTN
- Mother has DM and HTN
- Brother died at age 20 from complications of CF
- Two younger sisters are A&W

### ■ SH

The patient is a widower and lives alone. He has a 15-year-old son who lives with a maternal aunt. He has not spoken with his son for four years. The patient is an air traffic controller at the local airport. He smoked cigarettes for approximately 10 years but stopped smoking when he was diagnosed with HTN. He drinks "several beers every evening to relax" and does not pay particular attention to the sodium, fat, or carbohydrate content of the foods that he eats. He admits to "salting almost everything he eats, sometimes even before tasting it." He denies ever having dieted. He takes an occasional walk but has no regular daily exercise program.

*Patient Case Question 1.* Identify *six* risk factors for hypertension in this patient's history.

## Meds

- Hydrochlorothiazide 50 mg po QD
- Pseudoephedrine hydrochloride 60 mg po q6h PRN
- Beclomethasone dipropionate 1 spray into each nostril q6h PRN

*Patient Case Question 2.* Why is the patient taking hydrochlorothiazide and what is the primary pharmacologic mechanism of action of the drug?

*Patient Case Question 3.* Why is the patient taking pseudoephedrine hydrochloride and what is the primary pharmacologic mechanism of action of the drug?

*Patient Case Question 4.* Why is the patient taking beclomethasone dipropionate and what is the primary pharmacologic mechanism of action of the drug?

## All

Rash with penicillin use

## ROS

- States that his overall health has been fair to good during the past 12 months
- Weight has increased by approximately 20 pounds during the last year
- Denies chest pain, shortness of breath at rest, headaches, nocturia, nosebleeds, and hemoptysis
- Reports some shortness of breath with activity, especially when climbing stairs, and that breathing difficulties are getting worse
- Denies any nausea, vomiting, diarrhea, or blood in the stool
- Self-treats occasional right knee pain with OTC extra-strength acetaminophen
- Denies any genitourinary symptoms

*Patient Case Question 5.* What is the most clinically significant information related to HTN in this review of systems?

## Physical Exam and Lab Tests

### Gen

The patient is an obese black man in no apparent distress. He appears to be his stated age.

## Vital Signs

See Patient Case Table 5.1

| Patient Case Table 5.1 Vital Signs | | | |
|---|---|---|---|
| Average BP | 155/96 mm Hg (sitting) | Ht | 5'11" |
| HR | 73 and regular | Wt | 221 lb |
| RR | 15 and unlabored | BMI | 31.0 |
| T | 98.8°F | | |

*Patient Case Question 6.* Identify the *two* most clinically significant vital signs relative to this patient's HTN.

## HEENT

- TMs intact and clear throughout
- No nasal drainage
- No exudates or erythema in oropharynx
- PERRLA, pupil diameter 3.0 mm bilaterally
- Sclera without icterus
- EOMI
- Funduscopy reveals mild arteriolar narrowing with no nicking, hemorrhages, exudates, or papilledema

*Patient Case Question 7.* What is the significance of the HEENT examination?

## Neck

- Supple without masses or bruits
- Thyroid normal
- (−) lymphadenopathy

## Lungs

- Mild basilar crackles bilaterally
- No wheezes

## Heart

- RRR
- Prominent $S_3$ sound
- No murmurs or rubs

*Patient Case Question 8.* Which abnormalities in the heart and lung examinations may be related and why might these clinical signs be related?

## Abd

- Soft and ND
- NT with no guarding or rebound
- No masses, bruits, or organomegaly
- Normal BS

## Rectal/GU

- Normal size prostate without nodules or asymmetry
- Heme (−) stool
- Normal penis and testes

## Ext

- No CCE
- Limited ROM right knee

## Neuro

- No sensory or motor abnormalities
- CNs II–XII intact
- Negative Babinski
- DTRs = 2+
- Muscle tone = 5/5 throughout

**Patient Case Question 9.** Are there any abnormal neurologic findings and, if so, might they be caused by HTN?

## Laboratory Blood Test Results

See Patient Case Table 5.2

| Patient Case Table 5.2 Laboratory Blood Test Results | | | | | | | |
|---|---|---|---|---|---|
| Na | 139 meq/L | RBC | 5.9 million/mm³ | Mg | 2.4 mg/dL |
| K | 3.9 meq/L | WBC | 7,100/mm³ | PO$_4$ | 3.9 mg/dL |
| Cl | 102 meq/L | AST | 29 IU/L | Uric acid | 7.3 mg/dL |
| HCO$_3$ | 27 meq/L | ALT | 43 IU/L | Glu, fasting | 110 mg/dL |
| BUN | 17 mg/dL | Alk phos | 123 IU/L | T. cholesterol | 275 mg/dL |
| Cr | 1.0 mg/dL | GGT | 119 IU/L | HDL | 31 mg/dL |
| Hb | 16.9 g/dL | T. bilirubin | 0.9 mg/dL | LDL | 179 mg/dL |
| Hct | 48% | T. protein | 6.0 g/dL | Trig | 290 mg/dL |
| Plt | 235,000/mm³ | Ca | 9.3 mg/dL | PSA | 1.3 ng/mL |

**Patient Case Question 10.** Why might this patient's GGT be abnormal?

**Patient Case Question 11.** Identify *three* other clinically significant lab tests above.

## Urinalysis

See Patient Case Table 5.3

| Patient Case Table 5.3 Urinalysis | | | |
|---|---|---|---|
| *Appearance* | Clear and amber in color | *Microalbuminuria* | (+) |
| *SG* | 1.017 | *RBC* | 0/hpf |
| *pH* | 5.3 | *WBC* | 0/hpf |
| *Protein* | (−) | *Bacteria* | (−) |

***Patient Case Question 12.*** What is the clinical significance of the single abnormal urinalysis finding?

## ECG

Increased QRS voltage suggestive of LVH

## ECHO

Moderate LVH with EF = 46%

***Patient Case Question 13.*** What is the likely pathophysiologic mechanism for LVH in this patient?

***Patient Case Question 14.*** What does the patient's EF suggest?

# CASE STUDY

## 6

# HYPOVOLEMIC SHOCK

 *For the Disease Summary for this case study, see the CD-ROM.*

# PATIENT CASE

Ms. K.Z., a 22-year-old university coed, was rushed to the emergency room 35 minutes after sustaining multiple stab wounds to the chest and abdomen by an unidentified assailant. A witness had telephoned 911.

Paramedics arriving at the scene found the victim in severe acute distress. Vital signs were obtained: HR 128 (baseline 80), BP 80/55 (baseline 115/80), RR 37 and labored. Chest auscultation revealed decreased breath sounds in the right lung consistent with basilar atelectasis (i.e., collapsed lung). Pupils were equal, round, and reactive to light and accommodation. Her level of consciousness was reported as "awake, slightly confused, and complaining of severe chest and abdominal pain." Pedal pulses were absent, radial pulses were weak, and carotid pulses were palpable. The patient was immediately started on intravenous lactated Ringer's solution at a rate of 150 mL/hr.

---

**Patient Case Question 1.** With *two words*, identify the specific type of hypovolemic shock in this patient.

---

An electrocardiogram monitor placed at the scene of the attack revealed that the patient had developed sinus tachycardia. She was tachypneic, became short of breath with conversation, and reported that her heart was "pounding in her chest." She appeared to be very anxious and continued to complain of pain. Her skin and nail beds were pale but not cyanotic. Skin turgor was poor. Peripheral pulses were absent with the exception of a thready brachial pulse. Capillary refill time was approximately 7–8 seconds. Doppler ultrasound had been required to obtain an accurate BP reading. The patient's skin was cool and clammy. There was a significant amount of blood on her dress and on the pavement near where she was lying.

---

**Patient Case Question 2.** Based on the patient's clinical manifestations, approximately how much of her total blood volume has been lost?

---

During transport to the hospital, vital signs were reassessed: HR 138, BP 75/50, RR 38 with confusion. She was diagnosed with hypovolemic shock and IV fluids were doubled. Blood samples were sent for typing and cross-matching and for both chemical and hematologic analysis.

Laboratory test results are shown in Patient Case Table 6.1

## Patient Case Table 6.1 Laboratory Test Results

| Hb | 8 g/dL | $PaO_2$ | 53 mm Hg | pH | 7.31 |
|---|---|---|---|---|---|
| Hct | 25% | $PaCO_2$ | 52 mm Hg | $SaO_2$ | 84% on RA |

*Patient Case Question 3.* How many units of whole blood are minimally required?

*Patient Case Question 4.* Is it necessary that sodium bicarbonate be administered to the patient at this time?

Oxygen was started at 3 L/min by nasal cannula. Repeat arterial blood gases were: $PaO_2$ 82 mm Hg, $PaCO_2$ 38 mm Hg, pH 7.36, $SaO_2$ 95%.

*Patient Case Question 5.* Are arterial blood gas results improving or deteriorating?

ER physicians chose not to start a central venous line. An indwelling Foley catheter was inserted with return of 180 mL of amber-colored urine. Urine output measured over the next hour was 14 mL. Ms. Z's condition improved after resuscitation with 1 L lactated Ringer's solution and two units packed red blood cells over the next hour.

*Patient Case Question 6.* Based on urine output rate, in which class of hypovolemic shock can the patient be categorized at this time?

Laboratory blood test results are shown in Patient Case Table 6.2

## Patient Case Table 6.2 Laboratory Test Results

| Na | 136 meq/L | BUN | 37 mg/dL | PTT | 33 sec |
|---|---|---|---|---|---|
| K | 3.5 meq/L | Cr | 1.9 mg/dL | Ca | 9.0 mg/dL |
| Cl | 109 meq/L | Glu, random | 157 mg/dL | Plt | 178,000/mm³ |
| $HCO_3$ | 25 mg/dL | PT | 12.1 sec | WBC | 6,300/mm³ |

*Patient Case Question 7.* Explain the pathophysiology of the abnormal BUN and Cr.

*Patient Case Question 8.* Does the patient have a blood clotting problem?

*Patient Case Question 9.* Explain the pathophysiology of the abnormal serum glucose concentration.

The patient was taken to the operating room for surgical correction of lacerations to the right lung, liver, and pancreas. There, she received an additional six units of type B+ blood. Surgery was successful and the patient was admitted to the ICU for recovery with the following vital signs: HR 104, BP 106/70, RR 21, urinary output 29 mL/hr. A repeat BUN and Cr revealed that these renal function parameters had returned to near-normal values (23 mg/dL and 1.4 mg/dL, respectively).

---

***Patient Case Question 10.*** Based on clinical signs after surgery, in which class of hypovolemic shock can the patient be categorized at this time?

# 7 INFECTIVE ENDOCARDITIS

 *For the Disease Summary for this case study, see the CD-ROM.*

## PATIENT CASE

### ■ HPI

Mr. H.Y. is a 63-year-old male, who presents to the ER with a two-day history of high-grade fever with chills. "I don't feel well and I think that I may have the flu," he tells the ER nurse and physician. He also complains of "some painful bumps on my fingers and toes that came on last night." He denies IVDA. When asked about recent medical or dental procedures, he responded: "I had an infected tooth removed about two weeks ago." He does not recall receiving any antibiotics either prior to or after the procedure.

*Patient Case Question 1.* Which type of infective endocarditis is suggested by the patient's clinical manifestations—acute or subacute?

### ■ PMH

- Asthma since childhood
- Rheumatic fever as a child × 2 with mitral valve replacement 2 years ago
- HTN × 20 years
- DM type 2, × 9 years
- COPD × 4 years
- H/O tobacco abuse
- Alcoholic liver disease

*Patient Case Question 2.* Which *three* of the illnesses in this patient's medical history may be contributing to the onset of infective endocarditis and why are these diseases considered risk factors?

## FH

- Mother died from CVA at age 59; also had ovarian cancer
- Father had H/O alcohol abuse; suffered AMI at age 54; DM type 2; died in his 60s from pancreatic cancer that "spread to his bones"

## SH

- Married for 43 years, recently widowed and lives alone
- Father of 4 and grandfather of 10
- One son lives in same city, but his other children live in other states
- Insurance salesman who retired last year
- Monthly income is derived from social security, retirement account, and a small life insurance benefit following his wife's death (breast cancer)
- Manages his own medications, has no health insurance, and pays for his medications himself
- 45 pack-year smoking history, but quit when he was diagnosed with emphysema
- Has a history of alcohol abuse, but quit drinking 4 years ago; continues to attend AA meetings regularly and is active in his church as an usher and Prayer Warrior

## ROS

- Patient denies any pain other than the lesions on his fingers and toes
- Denies cough, chest pain, breathing problems, palmar or plantar rashes, and vision problems
- (+) for mild malaise and some loss of appetite

*Patient Case Question 3.* What is the significance of the absence of breathing problems, chest pain, rashes, and visual problems?

## Meds

- Theophylline 100 mg po BID
- Albuterol MDI 2 puffs QID PRN
- Atrovent MDI 2 puffs BID
- Nadolol 40 mg po QD
- Furosemide 20 mg po QD
- Metformin 850 mg po BID

*Patient Case Question 4.* For which *two* disease states might the patient be taking theophylline?

*Patient Case Question 5.* Which medication or medications is the patient taking for diabetes?

*Patient Case Question 6.* Which medication or medications is the patient taking for high blood pressure?

## ■ All

Penicillin (rash, shortness of breath, significant swelling "all over")

**Patient Case Question 7.** Why are the clinical manifestations of the penicillin allergy so significant?

## ■ PE and Lab Tests

### Gen

The patient is a significantly overweight, elderly male in moderate acute distress. His skin is pale and he is slightly diaphoretic. He is shivering noticeably.

### Vital Signs

See Patient Case Table 7.1

| Patient Case Table 7.1 Vital Signs | | | | | |
|---|---|---|---|---|---|
| BP | 150/92 | RR | 23 and unlabored | Ht | 5'10" |
| P | 118 | T | 102.5°F | Wt | 252 lb |

**Patient Case Question 8.** Is this patient technically considered *overweight* or *obese*?

### Skin/Nails

- Very warm and clammy
- No rashes
- No petechiae or splinter hemorrhages in nail beds
- Multiple tattoos
- No "track" marks

**Patient Case Question 9.** What is the significance of the absence of "track" marks?

### HEENT

- Anicteric sclera
- PERRLA
- EOMI
- Conjunctiva WNL
- No retinal exudates
- TMs intact
- Nares clear
- Oropharynx benign and without obvious lesions

- Mucous membranes moist
- Poor dentition

## Neck

- Supple
- (−) for lymphadenopathy, JVD, and thyromegaly

## Heart

- Tachycardia with regular rhythm
- Normal $S_1$ and $S_2$
- Diastolic murmur along the left sternal border (not previously documented in his medical records), suggestive of aortic regurgitation

---

**Patient Case Question 10.** What is the most significant and relevant clinical finding in the physical examination so far and what is the pathophysiology that explains this clinical sign?

---

## Chest

- CTA throughout
- Equal air entry bilaterally
- No wheezing or crackles
- Chest is resonant on percussion

## Abd

- Soft and non-tender
- (+) bowel sounds
- No organomegaly

## Genit/Rect

Deferred

## Ext

- No CCE
- Reflexes bilaterally 5/5 in all extremities
- Small, tender nodules that range in color from red to purple in the pulp spaces of the terminal phalanges of the fingers and toes ("Osler nodes")

## Neuro

- No focal deficits noted
- A & O × 3

## Laboratory Blood Test Results

See Patient Case Table 7.2

| **Patient Case Table 7.2 Laboratory Blood Test Results** | | | | | |
|---|---|---|---|---|---|
| Na | 135 meq/L | Glu, random | 145 mg/dL | Bands | 7% |
| K | 3.7 meq/L | Hb | 14.1 g/dL | Lymphs | 12% |
| Cl | 100 meq/L | Hct | 40% | Monos | 1% |
| HCO$_3$ | 22 meq/L | Plt | 213,000/mm$^3$ | Alb | 4.0 g/dL |
| BUN | 17 mg/dL | WBC | 19,500/mm$^3$ | ESR | 30 mm/hr |
| Cr | 1.0 mg/dL | Neutros | 80% | Ca | 8.9 mg/dL |

***Patient Case Question 11.*** Identify *five* elevated laboratory test results that are consistent with a diagnosis of bacterial endocarditis.

***Patient Case Question 12.*** Explain the pathophysiology for *any three* of the five elevated laboratory results identified in Question 11 above.

***Patient Case Question 13.*** Identify *two* subnormal laboratory results that are consistent with a diagnosis of bacterial endocarditis.

## Urinalysis

The urine was pale yellow, clear, and negative for proteinuria and hematuria. A urine toxicology screen was also negative.

***Patient Case Question 14.*** Explain the pathophysiology of proteinuria and hematuria in a patient with infective endocarditis.

## ECG

Normal

## Transthoracic ECHO

A 3-cm vegetation on the aortic valve was observed. No signs of ventricular hypertrophy or dilation were seen.

## Blood Cultures

3 of 3 sets (+) for *Streptococcus viridans* (collection times 1030 Tuesday, 1230 Tuesday, 1345 Tuesday)

***Patient Case Question 15.*** What are the *six* diagnostic Modified Duke University criteria that favor a diagnosis of infective endocarditis in this patient?

***Patient Case Question 16.*** What is the appropriate pharmacologic treatment for this patient?

# 8

# PERIPHERAL ARTERIAL DISEASE

 *For the Disease Summary for this case study, see the CD-ROM.*

# PATIENT CASE

## ■ History of Present Illness

Mrs. R.B. is a 52-year-old woman with a 40-year history of type 1 diabetes mellitus. Although she has been dependent on insulin since age 12, she has enjoyed relatively good health. She has been very careful about her diet, exercises daily, sees her primary care provider regularly for checkups, and is very conscientious about monitoring her blood glucose levels and self-administration of insulin. She is slightly overweight and was diagnosed with hypertension four years ago. Her high blood pressure has been well controlled with a thiazide diuretic. She does not smoke and rarely drinks alcoholic beverages.

Mrs. B. was planning to shop at the local supermarket on Saturday, but her son telephoned her at the last minute and apologized that he had to work and could not drive her. Since she had only a few necessary items to pick up, she decided to walk the five blocks to the store. Rather than wear her usual walking shoes, she wore a pair of more fashionable shoes. Upon her return home, Mrs. B. removed her shoes and noticed a small blister on the ball of her right foot. She felt no discomfort from the blister. However, two days later, she was alarmed when she found that the blister had developed into a large, open wound that was blue-black in color. For the next two days, she carefully cleansed the wound and covered it with sterile gauze each time. The wound did not heal and, in fact, became progressively worse and painful. Her son urged her to seek medical attention, and five days after the initial injury she made an appointment with her primary care provider.

***Patient Case Question 1.*** Identify this patient's *two* most critical risk factors for peripheral arterial disease.

## ■ Current Status

Mrs. B.'s foot wound is approximately 1 inch in diameter and contains a significant amount of necrotic tissue and exudate. Furthermore, there is a lack of pink granulation tissue—an indication that the wound is not healing. The patient has a history of bilateral intermittent claudication, but denies pain at rest and recent numbness, tingling, burning sensations, and pain in her buttocks, thighs, calves, or feet. Examination of the peripheral pulses revealed normal bilateral femoral and popliteal pulses. However, the right dorsalis pedis artery and right posterior tibial artery pulses were not palpable. The patient has no history of coronary artery disease or cerebrovascular disease.

*Patient Case Question 2.* What level of peripheral arterial disease is suggested by her pulse examination: iliac disease, femoral disease, superficial femoral artery disease, or tibial disease?

*Patient Case Question 3.* Briefly describe the locations of the dorsalis pedis artery and posterior tibial artery pulses.

# ■■■Physical Examination and Laboratory Tests

A pallor test revealed level 3 pallor in the right lower leg and foot and level 1 pallor in the left lower extremity. Ankle-brachial tests were conducted.

*Left brachial systolic pressure: 130 mm*
*Left ankle systolic pressure: 110 mm*
*Right brachial systolic pressure: 125 mm*
*Right ankle systolic pressure: 75 mm*

*Patient Case Question 4.* What conclusions can be drawn from the pallor and ankle-brachial test results?

A careful physical examination of the patient's feet and legs revealed that both feet were cool to the touch and the toes on her right foot were slightly cyanotic. However, there was no mottling of the skin and sensory, reflex, and motor functions of both legs were intact. Her vital signs are shown in Patient Case Table 8.1.

| Patient Case Table 8.1 Vital Signs | | | | | |
|---|---|---|---|---|---|
| BP | 130/90 sitting | RR | 18 | Ht | 62″ |
| P | 95 and regular | T | 99.8°F | Wt | 145 lb |

*Patient Case Question 5.* Why is it likely that the patient's body temperature is elevated?

A sample of the patient's blood was drawn and submitted for analysis.

## Laboratory Blood Test Results

See Patient Case Table 8.2

| Patient Case Table 8.2 Laboratory Blood Test Results | | | | | | | |
|---|---|---|---|---|---|
| Hb | 15.1 g/dL | *Monocytes* | 3% | ESR | 20 mm/hr |
| Hct | 41% | *Eosinophils* | 1% | BUN | 10 mg/dL |
| Plt | 318,000/mm$^3$ | Na | 139 meq/L | Creatinine | 0.7 mg/dL |
| WBC | 11,900/mm$^3$ | K | 4.3 meq/L | T cholesterol | 291 mg/dL |
| Neutrophils | 80% | Cl | 108 meq/L | LDL | 162 mg/dL |
| Lymphocytes | 16% | Glu, fasting | 210 mg/dL | HDL | 26 mg/dL |

*Patient Case Question 6.* What major conclusions can be drawn from the patient's blood work?

*Patient Case Question 7.* Does Mrs. B. have any signs of renal insufficiency, a common chronic complication of diabetes mellitus?

# ■ Clinical Course

The patient was hospitalized and both wound and blood cultures were started. Mrs. B. was treated with broad-spectrum antibiotics while waiting for culture reports. The wound was packed with saline-soaked Kerlix gauze to facilitate debridement of necrotic tissue. The patient was provided continuous insulin by IV with frequent monitoring of blood glucose concentrations. Serum glucose levels were maintained at 80–100 mg/dL. An electrocardiogram was normal. Wound and blood culture reports were eventually completed. The wound was contaminated with gram-positive bacteria, but the blood culture was negative.

Magnetic resonance angiography of the right lower extremity was subsequently performed and a right tibial artery obstruction was identified. The section of diseased vessel was short (3.0 cm), but there was 70% narrowing of the artery. The angiogram also showed some degree of collateral circulation around the obstructing lesion. The patient underwent successful percutaneous angioplasty of the diseased vessel and placement of a stent to restore blood flow. The foot wound showed significant signs of healing after several days of bedrest and continued antibiotic therapy. A decision to perform an amputation of the right foot was averted.

*Patient Case Question 8.* Based on the information provided in the patient's clinical workup, what type of medication is ultimately necessary?

*Patient Case Question 9.* Why is it unlikely that a thrombus or embolus contributed to arterial obstruction in this case?

*Patient Case Question 10.* What is "Legs for Life"?

# PULMONARY THROMBOEMBOLISM

 *For the Disease Summary for this case study, see the CD-ROM.*

## PATIENT CASE

### ■■■ Patient's Chief Complaints

"I have severe chest pain and I can't seem to catch my breath. I think that I may be having a heart attack."

### ■■■ History of Present Illness

Mrs. V.A. is a 30-year-old woman who presents to the hospital emergency room following 90 minutes of chest pain. She describes the severity of her pain as 8 on a scale of 10. An hour-and-a-half ago, she developed sharp and constant right-sided chest pain and right-sided mid-back pain. The pain became worse when she attempted to lie down or take a deep breath and improved a little when she sat down. She also has had difficulty breathing. She denies any fever, chills, or coughing up blood. She reports that she just returned home 36 hours ago following a 13-hour flight from Tokyo.

***Patient Case Question 1.*** What clinical manifestations, if any, suggest a pulmonary embolus in this patient?

### ■■■ Past Medical History

* Migraines with aura since age 23
* Mild endometriosis × 5 years
* Positive for Protein S deficiency
* One episode of deep vein thrombosis 2 years ago; treated with warfarin for 1 year
* Acute sinusitis 1 year ago

### ■■■ Past Surgical History

* Orthopedic surgery for leg trauma at age 7
* Ovarian cyst removed 10 months ago

## ◼◼ Family History

- Father has hypertension
- Mother died from metastatic cervical cancer at age 49
- Brother is alive and well
- No family history of venous thromboembolic disease

## ◼◼ Social History

- Patient lives with her husband and 8-year-old daughter
- Monogamous relationship with her husband of 10 years; sexually active
- 12 pack-year smoking history; currently smokes 1 pack per day
- Business executive with active travel schedule
- Negative for alcohol use or intravenous drug abuse
- Occasional caffeine intake

## ◼◼ Medications

- 30 µg ethinyl estradiol with 0.3 mg norgestrel × 4 years
- Amitriptyline 50 mg po Q HS
- Cafergot 2 tablets po at onset of migraine, then 1 tablet po every 30 minutes PRN
- Metoclopramide 10 mg po PRN
- Ibuprofen 200 mg po PRN for cramps
- Multiple vitamin 1 tablet po QD
- Denies taking any herbal products

***Patient Case Question 2.*** Identify *five* major risk factors of this patient for pulmonary thromboembolism.

***Patient Case Question 3.*** Why do you think this patient is taking amitriptyline at bedtime every evening?

***Patient Case Question 4.*** Why is this patient taking metoclopramide as needed?

***Patient Case Question 5.*** What condition is causing cramps in this patient for which she requires ibuprofen?

## ◼◼ Review of Systems

- (–) cough or hemoptysis
- (–) headache or blurred vision
- (–) auditory complaints
- (–) lightheadedness
- (–) extremity or neurologic complaints
- All other systems are negative

## ◼◼ Allergies

- Demerol ("makes me goofy")
- Sulfa-containing products (widespread measles-like, pruritic rash)

# ■ Physical Examination and Laboratory Tests

## General

The patient is a well-developed white woman who appears slightly anxious, but otherwise is in no apparent distress.

## Vital Signs

See Patient Case Table 9.1

| Patient Case Table 9.1 Vital Signs | | | | | | | |
|---|---|---|---|---|---|---|---|
| BP | 126/75 | RR | 40, labored | WT | 139 lb | O₂ SAT | 99% on room air |
| P | 105, regular | T | 98.6°F | HT | 5′5″ | | |

*Patient Case Question 6.* Are any of the patient's vital signs consistent with pulmonary thromboembolism?

*Patient Case Question 7.* Is this patient technically considered *underweight, overweight,* or *obese* or is this patient's weight considered *normal and healthy?*

## Skin

- Fair complexion
- Normal turgor
- No obvious lesions

## Head, Eyes, Ears, Nose, and Throat

- Pupils equal, round, and reactive to light and accommodation
- Extra-ocular muscles intact
- Fundi are benign
- Tympanic membranes clear throughout with no drainage
- Nose and throat clear
- Mucous membranes pink and moist

## Neck

- Supple with no obvious nodes or carotid bruits
- Normal thyroid
- Negative for jugular vein distension

*Patient Case Question 8.* If the clinician had observed significant jugular vein distension, what is a reasonable explanation?

## Cardiovascular

- Rapid but regular rate
- No murmurs, gallops, or rubs

## Chest/Lungs

- No tenderness
- Subnormal diaphragmatic excursion
- No wheezing or crackles

## Abdomen

* Soft with positive bowel sounds
* Non-tender and non-distended
* No hepatomegaly or splenomegaly

## Breasts

Normal with no lumps

## Genit/Rect

* No masses or discharge
* Normal anal sphincter tone
* Heme-negative stool

## Musculoskeletal/Extremities

* Prominent saphenous vein visible in left leg with multiple varicosities bilaterally
* Peripheral pulses 1+ bilaterally
* No cyanosis, clubbing, or edema
* Strength 5/5 throughout
* Both feet cool to touch

## Neurological

* Alert and oriented to self, time, and place
* Cranial nerves II–XII intact
* Deep tendon patellar reflexes 2+

## Laboratory Blood Test Results

See Patient Case Table 9.2

| Patient Case Table 9.2 Laboratory Blood Test Results | | | | | | | |
|---|---|---|---|---|---|---|---|
| Na | 141 meq/L | HCO$_3$ | 27 meq/L | Hb | 11.9 g/dL | WBC | 5,300/mm$^3$ |
| K | 4.3 meq/L | BUN | 17 mg/dL | Hct | 34.8% | PTT | 25.0 sec |
| Cl | 110 meq/L | Cr | 1.1 mg/dL | Plt | 306,000/mm$^3$ | PT | 14.0 sec |

***Patient Case Question 9.*** Are any of the patient's laboratory blood tests significantly abnormal? Provide a reasonable explanation for each abnormal test.

***Patient Case Question 10.*** What might the patient's chest x-ray reveal?

## Electrocardiography

Sinus tachycardia

## Echocardiography

Ventricular wall movements within normal limits

## Lower Extremity Venous Duplex Ultrasonography

Both right and left lower extremities show abnormalities of venous narrowing, prominent collateral vessels, and incompressibility of the deep venous system in the popliteal veins. These findings are consistent with bilateral DVT.

## V/Q Scan

Perfusion defect at right base. Some mismatch between perfusion abnormality and ventilation of right lung, suggesting an intermediate probability for pulmonary embolus.

## Pulmonary Angiogram

Abrupt arterial cutoff in peripheral vessel in right base

*Patient Case Question 11.* Which *single* clinical finding provides the strongest evidence for pulmonary embolus in this patient?

*Patient Case Question 12.* Which is a more appropriate duration of treatment with warfarin in this patient: 3 months, 6 months, or long-term anticoagulation?

*Patient Case Question 13.* Is the use of a thrombolytic agent in this patient advisable?

*Patient Case Question 14.* Would you suspect that this patient's plasma D-dimer concentration is negative or elevated? Why?

*Patient Case Question 15.* Is *massive pulmonary thromboembolism* an appropriate diagnosis of this patient?

*Patient Case Question 16.* What is a likely cause of respiratory alkalosis in this patient?

*Patient Case Question 17.* Areas of ischemia in the lung from a pulmonary embolus usually become hemorrhagic. The patient whose chest x-ray is shown in Patient Case Figure 9.1 presented with chest pain, hypoxia, and lower limb deep vein thrombosis. Where is the hemorrhagic area—upper right lung, lower right lung, upper left lung, or lower left lung?

*Patient Case Question 18.* In terms of thrombus development, what is the fundamental difference between heparin and alteplase?

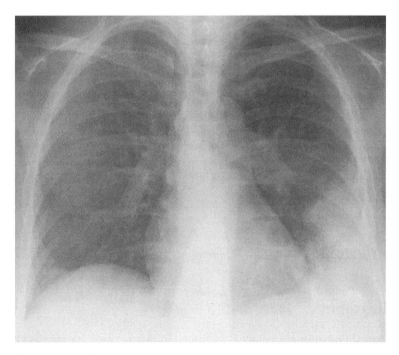

PATIENT CASE FIGURE 9.1

Chest x-ray from patient who presented with chest pain, hypoxia, and lower limb deep vein thrombosis. See Patient Case Question 17. (Reprinted with permission from Kahn GP and JP Lynch. Pulmonary Disease Diagnosis and Therapy: A Practical Approach. Philadelphia: Lippincott Williams & Wilkins, 1997.)

# 10 RHEUMATIC FEVER AND RHEUMATIC HEART DISEASE

 *For the Disease Summary for this case study, see the CD-ROM.*

# PATIENT CASE

## ▰▰ History of Present Illness

K.I. is a 14-year-old white female, who presents with her mother at the hospital emergency room complaining of a "very sore throat, a rash all over, and chills." She has had the sore throat for two days, but the rash and chills have developed within the past 12 hours.

## ▰▰ Past Medical History

- Negative for surgeries and hospitalizations
- Negative for serious injuries and bone fractures
- Measles, age 3
- Chickenpox, age 6
- Strep pharyngitis and severe case of rheumatic fever (arthritis, carditis, chorea), age 8, treated with ibuprofen and penicillin
- Has worn eyeglasses since age 12

## ▰▰ Family History

- Oldest of 6 siblings (3 sisters, 2 brothers)
- Father co-owns and manages tile company with his brother
- Mother is homemaker
- Youngest sister also developed strep pharyngitis and rheumatic fever 6 years ago

## ▰▰ Social History

- "A–B" student in 9th grade
- Would like to attend University of Wisconsin–Madison and major in computer science
- Enjoys reading, music, and using the internet

- Very active in various school activities, including soccer, chorus, journal club, and speech club
- Denies use of tobacco, alcohol, and illicit substances
- Denies sexual activity

# Medications

No prescribed or over-the-counter medicines

# Allergies

- No known drug allergies
- Hypersensitivity to poison ivy

# Physical Examination and Laboratory Tests

## General

The patient is a mildly nervous but cooperative, quiet, young, white female in no acute distress. Her face and hands are dirty and she is poorly dressed with regard to both clothing size and style. She has a slim build. Has difficulty engaging in conversation. Slightly guarded in responses and rarely makes eye contact. Answers all questions completely with a low speaking voice. Some fidgeting. No other odd or inappropriate motor behavior noted.

## Vital Signs

BP 103/75 lying down, right arm; P 89; RR 16; T 101.8°F; Wt 108 lb; Ht 5'3"

## Skin

- Very warm and slightly diaphoretic
- Widespread "scarlet" rash on arms, legs, chest, back, and abdomen
- Mild acne on forehead
- No bruises or other lesions

## HEENT

- Pupils equal, round, reactive to light and accommodation
- Extra-ocular muscles intact
- Fundi were not examined
- Tympanic membranes intact
- Teeth show no signs of erosion
- Throat shows erythema, tonsillar swelling/exudates/vesicles

## Neck/Lymph Nodes

- Neck supple
- Moderate bilateral cervical adenopathy
- Thyroid normal
- No carotid bruits
- No jugular vein distension

## Breasts

Normal without masses or tenderness

## Heart

- Regular rate and rhythm
- No murmurs, rubs, or gallops
- Normal $S_1$ and $S_2$
- No $S_3$ or $S_4$

## Lungs/Thorax

- Clear to auscultation
- No crackles or rales noted
- Patient denies any chest pain with deep breathing

## Abdomen

- Ticklish during exam
- Soft, supple, not tender, not distended
- No masses, guarding, rebound, or rigidity
- No hepatosplenomegaly
- Normal bowel sounds

## Genitalia/Rectal

- Normal external female genitalia
- Stool heme-negative

## Musculoskeletal/Extremities

- No cyanosis, clubbing, or edema
- Negative for joint pain
- Normal range of motion throughout
- Radial and pedal pulses 2+ bilaterally
- Grip strength 5/5 throughout

## Neurological

- Alert and oriented × 3
- Cranial nerves II → XII intact
- Deep tendon reflexes 2+
- No neurologic deficits noted

## Electrocardiogram

Normal

## Laboratory Blood Test Results

See Patient Case Table 10.1

### Patient Case Table 10.1 Laboratory Blood Test Results

| Na | 140 meq/L | Cl | 106 meq/L | Latex agglutination for group A strep | (+) |
|----|-----------|-----|-----------|---------------------------------------|-----|
| K | 4.2 meq/L | WBC | 16,500/mm³ | CRP | 19.5 mg/dL |
| Ca | 9.5 mg/dL | RBC | 5.3 million/mm³ | Anti-streptolysin O | (+) |

*Patient Case Question 1.* What is an appropriate diagnosis for this patient?

*Patient Case Question 2.* Identify *eleven* clinical manifestations that are consistent with your diagnosis above.

*Patient Case Question 3.* Why can rheumatic fever be ruled out as a diagnosis?

*Patient Case Question 4.* Does this patient have any signs of rheumatic heart disease?

*Patient Case Question 5.* What type of regular monitoring is necessary for this patient and why is this type of monitoring required?

*Patient Case Question 6.* Why is it expected that the patient's CRP is abnormal?

*Patient Case Question 7.* What is the pathophysiologic mechanism for cervical adenopathy in this patient?

*Patient Case Question 8.* What is the pathophysiologic mechanism for leukocytosis in this patient?

*Patient Case Question 9.* What is the drug of choice for this patient?

*Patient Case Question 10.* Identify *three* major risk factors for rheumatic fever in this patient.

# RESPIRATORY DISORDERS

# 11 ASBESTOSIS

 *For the Disease Summary for this case study, see the CD-ROM.*

# PATIENT CASE

## Patient's Complaints and History of Present Illness

Mr. R.I. is a 69-year-old man, who has been referred to the Pulmonary Disease Clinic by his nurse practitioner. He presents with the following chief complaints: "difficulty catching my breath and it is getting worse; a persistent, dry, and hacking cough; and a tight feeling in my chest." He is a retired construction contractor of 45 years, who primarily installed insulation materials in high-rise apartment and office buildings. He has been retired for four years and first began experiencing respiratory symptoms approximately six months ago. He has attributed those symptoms to "being a long-time smoker and it is finally catching up with me."

## Past Medical and Surgical History

- Appendectomy at age 13
- Osteoarthritis in left knee (high school football injury) × 30 years
- Status post-cholecystectomy, 16 years ago
- Benign prostatic hyperplasia, transurethral resection 7 years ago
- Hypertension × 7 years
- Hyperlipidemia × 4 years
- Gastroesophageal reflux disease × 4 years

## Family History

- Paternal history positive for coronary artery disease; father died at age 63 from "heart problems"
- Maternal history positive for cerebrovascular disease; mother died at age 73 "following several severe strokes"
- Brother died in a boating accident at age 17
- No other siblings

## Social History

- Previously divorced twice, but currently happily married for 23 years with 3 grown children (ages 40, 45, and 49)
- Enjoys renovating old houses as a hobby and watching NASCAR racing and football on television
- Smokes 1 pack per day × 45 years
- Rarely exercises
- Drinks "an occasional beer with friends on weekends" but has a history of heavy alcohol use
- Volunteers in the community at the food pantry and for Meals on Wheels
- No history of intravenous drug use
- May be unreliable in keeping follow-up appointments, supported by the remark "I don't like doctors"

## Review of Systems

- Denies rash, nausea, vomiting, diarrhea, and constipation
- Denies headache, chest pain, bleeding episodes, dizziness, and tinnitus
- Denies loss of appetite and weight loss
- Reports minor visual changes recently corrected with stronger prescription bifocal glasses
- Complains of generalized joint pain, but especially left knee pain
- Has never been diagnosed with chronic obstructive pulmonary disease or any other pulmonary disorder
- Denies paresthesias and muscle weakness
- Negative for urinary frequency, dysuria, nocturia, hematuria, and erectile dysfunction

## Medications

- Acetaminophen 325 mg 2 tabs po Q 6H PRN
- Ramipril 5 mg po BID
- Atenolol 25 mg po QD
- Pravastatin 20 mg po QD
- Famotidine 20 mg po Q HS

## Allergies

- Terazosin ("It makes me dizzy and I fell twice when I was taking it.")
- Penicillin (rash)

*Patient Case Question 1.* For which specific condition is the patient likely taking . . .

a. acetaminophen?

b. ramipril?

c. atenolol?

d. pravastatin?

e. famotidine?

# ■■ Physical Examination and Laboratory Tests

## General

The patient is a pleasant but nervous, elderly white gentleman. He appears pale but is in no apparent distress. He looks his stated age, has a strong Italian accent, and appears to be slightly overweight.

## Vital Signs

- Blood pressure (sitting, both arms) = average 131/75 mm Hg
- Pulse = 69 beats per minute
- Respiratory rate = 29 breaths per minute and slightly labored
- Temperature = 98.6°F
- Pulse oximetry = 95% on room air
- Height = 5'9"
- Weight = 179 lb

**Patient Case Question 2.** Does this patient have a *healthy* weight or is he technically considered *underweight, overweight,* or *obese?*

**Patient Case Question 3.** Which, if any, of the vital signs above is/are consistent with a diagnosis of asbestosis?

## Skin

- Pallor noted
- No lesions or rashes
- Warm and dry with satisfactory turgor
- Nail beds are pale

## Head, Eyes, Ears, Nose, and Throat

- Extra-ocular muscles intact
- Pupils equal at 3 mm with normal response to light
- Funduscopy within normal limits (no hemorrhages or exudates)
- No strabismus, nystagmus, or conjunctivitis
- Sclera anicteric
- Tympanic membranes within normal limits bilaterally
- Nares patent
- No sinus tenderness
- Oral pharyngeal mucosa clear
- Mucous membranes moist but pale
- Good dentition

**Patient Case Question 4.** What is the significance of an absence of hemorrhages and exudates on funduscopic examination?

## Neck and Lymph Nodes

- Neck supple
- Negative for jugular venous distension and carotid bruits
- No lymphadenopathy or thyromegaly

## Chest/Lungs

- Breathing labored with tachypnea
- Prominent end-inspiratory crackles in the posterior and lower lateral regions bilaterally
- Subnormal chest expansion
- Mild wheezing present

## Heart

- Regular rate and rhythm
- Normal $S_1$ and $S_2$
- Negative $S_3$ and $S_4$
- No murmurs or rubs noted

## Abdomen

- Soft, non-tender to pressure, and non-distended
- Normal bowel sounds
- No masses or bruits
- No hepatomegaly or splenomegaly

## Genitalia/Rectum

- Normal male genitalia, testes descended, circumcised
- Prostate normal in size and without nodules
- No masses or discharge
- Negative for hernia
- Normal anal sphincter tone
- Guaiac-negative stool

## Musculoskeletal/Extremities

- No clubbing, cyanosis, or edema
- Muscle strength 5/5 throughout
- Peripheral pulses 2+ throughout
- Decreased range of motion, left knee
- No inguinal or axillary lymphadenopathy

---

***Patient Case Question 5.*** What is the significance of the absence of jugular venous distension, hepato- and splenomegaly, extra cardiac sounds, and edema in this patient?

## Neurological

- Alert and oriented × 3
- Cranial nerves II–XII intact
- Sensory and proprioception intact
- Normal gait
- Deep tendon reflexes 2+ bilaterally

## Laboratory Blood Test Results

Blood was drawn for a standard chemistry panel and arterial blood gases. The results are shown in Patient Case Table 11.1.

**Patient Case Table 11.1 Laboratory Blood Test Results**

| Na | 142 meq/L | Cr | 0.9 mg/dL | WBC | 9,200/mm³ |
|----|-----------|-----|-----------|-----|-----------|
| K | 4.9 meq/L | Glu, fasting | 97 mg/dL | Plt | 430,000/mm³ |
| Cl | 105 meq/L | Ca | 9.1 mg/dL | pH | 7.35 |
| HCO₃ | 22 meq/L | Hb | 15.9 g/dL | PaO₂ | 83 mm Hg |
| BUN | 12 mg/dL | Hct | 41% | PaCO₂ | 47 mm Hg |

*Patient Case Question 6.* Is the patient *hypoxemic* or *hypercapnic?*

*Patient Case Question 7.* Is the patient *acidotic* or *alkalotic?*

## Pulmonary Function Tests (Spirometry)

- Vital capacity, 3200 cc
- Inspiratory reserve volume, 1700 cc
- Expiratory reserve volume, 1000 cc
- Tidal volume, 500 cc
- Total lung capacity, 4500 cc

*Patient Case Question 8.* Are the pulmonary function tests *normal*, consistent with *restrictive* respiratory disease, or consistent with *obstructive* respiratory disease?

*Patient Case Question 9.* Should supplemental oxygen be immediately given to this patient?

## Chest X-Ray

A posteroanterior radiograph showed coarse linear opacities at the base of each lung (more prominent on the left) that obscured the cardiac borders and diaphragm (*shaggy heart border sign*). These findings are consistent with asbestosis.

## High-Resolution CT Scan

Thickened septal lines and small, rounded, subpleural, intralobular opacities in the lower lung zone bilaterally suggest *fibrosis*. Ground-glass appearance involving air spaces in the upper lung zone bilaterally suggests *alveolitis*. Small, calcified diaphragmatic pleural plaques and mild "honeycomb" changes with cystic spaces less than 1 cm were seen bilaterally and are consistent with asbestosis.

*Patient Case Question 10.* What is the drug of choice for treating patients at this intermediate stage of asbestosis?

# CASE STUDY

# 12 | ASTHMA

 *For the Disease Summary for this case study, see the CD-ROM.*

# PATIENT CASE

## ■ Patient's Chief Complaints

With breathlessness: "Cold getting to me. Peak flow is only 65%. Getting worse."

## ■ History of Present Illness

D.R. is a 27 yo man, who presents to the nurse practitioner at the Family Care Clinic complaining of increasing SOB, wheezing, fatigue, cough, stuffy nose, watery eyes, and postnasal drainage—all of which began four days ago. Three days ago, he began monitoring his peak flow rates several times a day. His peak flow rates have ranged from 200 to 240 L/minute (baseline, 340 L/minute) and often have been at the lower limit of that range in the morning. Three days ago, he also began to self-treat with frequent albuterol nebulizer therapy. He reports that usually his albuterol inhaler provides him with relief from his asthma symptoms, but this is no longer sufficient treatment for this asthmatic episode.

## ■ Past Medical History

- Born prematurely at 6 months' gestation secondary to maternal intrauterine infection; weight at birth was 2 lbs, 0 ounces; lowest weight following delivery was 1 lb, 9 ounces; spent 2½ months in neonatal ICU and was discharged from hospital 2 weeks before mother's original due date
- Diagnosed with asthma at age 18 months
- Moderate persistent asthma since age 19
- Has been hospitalized 3 times (with 2 intubations) in the past 3 years for acute bronchospastic episodes and has reported to the emergency room twice in the past 12 months
- Perennial allergic rhinitis × 15 years

## ■ Family History

- Both parents living
- Mother 51 yo with H/O cervical cancer and partial hysterectomy
- Father 50 yo with H/O perennial allergic rhinitis and allergies to pets

- No siblings
- Paternal grandmother, step-grandfather and maternal grandmother are chain smokers but do not smoke around the patient

## Social History

- No alcohol or tobacco use
- Married with two biological children and one stepson
- College graduate with degree in business, currently employed as a business development consultant with private firm
- There are no pets in the home at this time

## Review of Systems

- Reports feeling unwell overall, "4/10"
- Denies H/A and sinus facial pain
- Eyes have been watery
- Denies decreased hearing, ear pain, or tinnitus
- Throat has been mildly sore
- (+) SOB and productive cough with clear, yellow phlegm for 2 days
- Denies diarrhea, N/V, increased frequency of urination, nocturia, dysuria, penile sores or discharge, dizziness, syncope, confusion, myalgias, and depression

## Medications

- Ipratropium bromide MDI 2 inhalations QID
- Triamcinolone MDI 2 inhalations QID
- Albuterol MDI 2 inhalations every 4–6 hours PRN

## Allergies

- Grass, ragweed, and cats → sneezing and wheezing

## Physical Examination and Laboratory Tests

### General

- Agitated, WDWN white man with moderate degree of respiratory distress
- Loud wheezing with cough
- Eyes red and watery
- Prefers sitting to lying down
- SOB with talking
- Speaks only in short phrases as a result of breathlessness

### Vital Signs

See Patient Case Table 12.1

| Patient Case Table 12.1 Vital Signs | | | | | |
|---|---|---|---|---|---|
| BP | 150/80 | RR | 24 | HT | 6'1" |
| P | 115 | T | 100.2°F | WT | 212 lbs |
| Pulsus paradoxus | 20 | Pulse ox | 92% (room air) | | |

***Patient Case Question 1.*** Based on the available clinical evidence, is this patient's asthmatic attack considered *mild, moderate,* or *bordering on respiratory failure?*

***Patient Case Question 2.*** What is the most likely trigger of this patient's asthma attack?

***Patient Case Question 3.*** Identify *three major* factors that have likely contributed to the development of asthma in this patient.

## Skin

- Flushed and diaphoretic
- No rashes or bruises

## HEENT

- EOMI
- PERRLA
- Fundi benign, no hemorrhages or exudates
- Conjunctiva erythematous and watery
- Nasal cavity erythematous and edematous with clear, yellow nasal discharge
- Hearing intact bilaterally
- TMs visualized without bulging or perforations
- Auditory canals without inflammation or obstruction
- Pharynx red with post-nasal drainage
- Uvula mid-line
- Good dentition
- Gingiva appear healthy

## Neck/Lymph Nodes

- Neck supple
- Trachea mid-line
- No palpable nodes or JVD noted
- Thyroid without masses, diffuse enlargement, or tenderness

## Chest/Lungs

- Chest expansion somewhat limited
- Accessory muscle use prominent
- Diffuse wheezes bilaterally on expiration and, occasionally, on inspiration
- Bilaterally decreased breath sounds with tight air movement

## Heart

- Tachycardia with regular rhythm
- No murmurs, rubs, or gallops
- $S_1$ and $S_2$ WNL

## Abdomen

- Soft, NT/ND
- No bruits or masses
- Bowel sounds present and WNL

## Genitalia/Rectum

Deferred

## Musculoskeletal/Extremities

- ROM intact in all extremities
- Muscle strength 5/5 throughout with no atrophy
- Pulses 2+ bilaterally in all extremities
- Extremities clammy but good capillary refill at 2 seconds with no CCE or lesions

## Neurological

- Alert and oriented to place, person, and time
- Thought content: *appropriate*
- Thought process: *appropriate*
- Memory: *good*
- Fund of knowledge: *good*
- Calculation: *good*
- Abstraction: *intact*
- Speech: *appropriate in both volume and rate*
- CNs II–XII: *intact*
- Fine touch: *intact*
- Temperature sensation: *intact*
- Vibratory sensation: *intact*
- Pain sensation: *intact*
- Reflexes 2+ in biceps, Achilles, quadriceps, and triceps bilaterally
- No focal defects observed

## Laboratory Blood Test Results

See Patient Case Table 12.2

| Patient Case Table 12.2 Laboratory Blood Test Results | | | | | |
|---|---|---|---|---|---|
| Na | 139 meq/L | Hb | 13.6 g/dL | Monos | 6% |
| K | 4.4 meq/L | Hct | 41% | Eos | 3% |
| Cl | 105 meq/L | Plt | $292 \times 10^3/mm^3$ | Basos | 1% |
| $HCO_3$ | 26 meq/L | WBC | $8.9 \times 10^3/mm^3$ | Ca | 8.8 mg/dL |
| BUN | 15 mg/dL | Segs | 51% | Mg | 2.5 mg/dL |
| Cr | 0.9 mg/dL | Bands | 2% | Phos | 4.1 mg/dL |
| Glu (non-fasting) | 104 mg/dL | Lymphs | 37% | | |

## Peak Flow

175 L/min

## Arterial Blood Gases

- pH 7.55
- $PaCO_2 = 30$ mm Hg
- $PaO_2 = 65$ mm Hg

## Chest X-Ray

Hyperinflated lungs with no infiltrates that suggest inflammation/pneumonia

---

***Patient Case Question 4.*** Do the patient's arterial blood gas determinations indicate that the asthmatic attack is *mild, moderate* or *bordering on respiratory failure*?

***Patient Case Question 5.*** Identify the metabolic state reflected by the patient's arterial blood pH.

***Patient Case Question 6.*** What is the cause of this metabolic state?

---

# ▄▄▄ Clinical Course

The patient is admitted for treatment with oxygen, inhaled bronchodilators, and oral prednisone (60 mg/day initially, followed by a slow taper to discontinuation over 10 days). However, the patient becomes increasingly dyspneic and more agitated despite treatment. Heart rate increases to 125 bpm, pulsus paradoxus increases to 30 mm Hg, respiratory rate increases to 35/min, and breathing becomes more labored. Wheezing becomes loud throughout both inspiratory and expiratory phases of the respiratory cycle. Signs of early cyanosis become evident. The extremities become cold and clammy and the patient no longer is alert and oriented. Repeat ABG are: pH 7.35, $PaO_2$ = 45 mm Hg, and $PaCO_2$ = 42 mm Hg (40% oxygen by mask).

---

***Patient Case Question 7.*** What do this patient's mental state, heart rate, pulsus paradoxus, respiratory rate, and wheezing suggest?

***Patient Case Question 8.*** Why are the patient's extremities cold?

***Patient Case Question 9.*** Why is the patient no longer alert and oriented?

***Patient Case Question 10.*** Why is the patient becoming cyanotic?

***Patient Case Question 11.*** Why has the skin become clammy?

***Patient Case Question 12.*** What do the patient's arterial blood gases indicate now?

---

# 13 BACTERIAL PNEUMONIA

 *For the Disease Summary for this case study, see the CD-ROM.*

## PATIENT CASE

### ■ Chief Complaints

Provided by patient's home caregiver: "Mrs. I. is confused and very sick. She was up most of last night coughing."

### ■ HPI

Mrs. B.I. is an 84-year-old white female, who is widowed and a retired bank manager. She owns her own home and has a 45-year-old female caregiver who lives in the home. Currently, Mrs. I. uses a walker and takes daily strolls to the park with her caregiver. She is able to perform most activities of daily living; however, the caregiver prepares all meals.

The patient presents to the clinic accompanied by her caregiver, who reports that Mrs. I. has a one-week history of upper respiratory symptoms and a two-day history of increasing weakness and malaise. Approximately three days ago, the patient developed a cough that has gradually become worse and she now has difficulty catching her breath. The caregiver also reports that the patient was confused last night and nearly fell while going to the bathroom. The patient has been coughing up a significant amount of phlegm that is thick and green in color. She has no fever. The caregiver has become concerned by the patient's reduction in daily activities and an inability to get rid of her "cold."

*Patient Case Question 1.* Based on the patient's history of illness, is this type of infection considered *community-acquired* or *nosocomial*?

### ■ PMH

- Tobacco dependence × 64 years
- Chronic bronchitis for approximately 13 years
- Urinary overflow incontinence × 10 years
- HTN × 6 years, BP has been averaging 140/80 mm Hg with medication

- Mild left hemiparesis caused by CVA 4 years ago
- Depression × 2 years
- Constipation × 6 months
- Influenza shot 3 months ago

# ▬▬ FH

- (+) for HTN and cancer
- (−) for CAD, asthma, DM

# ▬▬ SH

- Patient lives with caregiver in patient's home
- Smokes 1/2 ppd
- Some friends recently ill with "colds"
- Occasional alcohol use, none recently

# ▬▬ ROS

- Difficult to conduct due to patient's mental state (lethargy present)
- Caregiver states that patient has had difficulty sleeping due to persistent cough
- Caregiver has not observed any episodes of emesis but reports a decrease in appetite
- Caregiver denies dysphagia, rashes, and hemoptysis

***Patient Case Question 2.*** Provide a clinical definition for *lethargy*.

# ▬▬ Meds

- Atenolol 100 mg po QD
- HCTZ 25 mg po QD
- Aspirin 325 mg po QD
- Nortriptyline 75 mg po QD
- Combivent MDI 2 puffs QID (caregiver reports patient rarely uses)
- Albuterol MDI 2 puffs QID PRN
- Docusate calcium 100 mg po HS

# ▬▬ All

PCN (rash)

***Patient Case Question 3.*** Match the pharmacotherapeutic agents in the left-hand column directly below with the patient's health conditions in the right-hand column.

a. atenolol          _____ depression

b. HCTZ              _____ constipation

c. nortriptyline     _____ HTN

d. albuterol         _____ chronic bronchitis

e. docusate calcium

# ▰ PE and Lab Tests

## Gen

The patient's age appears to be consistent with that reported by the caregiver. She is well groomed and neat, uses a walker for ambulation, and walks with a noticeable limp. She is a lethargic, frail, thin woman who is oriented to self only. The patient is also coughing and using accessory muscles to breathe. She is tachypneic and appears to be uncomfortable and in moderate respiratory distress.

## Vital Signs

See Patient Case Table 13.1

| Patient Case Table 13.1 Vital Signs | | | |
|---|---|---|---|
| BP | 140/80, no orthostatic changes noted | HT | 5'10½" |
| P | 95 and regular | WT | 124 lbs |
| RR | 38 and labored | BMI | 17.6 |
| T | 98.3°F | $O_2$ saturation | 86% on room air |

## Skin

- Warm and clammy
- (–) for rashes

## HEENT

- NC/AT
- EOMI
- PERRLA
- Fundi without lesions
- Eyes are watery
- Nares slightly flared; purulent discharge visible
- Ears with slight serous fluid behind TMs
- Pharynx erythematous with purulent post-nasal drainage
- Mucous membranes are inflamed and moist

## Neck

- Supple
- Mild bilateral cervical adenopathy
- (–) for thyromegaly, JVD, and carotid bruits

## Lungs/Thorax

- Breathing labored with tachypnea
- RUL and LUL reveal regions of crackles and diminished breath sounds
- RLL and LLL reveal absence of breath sounds and dullness to percussion
- (–) egophony

## Cardiac

- Regular rate and rhythm
- Normal $S_1$ and $S_2$
- (–) for $S_3$ and $S_4$

## Abd

- Soft and NT
- Normoactive BS
- (–) organomegaly, masses, and bruits

## Genit/Rect

Examination deferred

## MS/Ext

- (–) CCE
- Extremities warm
- Strength 4/5 right side, 1/5 left side
- Pulses are 1+ bilaterally

## Neuro

- Oriented to self only
- CNs II–XII intact
- DTRs 2+
- Babinski normal

## Laboratory Blood Test Results

See Patient Case Table 13.2

| Patient Case Table 13.2 Laboratory Blood Test Results | | | | | |
|---|---|---|---|---|---|
| Na | 141 meq/L | Glu, fasting | 138 mg/dL | • Lymphs | 10% |
| K | 4.5 meq/L | Hb | 13.7 g/dL | • Monos | 3% |
| Cl | 105 meq/L | Hct | 39.4% | • Eos | 1% |
| $HCO_3$ | 29 meq/L | WBC | 15,200/mm³ | Ca | 8.7 mg/dL |
| BUN | 16 mg/dL | • Neutros | 82% | Mg | 1.7 mg/dL |
| Cr | 0.9 mg/dL | • Bands | 4% | $PO_4$ | 2.9 mg/dL |

## Arterial Blood Gases

See Patient Case Table 13.3

| Patient Case Table 13.3 Arterial Blood Gases | | | | | |
|---|---|---|---|---|---|
| pH | 7.50 | $PaO_2$ | 59 mm Hg on room air | $PaCO_2$ | 25 mm Hg |

## Urinalysis

See Patient Case Table 13.4

| Patient Case Table 13.4 Urinalysis | | | | | |
|---|---|---|---|---|---|
| Appearance: Light yellow and hazy | | Protein | (–) | Nitrite | (–) |
| SG | 1.020 | Ketones | (–) | Leukocyte esterase | (–) |
| pH | 6.0 | Blood | (–) | 2 WBC/RBC per HPF | |
| Glucose | (–) | Bilirubin | (–) | Bacteria | (–) |

## Chest X-Rays

- Consolidation of inferior and superior segments of RLL and LLL
- Developing consolidation of RUL and LUL
- (–) pleural effusion
- Heart size WNL

## Sputum Analysis

Gram stain: TNTC neutrophils, some epithelial cells, negative for microbes

## Sputum and Blood Cultures

Pending

*Patient Case Question 4.* Determine the patient's Pneumonia Severity of Illness score.

*Patient Case Question 5.* Should this patient be admitted to the hospital for treatment?

*Patient Case Question 6.* What is this patient's 30-day mortality probability?

*Patient Case Question 7.* Identify *two* clinical signs that support a diagnosis of "double pneumonia."

*Patient Case Question 8.* Identify *five* risk factors that have predisposed this patient to bacterial pneumonia.

*Patient Case Question 9.* Identify a minimum of *twenty* clinical manifestations that are consistent with a diagnosis of bacterial pneumonia.

*Patient Case Question 10.* Propose a likely microbe that is causing bacterial pneumonia in this patient and provide a strong rationale for your answer.

*Patient Case Question 11.* Identify *two* antimicrobial agents that might be helpful in treating this patient.

*Patient Case Question 12.* The patient has no medical history of diabetes mellitus, yet her fasting serum glucose concentration is elevated. Propose a reasonable explanation.

*Patient Case Question 13.* Why is this patient afebrile?

*Patient Case Question 14.* Is there a significant probability that bacterial pneumonia may have developed from a urinary tract infection in this patient?

*Patient Case Question 15.* Explain the pathophysiologic basis that underlies the patient's high blood pH.

***Patient Case Question 16.*** The chest x-ray shown in Patient Case Figure 13.1 reveals pneumonia secondary to infection with *Mucor* species in a patient with poorly controlled diabetes mellitus. Where is pneumonia most prominent: right upper lobe, right lower lobe, left upper lobe, or left lower lobe?

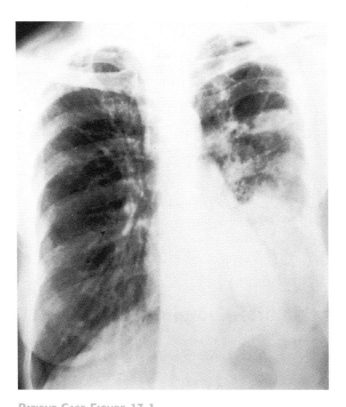

PATIENT CASE FIGURE 13.1
Chest x-ray from a patient with pneumonia due to infection with Mucor. See Patient Case Question 16. (Reprinted with permission from Crapo JD, Glassroth J, Karlinsky JB, King TE Jr. Baum's Textbook of Pulmonary Diseases, 7th ed. Philadelphia: Lippincott Williams & Wilkins, 2004.)

# CASE STUDY

## 14

# CHRONIC OBSTRUCTIVE PULMONARY DISEASE

 *For the Disease Summary for this case study, see the CD-ROM.*

## PATIENT CASE

### ■ Patient's Chief Complaints

"I'm falling apart. I've been having more trouble breathing, my cough has gotten worse in the past three days, and now my ankles are beginning to swell up."

### ■ History of Present Illness

J.T. is a 61 yo man with COPD who presents to the emergency room with a three-day history of progressive dyspnea, cough, and increased production of clear sputum. He usually coughs up only a scant amount of clear sputum daily, and coughing is generally worse after rising in the morning. The patient denies fever, chills, night sweats, weakness, muscle aches, joint aches, and blood in the sputum. He treated himself with albuterol MDI, but respiratory distress increased despite multiple inhalations.

Upon arrival at the emergency room, there were few breath sounds heard with auscultation, and the patient was so short of breath that he had difficulty climbing up onto the examiner's table and completing a sentence without a long pause. He was placed on 4 L oxygen via nasal cannulae and given nebulized ipratropium and albuterol treatments.

### ■ Past Medical History

- History of mental illness as a young adult; one suicide attempt at age 20
- HTN × 10 years
- COPD diagnosed 6 years ago
- Left lateral malleolus and first metatarsal fracture repair 17 months ago
- Occasional episodes of acute bronchitis treated as outpatient with antibiotics
- Mild CVA 4 months ago, appears to have no residual neurologic deficits
- (–) history of TB, asbestos exposure, occupational exposure, heart disease, or asthma

### ■ Family History

- Father died from lung cancer
- Mother is alive, age 80, also has COPD and is being treated with oxygen
- One sister, developed heart disease in her 50s
- One daughter and three grandchildren, alive and well

# Social History

- Patient is a recently retired beef products worker
- Married once and divorced at age 35, has not remarried
- Lives with elderly mother
- 2 pack/day Camel smoker for 37 years; has cut back to 5 cigarettes/day since he was diagnosed with COPD and is now willing to consider complete smoking cessation
- History of excessive alcohol use; has become a social drinker in last 15 years

# Review of Systems

- Denies recent weight loss but has lost 25 pounds during past 7 years
- Denies progressive fatigue, loss of libido, morning headaches, and sleeping problems

# Medications

- HCTZ 25 mg po Q AM
- Amlodipine 5 mg po QD
- Theophylline 200 mg po BID
- Albuterol 180 µg MDI 2 inhalations QID PRN
- Ipratropium 36 µg MDI 2 inhalations QID
- The patient has been compliant with his medications. However, he admits that he does not like to use ipratropium because it causes "dry mouth" and makes him feel "edgy."

*Patient Case Question 1.* Why is this patient taking amlodipine?

*Patient Case Question 2.* Why is this patient taking HCTZ?

# Physical Examination and Laboratory Tests

## General Appearance

Alert, thin, weak-appearing white male, who is somewhat improved and appears more comfortable after receiving oxygen and bronchodilator therapy

## Vital Signs

See Patient Case Table 14.1

| Patient Case Table 14.1 Vital Signs | | | | | | | |
|---|---|---|---|---|---|---|---|
| BP | 165/95 | RR | 32 and labored | HT | 5'10" |
| P | 110 and regular | T | 97.9°F | WT | 120 lb |

*Patient Case Question 3.* Is this patient technically *underweight, overweight, obese,* or is this patient's weight considered *healthy*?

## Skin

- Cold and dry
- (–) cyanosis, nodules, masses, rashes, itching, and jaundice
- (–) ecchymoses and petechiae
- Poor turgor

### Head, Eyes, Ears, Nose, and Throat

* PERRLA
* EOMs intact
* Eyes anicteric
* Normal conjunctiva
* Vision satisfactory with no eye pain
* Fundi without AV nicking, hemorrhages, exudates, and papilledema
* TMs intact
* (–) tinnitus and ear pain
* Nares clear
* (+) pursed lip breathing
* Oropharynx clear with no mouth lesions
* Yellowed teeth
* Oral mucous membranes very dry
* Tongue normal size
* No throat pain or difficulty swallowing

### Neck and Lymph Nodes

* Neck supple but thin
* (+) mild JVD
* (–) cervical lymphadenopathy, thyromegaly, masses, and carotid bruits

### Chest and Lungs

* Use of accessory muscles at rest
* "Barrel chest" appearance
* Poor diaphragmatic excursion bilaterally
* Percussion hyper-resonant
* Poor breath sounds throughout
* Prolonged expiration with occasional mild, expiratory wheeze
* (–) crackles and rhonchi
* (–) axillary and supraclavicular lymphadenopathy

### Heart

* Tachycardic with normal rhythm
* Normal $S_1$ and $S_2$
* Prominent $S_3$
* No rubs or murmurs

### Abdomen

* (+) hepatosplenomegaly, fluid wave, tenderness, and distension
* (–) masses, bruits, and superficial abdominal veins
* Normal BS

### Genitalia and Rectum

* Penis, testes, and scrotum normal
* Prostate slightly enlarged, but without nodules
* Heme (–) stool
* No internal rectal masses palpated

## Musculoskeletal and Extremities

- Cyanotic nail beds
- (−) clubbing
- 1+ bilateral ankle edema to mid-calf
- 2+ dorsalis pedis and posterior tibial pulses bilaterally
- (−) spine and CVA tenderness
- Denies muscle aches, joint pain, and bone pain
- Normal range of motion throughout

## Neurological

- Alert and oriented
- Cranial nerves intact
- Motor 5/5 upper and lower extremities bilaterally
- Strength, sensation, and deep tendon reflexes intact and symmetric
- Babinski downgoing
- Gait steady
- Denies headache and dizziness

## Laboratory Blood Test Results

See Patient Case Table 14.2

| Patient Case Table 14.2 Laboratory Blood Test Results | | | | | | |
|---|---|---|---|---|---|
| Na | 147 meq/L | Plt | $160 \times 10^3/mm^3$ | Bilirubin, total | 0.3 mg/dL |
| K | 4.1 meq/L | WBC | $9.1 \times 10^3/mm^3$ | PT | 14.2 sec |
| Cl | 114 meq/L | • PMNs | 62% | Alb | 4.0 g/dL |
| $HCO_3$ | 25 meq/L | • Lymphs | 27% | Protein, total | 6.8 g/dL |
| BUN | 29 mg/dL | • Eos | 3% | Alk phos | 78 IU/L |
| Cr | 1.1 mg/dL | • Basos | 1% | Ca | 8.8 mg/dL |
| Glu, fasting | 98 mg/dL | • Monos | 7% | $PO_4$ | 3.5 mg/dL |
| Hb | 19.3 g/dL | AST | 14 IU/L | Mg | 2.5 mg/dL |
| Hct | 55% | ALT | 31 IU/L | AAT | 137 mg/dL |

## Arterial Blood Gases (on 4 L $O_2$ by Cannulae)

- pH          7.32
- $PaO_2$          65 mm Hg
- $PaCO_2$          54 mm Hg
- $SaO_2$          90%

## Pulmonary Function Tests

- $FEV_1$ = 1.67 L (45% of expected)
- FVC = 4.10 L (85% of expected)
- $FEV_1$/FVC = 0.41 (expected = 0.77)

## Chest X-Rays

- Hyperinflation with flattened diaphragm
- Large anteroposterior diameter
- Diffuse scarring and bullae in all lung fields but especially prominent in lower lobes bilaterally
- No effusions or infiltrates
- Large pulmonary vasculature

***Patient Case Question 4.*** Identify all of this patient's risk factors for chronic obstructive pulmonary disease and note which of them is the single most significant risk factor.

***Patient Case Question 5.*** Identify all of the clinical manifestations in this patient that are consistent with *chronic bronchitis.*

***Patient Case Question 6.*** Identify all of the clinical manifestations in this patient that are consistent with *emphysema.*

***Patient Case Question 7.*** Identify all of the clinical manifestations in this patient that are consistent with *pulmonary hypertension* and *cor pulmonale.*

***Patient Case Question 8.*** To which stage of development has this patient's COPD progressed?

***Patient Case Question 9.*** Which serious condition is indicated by the patient's arterial blood gas analysis?

***Patient Case Question 10.*** The patient has a strong history of alcohol abuse, which can cause liver dysfunction. Are there any indications that liver function has been compromised?

***Patient Case Question 11.*** Explain the apparent disparity in this patient's two major renal function tests (i.e., BUN and Cr).

***Patient Case Question 12.*** Would this patient benefit from home oxygen therapy?

***Patient Case Question 13.*** Is there any reason to believe that an infection caused this patient's relapse of chronic obstructive pulmonary disease?

***Patient Case Question 14.*** Is the patient in this case study alpha-1-antitrypsin deficient?

***Patient Case Question 15.*** Create a figure legend for the illustrations shown in Patient Case Figure 14.1.

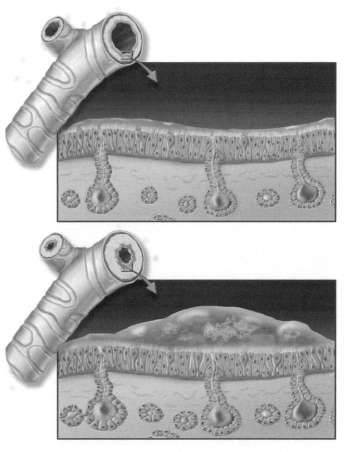

PATIENT CASE FIGURE 14.1

See Patient Case Question 15. (Image provided by the Anatomical Chart Company.)

# CASE STUDY

# 15

# CYSTIC FIBROSIS

 *For the Disease Summary for this case study, see the CD-ROM.*

# PATIENT CASE

## ■■■ Patient's Chief Complaints

Provided by patient's mother: "I noticed a let-down in T's exercise tolerance level a week ago, and the last couple of days his cough and sputum production have gotten much worse. When he started having breathing problems, I brought him in immediately. T is normally a bubbly and lively little boy and it is obvious when he isn't feeling well. I think that he has another infection."

## ■■■ HPI

T.B. is a 6 yo Caucasian male with a history of CF. He was diagnosed with CF at 8 months of age. He had been doing well until five days ago, when his mother noticed that he became tired very easily while playing. She also reported an increasing cough productive of very dark-colored sputum but that he had no fever. The patient also has not had much of an appetite during the past week and has lost 2½ pounds. His oxygen saturation is currently 87% and he was immediately placed on oxygen via nasal cannula.

## ■■■ PMH

T.B. was born (74 months ago) a 6 lb-7 oz white male to a 23 yo mother. A normal vaginal delivery followed an uncomplicated pregnancy. The infant had Apgar scores of 8 and 9 at 1 and 5 minutes, respectively. The initial physical examination was unremarkable, but at 30 hours following delivery, the infant developed abdominal distension and began vomiting bile. No bowel movements had occurred since birth. A second physical exam disclosed an afebrile, well-developed infant with a tense abdomen from which only occasional faint bowel sounds were heard. The anus was patent, lungs were clear to auscultation, and the cardiac exam was unremarkable. There were no neurologic abnormalities. Radiography of the abdomen revealed distended loops of bowel without air. Both the CBC and serum chemistry panel were normal. Exploratory laparotomy disclosed meconium ileus and atresia of the distal ileum. The narrowed segment of ileum was successfully resected and the infant recovered without complications. An attempt to collect a sweat sample for chloride analysis was unsuccessful. After discharge, the infant was lost to follow-up.

At 8 months of age, the child presented with failure to thrive characterized by poor weight gain. His appetite had been good, but for several months he had been having up to 6 pale and foul-smelling bowel movements daily. During that time, he had also experienced several episodes of bronchitis. Physical examination revealed a small, frail-looking, pale child who appeared malnourished with little subcutaneous fat and a protuberant abdomen. There was a scattering of crackles in both lungs consistent with pulmonary edema or pneumonia. The cardiac exam was normal. Chest x-rays showed markings in all lung fields. The patient's WBC was $8.3 \times 10^3/mm^3$, serum albumin was 1.9 g/dL, sweat chloride was 99 meq/L, and a stool smear was positive for fat. The child was hospitalized and 24 hours later became febrile with tachypnea and increasing signs of respiratory distress. Auscultation revealed poor breath sounds in the right lung. Radiographs of the chest revealed consolidation of the right lung consistent with pneumonia. The WBC had increased to $19.3 \times 10^3/mm^3$ with an increase in band forms (i.e., immature neutrophils) in the peripheral blood to 16%. Sputum cultures were positive for both *Pseudomonas aeruginosa* and *Staphylococcus aureus*. With intensive support and aggressive intravenous antibiotic therapy, the infection resolved and the patient recovered fully. A diagnosis of CF was established and the patient was referred to the regional CF center for follow-up.

During the next six years, the patient was hospitalized three times for respiratory infections and one episode of hemoptysis. The infections required hospitalization for up to two weeks at a time and IV antibiotics. He was also diagnosed with bronchiectasis and pancreatic insufficiency. His mother has been administering postural drainage to her son three times daily for approximately 30 minutes each. Some of the positions are obviously uncomfortable, but T never complains. He is being maintained on a high-calorie, high-protein, and unrestricted fat diet that is supplemented with fat-soluble vitamins and iron.

## ▬ FH

- Father has HTN; mother is well
- Mother knew that she was a carrier for CF when they married, but father did not
- The patient is the only child born to a 24 yo father and 23 yo mother
- A maternal uncle died at age 16 from pneumonia secondary to CF
- The remainder of the FH is unremarkable

## ▬ SH

- Patient lives at home with his father and mother and attends first grade; he is doing well in school
- Father is a full-time evening custodian at a local community college
- Mother is currently a "stay-at-home mom," but is also a registered nurse
- Family has city water and no pets
- Father smokes but only outside of the home

## ▬ ROS

- Patient complains of chest pain when coughing
- Reduced ability to perform usual daily activities due to SOB
- (–) vomiting, abdominal discomfort/pain, diarrhea, constipation, change in urinary frequency, increase in thirst

## ▬ Meds

- Aerosolized tobramycin 300 mg BID
- Albuterol 2.5 mg via nebulizer TID
- Dornase alfa 2.5 mg via nebulizer QD

- Fluticasone propionate 100 µg, 1 puff BID
- Prednisone 4 mg po Q 6h
- Pancrelipase: 8000 USP units lipase + 30,000 USP units amylase + 30,000 USP units protease with each meal; 4000 USP units lipase + 12,000 USP units amylase + 12,000 USP units protease with each snack
- Ferrous sulfate 15 mg po Q 8h
- ADEK Multivitamin Pediatric Chewable Tablets 1 tab po BID

 **All**

NKDA

 **PE and Lab Tests**

## Gen

The patient is a pleasant, thin, 6 yo white male who has difficulty breathing and gasps for air when his oxygen cannula is removed. He seems small for his age. His color is pale and he appears frail and tired. The patient is sitting up on the examiner's table in the emergency room.

## Vital Signs

See Patient Case Table 15.1

| Patient Case Table 15.1 Vital Signs | | | | | |
|---|---|---|---|---|---|
| BP | 105/68 (*sitting*) | T | 98.4°F | SaO$_2$ | 95% with 1.5 L O$_2$<br>88% on room air |
| P | 122 (*regular*) | WT | 29 lb<br>(*normal for age: 36–60 lbs*) | | |
| RR | 33 (*labored*) | HT | 3'4"<br>(*normal for age: 3'6"–4'1"*) | | |

## Skin

- Color pale
- Cool to the touch, dry, and intact
- (–) rashes, bruises, and other unusual lesions
- Good turgor

## HEENT

- Pupils equal at 3 mm, round, and reactive to light and accommodation
- Extra-ocular muscles intact
- Funduscopic exam unremarkable
- White sclera
- Conjunctiva pale and non-edematous
- TMs clear throughout, translucent, and without drainage
- Nares with dried mucus in both nostrils

- No oral lesions or erythema
- Secretions noted in posterior pharynx

## Neck/LN

- Neck supple without masses
- (–) lymphadenopathy, thyromegaly, JVD, and carotid bruits

## Lungs

- Crackles heard bilaterally in upper lobes
- Decreased breath sounds in lower lobes
- Wheezing noted without auscultation
- RLL and LLL dull to percussion posteriorly

## Heart

- Tachycardic with regular rhythm
- (–) murmurs and rubs
- $S_1$ and $S_2$ normal
- (–) $S_3$ and $S_4$

## Abd

- Abdomen soft, NT/ND
- (+) BS
- (–) HSM, masses, and bruits

## Genit/Rect

- Stool heme negative
- Normal penis and testes

## MS/Ext

- Mild clubbing noted
- (–) cyanosis, edema, and femoral bruits
- Capillary refill WNL at < 2 sec
- Age-appropriate strength and ROM
- Radial and pedal pulses WNL at 2+ throughout

## Neuro

- Awake, alert, and oriented
- CNs intact
- DTRs 2+
- No gross motor or sensory deficits present
- Somewhat uncooperative with full neurologic exam

## Laboratory Blood Test Results

See Patient Case Table 15.2

**Patient Case Table 15.2 Laboratory Blood Test Results**

| | | | | | |
|---|---|---|---|---|---|
| Na | 137 meq/L | MCHC | 29 g/dL | AST | 16 IU/L |
| K | 3.8 meq/L | Plt | 187,000/mm³ | ALT | 20 IU/L |
| Cl | 102 meq/L | WBC | 18,900/mm³ | T Bilirubin | 1.0 mg/dL |
| HCO₃ | 24 meq/L | • PMNs | 74% | T Protein | 7.3 g/dL |
| BUN | 19 mg/dL | • Bands | 6% | Alb | 3.8 g/dL |
| Cr | 0.7 mg/dL | • Lymphs | 17% | Vitamin A | 40 mg/dL |
| Glu, fasting | 109 mg/dL | • Monos | 3% | Vitamin D, 25OH | 43 ng/mL |
| Hb | 11.8 g/dL | Ca | 8.3 mg/dL | Vitamin E | 0.2 mg/dL |
| Hct | 35.1% | PO₄ | 2.9 mg/dL | PT | 11.4 sec |
| MCV | 77 fL | Mg | 2.1 mg/dL | PTT | 34.8 sec |

## Sputum Culture Results

(+) *Pseudomonas aeruginosa, Stenotrophomonas maltophilia,* and *Staphylococcus aureus*

## Pulmonary Function

$FEV_1$ 63% of predicted

## Chest X-Rays

Consolidation of lower lobes of both lungs consistent with double pneumonia

## Peripheral Blood Smear

Microcytic hypochromic red blood cells

---

***Patient Case Question 1.*** Which of the following best explains why the patient in this case study has cystic fibrosis?

a. development of meconium ileus soon after birth

b. failure to thrive

c. both parents are carriers of a mutation for cystic fibrosis

d. frequent infections early in life

e. malabsorption of fats and proteins

***Patient Case Question 2.*** Why would you expect the patient in this case study to be malnourished?

a. malabsorption of fats and proteins

b. deficiency of vitamins and minerals

c. significant use of calories to maintain breathing

d. both a and b

e. a, b, and c

***Patient Case Question 3.*** Why does the patient in this case study receive postural drainage?

a. to loosen secretions from the lungs and remove them from the airways

b. to facilitate the exchange of gases

c. to strength chest muscles

d. both a and b

e. a, b, and c

***Patient Case Question 4.*** Which of the following clinical manifestations might the patient demonstrate with the development of cor pulmonale?

a. jugular venous distension

b. edema of the ankles and feet

c. hepatomegaly

d. both a and b

e. a, b, and c

***Patient Case Question 5.*** Based on laboratory test results, which types of nutritional supplementation should be enhanced?

***Patient Case Question 6.*** List *three* specific laboratory test results that are consistent with development of a bacterial infection.

***Patient Case Question 7.*** Which *two* specific laboratory test results above suggest that the patient is not vitamin K deficient?

***Patient Case Question 8.*** Describe the pathophysiology that is causing *pallor* in this patient.

***Patient Case Question 9.*** Which clinical evidence indicates that cirrhosis has not developed in this patient as a result of cystic fibrosis?

***Patient Case Question 10.*** Which clinical evidence indicates that hypoproteinemia secondary to cystic fibrosis is not an issue in this patient?

***Patient Case Question 11.*** Which clinical evidence indicates that diabetes mellitus has not developed in this patient as a result of cystic fibrosis?

***Patient Case Question 12.*** Is this patient *hyponatremic* or *hypochloremic?*

# CASE STUDY

# 16

# LUNG CANCER

 *For the Disease Summary for this case study, see the CD-ROM.*

# PATIENT CASE

## ◼◼ Patient's Chief Complaints

"My voice has been hoarse and husky for about two weeks. I've been gargling with salt water, but the problem doesn't seem to be getting any better. There's no pain or tenderness in my throat. I'm a TV news anchorman and my voice is important to my livelihood. I haven't been able to anchor the nightly news now for 10 days."

## ◼◼ HPI

P.J. is a 54-year-old African American male, who presents to the ED with a complaint of a two-week history of hoarseness that is not getting better. When questioned further, he admits that his usual morning "smoker's cough" is getting worse and that he has "given serious thought lately to quitting smoking in the near future."

## ◼◼ PMH

- Hypothyroidism × 27 years
- Bilateral osteoarthritis of knees × 8 years
- Depression × 2 years
- Iron deficiency anemia of unknown cause, 8 months
- Seasonal allergic rhinitis since adolescence
- Several episodes of mildly bloody sputum in past year that resolved in a few days; patient did not seek medical help
- No prior history of trauma or surgeries
- Had influenza vaccine last year
- Last tetanus booster, 6 years ago

## ◼◼ FH

- Family history is negative for lung cancer; however, there is a positive family history for other types of cancer—paternal uncle with colorectal cancer, one niece with non-Hodgkin's lymphoma, and one niece with malignant melanoma

- Father was a mine worker and died at age 66 from complications of anthracosis
- Mother, age 77, is alive and suffers from diabetes mellitus and arthritis
- Patient is second child of four siblings
- All close family members live nearby, visit often, and are cigarette smokers; his wife has also been a long-term smoker

## ■ SH

- Married and lives with wife of 33 years
- Has 2 adult biological children and one adopted child
- Has been a 1–1½ ppd cigarette smoker since age 17
- Occasionally uses alcohol (3–4 drinks/week, usually beer)
- Vietnam War veteran with Congressional Medal of Honor
- Denies IV drug use, although he last snorted heroin 2 years ago
- Has resided for approximately 25 years near a site with a history of radioactive contamination

## ■ Meds

- Ferrous sulfate 325 mg po TID
- Levothyroxine 88 μg po QD
- Acetaminophen 500 mg po PRN
- Intra-articular cortisone injections of knees, PRN
- Nortriptyline 50 mg po QD
- OTC antihistamine, April–August every year PRN for seasonal allergic rhinitis

## ■ All

PCN → diarrhea

## ■ ROS

- Patient is positive for worsening cough and recent onset of shortness of breath with moderate exertion (e.g., climbing one flight of stairs)
- Patient denies all of the following: fever and chills; fatigue; weakness; poor appetite; unintentional weight loss; difficulty or pain with swallowing; pain in chest, abdomen, shoulders, or back; recent onset of vision problems; headache; nausea or vomiting; dizziness; significant swelling; bowel or bladder problems

## ■ PE and Lab Tests

### Gen

- Patient is an A & O, middle-aged, slightly overweight African American male in NAD
- Well groomed and well dressed and appears older than stated age and somewhat restless
- He is not guarded in his responses
- No odd or inappropriate motor behavior noted
- Speech is normal in both volume and rate
- Appears to have good attention span and concentration

### Vital Signs

See Patient Case Table 16.1

| **Patient Case Table 16.1 Vital Signs** | | | | | |
|---|---|---|---|---|---|
| BP | 125/70 sitting, left arm | RR | 24 and slightly labored | HT | 5'9½" |
| P | 95 and regular | T | 99.0°F | WT | 185 lbs (187 lb 10 months ago) |

## Skin

- Warm and dry
- No bruising or discoloration
- Overall good-to-fair skin turgor
- Marked "crow's feet" periorbital wrinkling

## HEENT

- NC/AT
- (−) facial swelling
- EOM intact
- (–) nystagmus and photophobia
- PERRLA
- Normal funduscopic exam without retinopathy
- Normal sclera
- Ear canals clear and eardrums negative; good auditory acuity
- Nose unremarkable
- Significant repair of dental caries—original teeth present
- Oral mucosa soft and moist
- Tongue midline and normal
- Tonsils intact and normal

## Neck/LN

- Normal motion of neck without masses
- Normal thyroid
- (–) JVD and bruits
- (–) cervical, supraclavicular, and axillary lymphadenopathy

## Lungs

- Wheeze auscultated in right upper lobe on inspiration
- Percussion reveals area of resonance to dullness over right upper lobe

## Heart

- Apical pulse normally located at 5th intercostal space at mid-clavicular line
- Regular rate and rhythm
- Normal $S_1$ and $S_2$
- (–) murmurs, rubs, $S_3$ and $S_4$

## Abd

- Soft, non-distended, and non-tender to palpation
- No masses or bruits
- Normal peristaltic activity

- No hepatomegaly or splenomegaly
- No CVA tenderness

## Genit/Rect

- Normal penis, scrotum, and testicles
- Slightly enlarged prostate but (–) for nodules
- Rectal exam: good sphincter tone and guaiac (–) stool

## MS/Ext

- Pulses 2+ throughout
- (−) CCE
- Joint enlargement and limited ROM, both knees, consistent with DJD

## Neuro

- CNs II–XII grossly intact
- DTRs 2+
- Memory intact
- Normal gait
- A & O × 3
- No sensory deficits
- Coordination intact
- Muscle tone equal at 5/5 throughout
- Babinski normal and downgoing bilaterally

## Laboratory Blood Test Results

See Patient Case Table 16.2

### Patient Case Table 16.2 Laboratory Blood Test Results

| | | | | | |
|---|---|---|---|---|---|
| Na | 142 meq/L | Glu, fasting | 94 mg/dL | ALT | 30 IU/L |
| K | 3.9 meq/L | Hb | 13.8 g/dL | AST | 20 IU/L |
| Cl | 102 meq/L | Hct | 39.6% | Total Bilirubin | 1.2 mg/dL |
| $HCO_3$ | 28 meq/L | Plt | $250 \times 10^3/mm^3$ | Total Protein | 6.3 g/dL |
| BUN | 20 mg/dL | WBC | $5.5 \times 10^3/mm^3$ | Alk Phos | 78 IU/L |
| Cr | 1.2 mg/dL | Ca | 11.4 mg/dL | TSH | 2.4 µU/mL |

## Chest X-Rays

- Anteroposterior and lateral views show a 3.5-cm mass located centrally in right upper lobe displacing the right bronchus, roughly corresponding to the area of dullness and wheezing heard by auscultation
- Left lung is clear
- No signs of pleural effusion were noted

## CT Scans

- Chest: Reveals the lesion seen on x-rays plus mediastinal widening and moderately enlarged right-sided hilar nodes; left-sided hilar nodes and all mediastinal nodes appear normal

- Abdomen: Normal—no unusual lesions noted
- Brain: Normal—no pathology evident

## Bone Scan

WNL

## Fluorescence Bronchoscopy with Lung and Lymph Node Biopsies

- Lung mass: Squamous cells with prominent nucleoli plus keratin pearls
- Hilar nodes (ipsilateral): Squamous cells with distinct nucleoli, tissue is (+) for keratin
- Mediastinal nodes (ipsilateral): Negative

## Pulmonary Function Testing

$FEV_1$ = 1.8 L

---

***Patient Case Question 1.*** Identify this patient's *five* prominent risk factors for lung cancer.

***Patient Case Question 2.*** Why is this patient taking nortriptyline?

***Patient Case Question 3.*** Cite all the clinical evidence that either *supports* or *excludes* metastasis of lung cancer to the brain in this patient.

***Patient Case Question 4.*** Cite all the clinical evidence that either *supports* or *excludes* metastasis of lung cancer to bone in this patient.

***Patient Case Question 5.*** Cite all the clinical evidence that either *supports* or *excludes* metastasis of lung cancer to the liver in this patient.

***Patient Case Question 6.*** Which *type* of lung cancer does this patient have?

***Patient Case Question 7.*** To which *stage* has this lung cancer progressed?

***Patient Case Question 8.*** What is an appropriate treatment for this patient—surgery, chemotherapy, and/or radiation therapy?

***Patient Case Question 9.*** For which type of surgery is this patient a candidate?

***Patient Case Question 10.*** What might have caused this patient's iron deficiency anemia 8 months ago?

***Patient Case Question 11.*** Why is *wheezing* a consistent finding with this patient's diagnosis?

***Patient Case Question 12.*** Identify this patient's *single* abnormal laboratory blood test and briefly explain why this finding is consistent with the diagnosis.

***Patient Case Question 13.*** What is the significance of the patient's serum TSH laboratory test?

***Patient Case Question 14.*** Is the patient's anemia currently well controlled?

# GASTROINTESTINAL DISORDERS

# ACUTE PANCREATITIS

 *For the Disease Summary for this case study, see the CD-ROM.*

# PATIENT CASE

## ■ Patient's Chief Complaint

"It feels like I have a knife in my stomach."

## ■ HPI

F.C. is a 63 yo African American male, who presents to the emergency room at the hospital with intense left upper quadrant pain radiating to his back and under his left shoulder blade. He states that he has had intermittent, upper abdominal pain for approximately three weeks, but that the pain has been increasing in severity during the last four days.

## ■ PMH

- CAD; S/P angioplasty 1 year ago; denies any chest pain since
- HTN; does not remember exactly how long; he states "for years"
- S/P cholecystectomy
- S/P appendicitis
- (+) for hepatitis C × 5 years
- Generalized anxiety disorder, 18 months

## ■ FH

- Father was an alcoholic and died at age 49 from MI
- Mother alive at 83 with CAD
- Brother, age 60, alive and healthy
- No family history of gastrointestinal disease reported

# ▬▬ SH

- Married with 8 children
- Retired high school math teacher and wrestling coach
- Alcohol abuse with 10–12 cans of beer per day for 15 years
- Denies use of tobacco or illicit drugs

# ▬▬ Meds

- Nifedipine 90 mg po QD
- Lisinopril 20 mg po QD
- Paroxetine 20 mg po QD
- Tylenol #3, 2 tablets po QD PRN for back pain that started recently

---

*Patient Case Question 1.* For which condition is this patient likely taking nifedipine?

*Patient Case Question 2.* For which condition is this patient likely taking lisinopril?

*Patient Case Question 3.* For which condition is this patient likely taking paroxetine?

# ▬▬ All

- PCN → rash
- Aspirin → hives and wheezing
- Cats → wheezing

# ▬▬ ROS

- States that he has been feeling "very warm" and has experienced several episodes of nausea and vomiting during the past 72 hours
- Also describes an approximate 8- to 10-lb weight loss over the past 1½ months secondary to intense post-prandial pain and some loss of appetite
- He has noted a reduction in frequency of bowel movements
- No complaints of diarrhea or blood in the stool
- No knowledge of any previous history of poor blood sugar control

# ▬▬ PE and Lab Tests

## Gen

The patient is a black male who looks his stated age. He seems restless and in acute distress. He is sweating profusely and appears ill. He is bent forward on the examiner's table.

## Vital Signs

See Patient Case Table 17.1

| Patient Case Table 17.1 Vital Signs | | | | | |
|---|---|---|---|---|---|
| BP | 85/60 | RR | 35 | WT | 154 lb |
| HR | 120 | T | 101.4°F | HT | 5′ 7½″ |

## HEENT

- PERRLA
- EOMI
- (−) jaundice in sclera
- TMs intact
- Oropharynx pink and clear
- Oral mucosa dry

## Skin

- Dry with poor skin turgor
- Some tenting of skin noted
- No lesions noted
- (−) Grey Turner sign
- (−) Cullen sign

---

*Patient Case Question 4.* What is meant by "tenting of the skin" and what does this clinical sign suggest?

*Patient Case Question 5.* Are the negative Grey Turner and Cullen signs evidence of a *good* or *poor* prognosis?

---

## Neck

- Supple
- (−) carotid bruits, lymphadenopathy, thyromegaly, and JVD

## Heart

- Sinus tachycardia
- Normal $S_1$ and $S_2$ and (−) for additional cardiac sounds
- No m/r/g

## Lungs

Clear to auscultation bilaterally

## Abd

- Moderately distended with diminished bowel sounds
- (+) guarding
- Pain is elicited with light palpation of left upper and mid-epigastric regions
- (−) rebound tenderness, masses, HSM, and bruits

## Ext

- No CCE
- Cool and pale
- Slightly diminished pulses in all extremities
- Normal ROM throughout
- Diaphoretic

## Rect

- Normal sphincter tone
- No bright red blood visible
- Stool is guaiac-negative
- (−) hemorrhoids
- Prostate WNL with no nodules

## Neuro

- A & O × 3 (person, place, time)
- Able to follow commands
- CNs II–XII intact
- Motor, sensory, cerebellar, and gait WNL
- Strength is 5/5 in all extremities
- DTRs 2+ throughout

## Laboratory Blood Test Results

See Patient Case Table 17.2

| Patient Case Table 17.2 Laboratory Blood Test Results | | | | | | | |
|---|---|---|---|---|---|---|---|
| Na | 134 meq/L | • Neutrophils | 73% | T bilirubin | 0.9 mg/dL |
| K | 3.5 meq/L | • Bands | 3% | Alb | 3.3 g/dL |
| Cl | 99 meq/L | • Eosinophils | 1% | Amylase | 1874 IU/L |
| $HCO_3$ | 25 meq/L | • Basophils | 1% | Lipase | 2119 IU/L |
| BUN | 34 mg/dL | • Lymphocytes | 20% | Ca | 8.3 mg/dL |
| Cr | 1.5 mg/dL | • Monocytes | 2% | Mg | 1.7 mg/dL |
| Glu, fasting | 415 mg/dL | AST | 291 IU/L | $PO_4$ | 2.4 mg/dL |
| Hb | 18.3 g/dL | ALT | 161 IU/L | Trig | 971 mg/dL |
| Hct | 53% | Alk phos | 266 IU/L | Repeat Trig | 969 mg/dL |
| WBC | 16,400/mm³ | LDH | 411 IU/L | $SaO_2$ | 96% |

## Urinalysis

See Patient Case Table 17.3

| Patient Case Table 17.3 Urinalysis | | | | | |
|---|---|---|---|---|---|
| Appearance: | yellow, clear | SG | 1.023 | pH | 6.5 |
| Glucose | + | Bilirubin | − | Bacteria | − |
| Ketones | − | Nitrite | − | Urobilinogen | − |
| Hemoglobin | − | Crystals | − | WBC | 2/HPF |
| Protein | − | Casts | − | RBC | 1/HPF |

## Chest X-Ray

- Anteroposterior view shows heart to be normal in size
- Lungs are clear without infiltrates, masses, effusions, or atelectasis

## Abdominal Ultrasound

- Non-specific gas pattern
- No regions of dilated bowel

## Abdominal CECT

Grade C

---

*Patient Case Question 6.* Identify *three* major risk factors for acute pancreatitis in this patient.

*Patient Case Question 7.* Identify *two* abnormal laboratory tests that suggest that acute renal failure has developed in this patient.

*Patient Case Question 8.* Why are hemoglobin and hematocrit abnormal?

*Patient Case Question 9.* How many Ranson criteria does this patient have and what is the probability that the patient will die from this attack of acute pancreatitis?

*Patient Case Question 10.* Does the patient have a significant electrolyte imbalance?

*Patient Case Question 11.* Why was no blood drawn for an ABG determination?

# 18

## CIRRHOSIS

 *For the Disease Summary for this case study, see the CD-ROM.*

# PATIENT CASE

## ▬ Patient's Chief Complaints

Provided by wife: "My husband's very confused and he has been acting strangely. This morning, he couldn't answer my questions and seemed not to recognize me. I think that his stomach has been swelling up again, too. He stopped drinking four years ago, but his cirrhosis seems to be getting worse."

## ▬ HPI

S.G. is a 46 yo white male with a history of chronic alcoholism and alcoholic cirrhosis. He was admitted to the hospital from the outpatient clinic with abdominal swelling and confusion. He has unintentionally gained 15 lbs during the past four weeks. According to his wife, the patient has not been sleeping well for several weeks, has been feeling very lethargic for the past three days, can't seem to remember appointments lately, and, uncharacteristically, has lost his temper with her several times in the last month. S.G.'s boss at work had also telephoned her last week concerned about his "unusual and violent behavior on the job."

## ▬ PMH

* Pneumonia 9 years ago that resolved with antimicrobial therapy
* Cirrhosis secondary to heavy alcohol use diagnosed 4 years ago with ultrasound and liver biopsy (micronodular cirrhosis)
* H/O uncontrolled ascites and peripheral edema
* H/O two upper GI hemorrhages from esophageal varices
* H/O anemia
* H/O *E. coli*-induced bacterial peritonitis 4 years ago
* H/O acute pancreatitis secondary to alcohol abuse
* No history to suggest cardiac or gallbladder disease
* No previous diagnosis of viral or autoimmune hepatitis

## ■ SURG

- S/P appendectomy requiring blood transfusions 30 years ago
- S/P open-reduction internal fixation of right femur secondary to MVA 5 years ago

## ■ FH

- Father died at age 52 from liver disease of unknown etiology
- Mother had rheumatoid arthritis and ulcerative colitis, died from massive stroke at age 66
- Maternal aunt, age 71, with Graves disease
- Patient has no siblings

## ■ SH

- Educated through eighth grade
- Department store men's clothing manager and salesman, 17-year career
- Married for 19 years with 1 daughter, age 10
- H/O ethanol abuse, quit 5 years ago following MVA, previously drank 3 cases of beer/week × 15 years
- H/O IVDA (heroin) and intranasal cocaine, quit 5 years ago
- Has smoked approximately 1/2 ppd for many years

## ■ Meds

- Propranolol 10 mg po TID
- Spironolactone 50 mg po QD
- Furosemide 20 mg po QD
- MVI 1 tablet po QD
- Occasional ibuprofen or acetaminophen for headache
- Patient has H/O non-compliance with his medications

## ■ All

NKDA

## ■ ROS

- Increasing abdominal girth
- (–) complaints of abdominal pain, fever, chills, nausea, vomiting, hematemesis, tarry stools, loss of appetite, cough, chest pain, SOB, lightheadedness, weakness, blood in the urine, diarrhea, constipation, and dry mouth

***Patient Case Question 1.*** Hematemesis and tarry stools are clinical signs of which serious potential complication of cirrhosis?

# ■■■ PE and Lab Tests

## Gen

The patient is restless, mildly jaundiced, and disoriented to time, place, and people. He is slow to answer questions and his answers make little sense. He is ill-appearing but in no obvious distress.

## VS

- BP 120/75, P 83 and regular (supine)
- BP 118/70, P 80 and regular (standing)
- RR 14 and unlabored
- T 98.8°F orally
- WT 171 lbs
- HT 5 ft-7 in
- $SaO_2$ = 97%

## Skin

- Warm, dry, and well perfused with normal turgor
- Mild jaundice
- (+) spider nevi on chest
- (−) palmar erythema
- Several ecchymoses on lower extremities
- Large "cobra" tattoo on right upper arm

## HEENT

- (−) bruises, masses, and deformities on head
- (+) icteric sclera
- Pupils at 3 mm and reactive to light
- EOMI
- Funduscopic exam WNL
- TMs clear and intact
- O/P pink, clear, and moist without erythema or lesions

## Neck/LN

- Supple
- (−) JVD
- (−) goiter, thyroid nodules, carotid bruits, and adenopathy

## Chest

- Lungs CTA bilaterally without wheezes or crackles
- Diaphragmatic excursions WNL
- Good air exchange
- (+) gynecomastia

## Heart

- RRR
- Normal $S_1$ and $S_2$ with no $S_3$ or $S_4$
- No m/r/g heard

## Abd

- Moderately distended, firm, and slightly tender
- (+) prominent veins observed around umbilicus
- (+) HSM
- Active BS
- (−) guarding, rebound tenderness, palpable masses, and aortic, iliac, and renal bruits

## Genit/Rect

- Heme-negative stool
- Penis normal, testicles moderately atrophic but without masses
- Normal sphincter tone
- (+) hemorrhoids
- Prostate may be slightly enlarged but (−) for nodules and tenderness

## MS/Ext

- No clubbing or edema
- Good peripheral pulses at 2+ throughout
- Normal range of motion throughout

## Neuro

- CNs grossly intact
- Brisk DTRs at 2+
- Slight asterixis noted
- Strength is equal bilaterally
- Confused and disoriented
- Negative Babinski
- Sensory grossly intact

***Patient Case Question 2.*** Identify a *minimum of 15* clinical signs and symptoms that are consistent with a diagnosis of cirrhosis.

## Laboratory Blood Test Results

See Patient Case Table 18.1

### Patient Case Table 18.1 Laboratory Blood Test Results

| | | | | | |
|---|---|---|---|---|---|
| Na | 135 meq/L | WBC | 4,700/mm³ | Mg | 1.7 mg/dL |
| K | 3.5 meq/L | PT | 15.6 sec | AFP | 90 ng/mL |
| Cl | 101 meq/L | PTT | 45.1 sec | HBsAg | (−) |
| HCO$_3$ | 25 meq/L | NH$_3$ | 250 µg/dL | HIV | (−) |
| BUN | 12 mg/dL | AST | 107 IU/L | Anti-HCV | (+) |
| Cr | 0.6 mg/dL | ALT | 86 IU/L | HCV RNA | 2.8 million/mL |
| Glu, fasting | 90 mg/dL | Alk Phos | 224 IU/L | ANA | (−) |
| Hb | 14.0 g/dL | Bilirubin | 2.4 mg/dL | Fe | 75 µg/dL |
| Hct | 39.7% | Protein | 6.6 g/dL | Ferritin | 200 ng/mL |
| MCV | 90 fL | Alb | 2.7 g/dL | Transferrin saturation | 38% |
| Plt | 34,500/mm³ | Ca | 8.5 mg/dL | Ceruloplasmin | 37 mg/dL |

***Patient Case Question 3.*** Is the patient anemic at this time and, if so, is the anemia *normocytic, microcytic,* or *macrocytic?*

***Patient Case Question 4.*** What is the most significant abnormality that this patient's CBC has revealed?

***Patient Case Question 5.*** Based on the laboratory data, why has this patient's cirrhosis shown a sudden and unexpected progression?

***Patient Case Question 6.*** Identify *four* risk factors that may have contributed to this patient's current condition.

***Patient Case Question 7.*** Why can bacterial peritonitis be ruled out as a current potential diagnosis?

***Patient Case Question 8.*** What justification might the patient's primary health care provider have for conducting an ANA test?

***Patient Case Question 9.*** Why can hemochromatosis be ruled out as a contributing factor to this patient's condition?

***Patient Case Question 10.*** Why can Wilson disease be ruled out as a contributing factor to this patient's condition?

***Patient Case Question 11.*** Why can autoimmune hepatitis and primary biliary cirrhosis be ruled out as contributing factors to this patient's condition?

***Patient Case Question 12.*** Is there any evidence that this patient is at high risk for osteoporosis?

***Patient Case Question 13.*** Identify *two* abnormal laboratory tests that are consistent with ascites.

***Patient Case Question 14.*** Which *single* laboratory test strongly suggests that the patient has developed hepatic encephalopathy?

***Patient Case Question 15.*** How would you grade this patient's encephalopathy?

***Patient Case Question 16.*** What is this patient's CTP score?

***Patient Case Question 17.*** What is the probability that this patient will live for one year?

***Patient Case Question 18.*** Does this patient have any signs of *dehydration* or *hepatorenal syndrome?*

***Patient Case Question 19.*** The patient's primary care provider has decided to conduct extensive clinical studies for the diagnosis of liver cancer. Which *single* abnormal laboratory value has raised a concern that hepatocellular carcinoma may have developed?

*For the Disease Summary for this case study,
see the CD-ROM.*

## PATIENT CASE

### ■ Patient's Chief Complaint

"My colon cancer is back, I've had another surgery, and I'm ready to start another round of chemotherapy."

### ■ HPI

Dr. H.U. is a 53 yo old Asian American male, who was diagnosed with colon cancer 18 months ago. He had been completely asymptomatic until the onset of RLQ discomfort. Four days after the initial onset of symptoms, he experienced severe abdominal pain (9/10 on the standard pain scale) and presented at the emergency room. An abdominal CT scan revealed a mass in the RLQ involving the colon. A 4.5-cm tumor was surgically resected and all signs of visible disease were cleared. There was no sign of liver or lung involvement on CT scan or upon gross examination by the surgical team. Abdominal lymph nodes were biopsied to determine the extent of the disease. The pathology report revealed that the colon tumor was a poorly differentiated adenocarcinoma. The tumor had penetrated deep through the entire width of the wall of the ascending colon and perforated the visceral peritoneal membrane. Extent of the cancer was consistent with stage IIB.

*Patient Case Question 1.* What is the probability that the patient will still be alive in 5 years?

Serum CEA was 15.9 ng/mL. The patient underwent six cycles of fluorouracil (425 mg/m² IV QD × 5 days) plus leucovorin (20 mg/m² IV QD × 5 days) administered every 4–5 weeks as the patient was able to tolerate. After adjuvant chemotherapy was completed, chest and abdominal CT scans were negative and serum CEA was 3.4 ng/mL. The serum CEA level indicated that the patient had achieved a remission.

Last month, however, the patient noticed bright red blood on the surface of the stool and immediately contacted his oncologist. He reported that he was not experiencing any pain, fatigue, bloating, vomiting, constipation, or diarrhea. His serum CEA had increased to 23.2 ng/mL and exploratory laparotomy revealed recurrent cancer in the terminal ileum and a large segment of the descending colon that extended into the rectosigmoid colon. There were no signs of disease in the rectum. A chest CT scan was normal, but an abdominal CT scan and ultrasound revealed evidence of multiple (12–15), small, hepatic metastases. All regions of tumor involvement in the ileum, descending colon, and rectosigmoid colon were resected and a colostomy was performed.

---

***Patient Case Question 2.*** What is the probability that the patient will still be alive in five years?

---

## ◼◼ PMH

- Chickenpox at age 6
- Asthma $\times$ 35 years
- Crohn disease $\times$ 8 years
- Portion of jejunum resected 6 years ago (scarring and stricture from Crohn disease → obstruction)
- Type 2 DM $\times$ 6 years
- Bilateral osteoarthritis of the knees $\times$ 3 years
- Intra-articular cortisone injection, both knees, 5 months and 2 months ago
- Negative for serious injuries or bone fractures

## ◼◼ FH

- Father, age 75, is alive but has type 2 DM, CAD, and several episodes of severe depression with suicide attempts
- Mother, age 72, has traits of OCD but has not been diagnosed or treated
- Patient has 7 siblings—two sisters with HTN, one brother with Addison disease, one brother with type 2 DM and hypothyroidism, one sister with Down syndrome
- No family history of cancer
- He is married with one son, age 35, who is alive and well

## ◼◼ SH

- Patient is a university professor of pathology and primate research
- Has smoked 3–4 cigars/day for 20 years
- Drinks 2–3 cans of beer and 1 glass of sake daily
- Sedentary lifestyle

## ◼◼ Meds

- Metformin 500 mg po BID
- Budesonide 9 mg po QD
- Vitamin B12 1000 µg IM Q month
- Albuterol inhaler PRN (recently less than 1$\times$/week)

## ◼◼ All

Adhesive tape and latex (rash)

*Patient Case Question 3.* Why is the patient taking budesonide?

# ROS

The patient lost weight, but he is finally getting his strength back after his second surgery. No chest pain, headaches, SOB, DOE, weakness, fatigue, or wheezing. Complains of mild irritation around the colostomy site but states that the "bag is working well" with no current malodorous problems. He has had some diarrhea with fluorouracil and leucovorin therapy in the past but took loperamide and tolerated side effects "fairly well." He still has a few aches and pains in his knees.

# PE and Lab Tests

## Gen

- Middle-aged Asian-American male
- Appears stated age of 53
- Cooperative but mildly anxious, oriented, attentive, and in NAD

## Vital Signs

See Patient Case Table 19.1

| Patient Case Table 19.1 Vital Signs | | | | | |
|---|---|---|---|---|---|
| BP 120/65 | (sitting, L arm) | RR | 17 and unlabored | HT | 5′10½″ |
| P | 70 and regular | T | 98.3°F | WT | 179 lbs |

## Skin

Warm with normal turgor and no lesions

## HEENT

- PERRLA
- EOMI
- Mildly icteric sclera
- Fundi benign
- TMs intact
- OP clear with moist mucous membranes

## Neck/LN

- Neck supple
- (−) cervical or axillary lymphadenopathy

## Thorax

Lungs are clear to auscultation and resonant throughout all lung fields

## Heart

- RRR
- Normal $S_1$ and $S_2$
- $(-)$ murmurs, rubs, or gallops

## Abd

- Colostomy in LLQ
- Tender at both costal margins
- Hepatomegaly prominent
- Mild distension with some ascites

## Genit/Rect

- Normal male genitalia
- Slightly enlarged prostate with no distinct nodules
- Heme-negative stool
- No rectal wall tenderness or masses

## Ext

- $(-)$ CCE
- Pulses intact throughout

## Neuro

- Speech normal
- CNs II–XII intact
- Motor: normal strength throughout
- Sensation normal
- Reflexes 2+ and symmetric throughout
- Babinski negative bilaterally
- Rapid movements, gross and fine motor coordination are normal
- Good sitting and standing balance
- Gait normal in speed and step length
- Alert and oriented $\times$ 3
- Able to do serial 7's
- Able to abstract
- Short- and long-term memories intact
- No peripheral neurologic deficits secondary to DM

*Patient Case Question 4.* Provide a reasonable explanation for the rather comprehensive neurologic exam performed by the oncologist.

*Patient Case Question 5.* Identify the *single major risk factor* associated with the patient's first occurrence of colon cancer.

*Patient Case Question 6.* Identify *four* more risk factors that may have contributed to the patient's first occurrence of colon cancer.

*Patient Case Question 7.* Identify the *single major risk factor* associated with the patient's recurrence of colon cancer.

## Laboratory Blood Test Results

See Patient Case Table 19.2

| Patient Case Table 19.2 Laboratory Blood Test Results | | | | | |
|---|---|---|---|---|---|
| Na | 140 meq/L | Hb | 14.2 g/dL | ALT | 169 IU/L |
| K | 4.0 meq/L | Hct | 44% | LDH | 469 IU/L |
| Cl | 101 meq/L | RBC | $5.3 \times 10^6/mm^3$ | Total bilirubin | 1.9 mg/dL |
| $HCO_3$ | 26 meq/L | Plt | $429 \times 10^3/mm^3$ | Alb | 2.9 g/dL |
| BUN | 9 mg/dL | WBC | $6.5 \times 10^3/mm^3$ | Total protein | 4.5 g/dL |
| Cr | 0.7 mg/dL | CEA | 16.1 ng/mL | Ca | 9.2 mg/dL |
| Glu, fasting | 161 mg/dL | AST | 78 IU/L | $PO_4$ | 3.5 mg/dL |

*Patient Case Question 8.* Identify *seven* abnormal laboratory test results that are consistent with a diagnosis of colorectal cancer.

*Patient Case Question 9.* Why might liver function tests be abnormal?

*Patient Case Question 10.* Can you find any explanation among laboratory data for the development of ascites in this patient?

*Patient Case Question 11.* Based on the laboratory data, should chronic bleeding be a concern in this patient?

# CASE STUDY

## 20

# CONSTIPATION

 *For the Disease Summary for this case study, see the CD-ROM.*

# PATIENT CASE

## ■ Patient's Chief Complaint

"I've been having some problems moving my bowels lately. I was hoping that you might prescribe something to help me that my Medicare plan will cover."

## ■ History of Present Illness

R.H. is a 74 yo black woman, who presents to the family practice clinic for a scheduled appointment. She complains of feeling bloated and constipated for the past month, sometimes going an entire week with only one bowel movement. Until this episode, she has been very regular all of her life, having a bowel movement every day or every other day. She reports straining most of the time and it often takes her 10 minutes at a minimum to initiate a bowel movement. Stools have been extremely hard. She denies pain during straining. A recent colonoscopy was negative for tumors or other lesions. She has not yet taken any medications to provide relief for her constipation.

Furthermore, she reports frequent heartburn (3–4 times each week), most often occurring soon after retiring to bed. She uses three pillows to keep herself in a more upright position during sleep. On a friend's advice, she purchased a package of over-the-counter aluminum hydroxide tablets to help relieve the heartburn. She has had some improvement since she began taking the medicine. She reports using naproxen as needed for arthritic pain in her hands and knees. She states that her hands and knees are extremely stiff when she rises in the morning. Because her arthritis has been getting worse, she has stopped taking her daily walks and now gets very little exercise.

## ■ Past Medical History

- Menopause occurred 23 years ago
- Cystocele 12 years ago
- Osteoarthritis × 7 years
- HTN × 5 years
- S/P cholecystectomy 4 years ago

- Arthroscopy of right knee 4 years ago, complicated 1 week later by invasive staphylococcal infection for which she received 6 weeks of IV vancomycin therapy
- Depressive affective mood disorder × 3 years
- GERD with recurrent symptoms × 30 months

## ■ Family History

- She has one child who is alive and well
- Her mother died in her 80s from diabetes and stroke
- Her father died at age 60 from acute MI
- Two brothers, 68 and 70 yo, are alive and both have HTN
- No known family history of colorectal disease

## ■ Social History

- She is widowed and living alone but is presently engaged; husband of 41 years passed away 4 years ago
- (−) alcohol and tobacco use
- (+) caffeine use, 2 cups of coffee with each meal
- She does not pay attention to sodium, fat, or carbohydrate content of foods; she prepares her own meals and eats few fresh fruits, vegetables, and whole grains
- (−) history of sexual abuse, eating disorders, or psychological problems
- Denies non-compliance with her medications ("I always take my medicines on time.")

## ■ Review of Systems

- (+) for constipation, lower abdominal fullness, frequent sense of incomplete evacuation, heartburn, occasional arthritic pain in hands and knees with movement, frequent insomnia
- (−) for abdominal pain, nausea, vomiting, malaise, tendency to suppress bowel movements, alternating bouts of diarrhea and constipation, fatigue, fecal incontinence
- (−) history for endocrine and neurologic disorders

## ■ Medications

- Nifedipine 30 mg po QD
- Hydrochlorothiazide 50 mg po QD
- Imipramine 100 mg po QD
- Multiple vitamin 1 tablet po QD
- Aluminum hydroxide 300 mg po PRN
- Glucosamine hydrochloride 500 mg po TID
- Conjugated estrogens 0.625 mg po QD
- Medroxyprogesterone acetate 2.5 mg po QD
- Zolpidem tartrate 5 mg po HS PRN

## ■ Allergies

- Penicillin and cephalexin → severe hives
- Sulfa drugs → confusion
- Citrus fruits and juices → upset stomach

*Patient Case Question 1.* For which condition is this patient taking nifedipine?

*Patient Case Question 2.* For which condition is this patient taking hydrochlorothiazide?

*Patient Case Question 3.* Why is this patient taking glucosamine?

*Patient Case Question 4.* Why is this patient taking medroxyprogesterone acetate?

*Patient Case Question 5.* For which condition is this patient taking zolpidem tartrate?

# ■■■ Physical Examination and Laboratory Tests

## General Appearance

- Patient is a well-developed, well-nourished, pleasant, talkative, cooperative, and slightly anxious, elderly African American female
- She is well dressed in a suit, well groomed, and appears younger than her stated age
- She is sitting up on the examination table in no apparent distress and appears both alert and oriented

## Vital Signs

See Patient Case Table 20.1

| Patient Case Table 20.1 Vital Signs | | | | | |
|---|---|---|---|---|---|
| BP average (sitting) | 115/70 | RR | 16 and unlabored | HT | 5′4″ |
| P | 82 and regular | T | 98.9°F | WT | 143 lbs |

## Skin

- Normal skin turgor and color
- Warm, moist, and soft
- (−) rashes, bruises, or other lesions

## Head, Eyes, Ears, Nose, and Throat

- Normocephalic and atraumatic
- Pupils equal at 3 mm, round, and reactive to light and accommodation
- Extra-ocular muscles intact without nystagmus
- Sclera clear and without icterus
- Fundi within normal limits and without arteriolar narrowing or nicking, hemorrhages, exudates, or papilledema
- External auricular canals clear
- Tympanic membranes within normal limits and without drainage
- Oropharynx well hydrated with moist mucous membranes

*Patient Case Question 6.* Why is a funduscopic exam appropriate in this patient?

## Neck/Lymph Nodes

- Supple
- (−) jugular venous distension, thyromegaly, and carotid bruits
- No nodal involvement

## Heart

- Regular rate and rhythm
- Normal $S_1$ and $S_2$
- No murmur or extra cardiac sounds

## Chest/Lungs

- Chest clear to auscultation
- Normal breath sounds
- Normal diaphragmatic excursions

## Abdomen

- (−) hepatosplenomegaly, masses, tenderness, and guarding
- (+) slight distension
- Normoactive bowel sounds

## Breasts

- Exam deferred
- (−) mammogram 2 months ago

## Rectal

- (−) fissures, hemorrhoids, prolapse, obstructive lesions, and bleeding
- Large amount of stool in rectal vault
- (−) occult blood in stool

## Extremities/Muscles

- (+) tenderness in hands bilaterally
- (−) cyanosis, clubbing, and edema
- Capillary refill within normal limits at 2 secs
- 2+ peripheral pulses throughout
- Subnormal strength and limited range of motion in both lower extremities
- Patellar crepitus of both knees
- Right knee incision from prior arthroscopy is well healed with minimal scarring

## Neurological

- Alert and oriented to person, place, and time
- Cranial nerves II–XII symmetric and intact
- Deep tendon reflexes normal at 2+

- Normal plantar flexion
- Sensation not impaired

## Laboratory Blood Test Results

See Patient Case Table 20.2

| Patient Case Table 20.2 Laboratory Blood Test Results | | | | | |
|---|---|---|---|---|---|
| Na | 140 meq/L | Cr | 0.8 mg/dL | PTH | 228 pg/mL |
| K | 4.1 meq/L | Glu, fasting | 98 mg/dL | Hb | 13.8 g/dL |
| Cl | 105 meq/L | Ca | 11.9 mg/dL | Hct | 41.5% |
| $HCO_3$ | 25 meq/L | TSH | 3.71 μU/mL | WBC | $9.8 \times 10^3/mm^3$ |
| BUN | 18 mg/dL | $FT_4$ | 17 pmol/L | Plt | $250 \times 10^3/mm^3$ |

*Patient Case Question 7.* List a minimum of *nine* risk factors that may be contributing to constipation.

*Patient Case Question 8.* List *eight* clinical signs and symptoms that are consistent with constipation.

*Patient Case Question 9.* Why is anemia not a suspected complication of this condition?

*Patient Case Question 10.* Would a *urinalysis, series of liver function tests,* or *serum uric acid level* be appropriate for this patient?

*Patient Case Question 11.* Should there be any concern at this time that the patient's hypertension is "out of control"?

*Patient Case Question 12.* Identify *two* clinical signs that strongly negate the possibility that hypothyroidism is contributing to constipation.

*Patient Case Question 13.* Why is constipation in this patient not likely the result of irritable bowel syndrome?

# CROHN DISEASE

 *For the Disease Summary for this case study, see the CD-ROM.*

# PATIENT CASE

## ■ HPI

C.D. is a 32 yo woman with a 14-year Hx of Crohn disease who presents with a three-day Hx of diarrhea and steady abdominal pain. She has been referred by her PCP to the GI clinic. The clinical course of her disease has included obstruction due to small intestine stricture and chronic steroid dependency with disease relapse when attempting to taper steroids. Endocrine tests reveal that she has developed adrenal insufficiency as a result of steroid use and a DEXA scan has demonstrated significant demineralization of bone.

> *Patient Case Question 1.* What is the pathophysiologic mechanism for adrenal insufficiency in this patient?
>
> *Patient Case Question 2.* What is a potential cause of the abnormal DEXA scan in this patient?

## ■ PSH

- Portion of small bowel resected 5 years ago (obstruction from scarring and stricture)
- Ovarian cyst drained, age 18
- Appendectomy, age 13

## ■ PMH

- Crohn disease diagnosed 14 years ago (weight loss, severe diarrhea with multiple bowel movements, abdominal pain, dehydration)
- Major depression

# ▬▬ FH

No family Hx of IBD

# ▬▬ SH

- Has been married for 11 years and has two daughters who are healthy
- Works as a nurse with a local home healthcare agency
- Non-smoker and non-drinker

# ▬▬ ROS

- Up to 10 loose to semi-solid stools/day, non-bloody
- Denies chills and canker sores
- Stable weight with good appetite
- Denies joint pain, skin lesions, blurred vision, and eye pain
- Some mild fatigue

# ▬▬ Meds

- Prednisone, 40 mg po QD
- Trazodone, 100 mg po BID
- Cyanocobalamin, 250 μg IM Q month

*Patient Case Question 3.* For which condition has trazodone been prescribed for this patient?

*Patient Case Question 4.* Why is this patient taking cyanocobalamin IM?

*Patient Case Question 5.* Based on your analysis of this patient's medication profile alone, what can you deduce about the degree of severity (*mild to moderate* or *severe*) of Crohn disease in this patient?

# ▬▬ All

- Codeine → nausea and vomiting
- IV dye → acute renal failure

# ▬▬ PE and Lab Tests

## Gen

- Overweight white female, somewhat anxious, moderate acute distress from chronic pain
- Cushingoid facial appearance

*Patient Case Question 6.* What is likely the cause of this patient's cushingoid facial appearance?

*Patient Case Question 7.* Briefly describe a cushingoid facial appearance.

## VS

BP 165/95, P 69, RR 15, afebrile, Ht 61 in, Wt 154 lbs

---

***Patient Case Question 8.*** What is the most likely cause of the abnormal vital sign of most concern above?

---

## Skin

* Warm and dry with flakiness
* Poor turgor

---

***Patient Case Question 9.*** What do the examination findings in the skin suggest?

---

## HEENT

* PERRLA
* EOMI
* Mild arteriolar narrowing on funduscopic exam without hemorrhages, exudates, or papilledema
* Sclera without icterus
* TMs intact and clear throughout with no drainage
* Dry mucous membranes

---

***Patient Case Question 10.*** What does the phrase "sclera without icterus" suggest?

***Patient Case Question 11.*** Identify the two abnormal HEENT findings above and provide a pathophysiologic explanation for each of them.

---

## Neck

* Supple
* No masses, JVD, lymphadenopathy, or thyromegaly

## Lungs

CTA, no crackles or rales noted

## Heart

RRR with no murmurs, rubs, or gallops

## Abdomen

* Truncal obesity with abdominal striae
* Soft abdomen, not distended, and without bruits
* Guarding with pressure to right lower quadrant
* BS hyperactive

*Patient Case Question 12.* What is a likely cause of "truncal obesity with striae"?

*Patient Case Question 13.* What are *striae?*

*Patient Case Question 14.* What is meant by *guarding?*

## Rectal

- No perianal lesions or internal masses
- Stool is heme-negative

## MS/Ext

- No clubbing, cyanosis, or edema
- Appropriate strength and ROM
- Pulses 2+ throughout
- No femoral bruits

## Neuro

- A & O × 3
- No gross motor or sensory deficits noted
- CNs II–XII intact
- DTRs 2+

## Laboratory Blood Test Results

See Patient Case Table 21.1

| Patient Case Table 21.1 Laboratory Blood Test Results | | | |
|---|---|---|---|
| Sodium | 141 meq/L | Aspartate aminotransferase | 22 IU/L |
| Potassium | 3.0 meq/L | Alanine aminotransferase | 54 IU/L |
| Chloride | 106 meq/L | Total bilirubin | 0.8 mg/dL |
| Bicarbonate | 23 meq/L | Total protein | 3.9 g/dL |
| Blood urea nitrogen | 19 mg/dL | Albumin | 2.4 g/dL |
| Creatinine | 1.0 mg/dL | Calcium | 8.7 mg/dL |
| Glucose, fasting | 120 mg/dL | Magnesium | 2.9 mg/dL |
| Hemoglobin | 13.8 g/dL | Phosphorus | 3.3 mg/dL |
| Hematocrit | 39% | Adrenocorticotropic hormone | 2 pg/mL |
| Platelets | 180,000/mm$^3$ | Erythrocyte sedimentation rate | 24 mm/hr |
| White blood cells | 11,700/mm$^3$ | C-reactive protein | 1.6 mg/dL |

*Patient Case Question 15.* Identify the *four abnormally elevated* laboratory findings above and provide a brief and reasonable pathophysiologic explanation for each of them.

*Patient Case Question 16.* Identify the *four abnormally low* laboratory findings above and provide a brief and reasonable pathophysiologic explanation for each of them.

*For the Disease Summary for this case study,
see the CD-ROM.*

# PATIENT CASE

## ■ Mother's Chief Complaints

"Our daughter has been vomiting and has had diarrhea for three days. She also has had a
fever, but I've been giving her acetaminophen every six hours. The clear liquids and Pedialyte
that she has been drinking don't seem to be helping much and she looks so sickly."

## ■ HPI

J.L. is a 4½-month-old Asian American female infant who was taken to the emergency room
of a local hospital because her parents were concerned about vomiting, diarrhea, fever, and
irritability. The patient was in good health until four days prior to presentation when she felt
warm to her mother. The patient attends daycare, and other children at the daycare center
have had similar symptoms recently.

During the first day of her illness, she continued to take normal feedings of Similac with
iron formula (approximately 6 ounces every six hours) and an occasional feeding of rice
cereal. However, by the second day, her appetite had decreased significantly and she began
to have frequent, loose, and watery stools (i.e., 6–8/day). During the 12 hours prior to presentation, J.L. had eight watery stools. The stools did not appear to contain blood. Early on
the morning of the second day of illness, the patient vomited shortly after feeding. The vomitus was non-bloody. She continued to vomit after each feeding for the next two meals and
became increasingly more irritable. The mother called her pediatrician, who recommended
12 hours of clear liquids, including weak tea with sugar, Pedialyte, and warm 7-Up. Except
for one episode in the past 48 hours, vomiting improved but diarrhea continued despite these
measures. Over the following two days, fever was intermittent and the child became more
lethargic. The parents continued the clear liquids that the doctor had ordered.

On the day of presentation at the hospital, the mother stated that her daughter had a
temperature of 101.5°F, was sleepy but very irritable when awake, and had fewer wet diapers
than normal. She also noted that her daughter's skin was cool to the touch, her lips were dry
and cracked, and her eyes appeared sunken with dark circles around them. At a doctor's
appointment 10 days prior to presentation, the patient's weight was 14.5 lbs.

***Patient Case Question 1.*** Is this patient's diarrhea considered *acute* or *chronic*?

## ■■■ PMH

- Born at 37 weeks' gestation following uncomplicated labor and spontaneous vaginal delivery to a 23 yo Asian American female
- Apgar scores were normal at 9 and 9 at one and five minutes after birth
- Weighed 7.7 lbs at birth
- Benign heart murmur observed at birth; no other complications

## ■■■ Maternal History

- Uncomplicated delivery
- During her pregnancy, she experienced one episode of bacterial vaginosis that responded to metronidazole
- Prenatal medications: prenatal vitamins and iron supplement
- Denies use of alcohol, tobacco, and illicit drugs

## ■■■ Immunizations

Shots are up-to-date, including hepatitis B vaccine

## ■■■ All

NKDA

## ■■■ FH

- Asian American mother (23 yo) and father (35 yo), both in good health
- No siblings

## ■■■ SH

- Both parents work outside of the home and patient attends daycare regularly
- Family has one cat, and their home is supplied with city water

## ■■■ PE and Lab Tests

### Gen

Patient is ill-appearing and lethargic but is arousable with stimulation. There is no muscle twitching. The anterior fontanelle is depressed and the eyes are sunken and dark. The skin is cool. Abdominal skin shows poor elasticity (skin remained in folds when pinched).

### VS

See Patient Case Table 22.1

| Patient Case Table 22.1 Vital Signs | | | | | | |
|---|---|---|---|---|---|---|
| BP | 85/55 | RR | 51 | WT | 13.0 lbs (10% weight loss in past 10 days) | |
| P | 156 | T (rectal) | 101.1°F | SaO$_2$ | 98% | |

## Skin

- No rashes or lesions
- Skin turgor subnormal
- Capillary refill time delayed to 5 seconds

## HEENT

- Pupils equal, round, and responsive to light
- TMs gray and translucent
- Nose clear
- Tongue dry and rugged

## Neck/LN

Supple and otherwise normal with no enlarged nodes

## Lungs/Thorax

- Tachypneic
- No crackles or wheezes

## Heart

- Tachycardic
- No murmurs noted

## Abd

- Anterior abdominal wall is sunken and presents a concave (rather than normal convex) contour
- (+) BS
- Soft, NT/ND
- No masses or HSM

## Genit/Rect

- Normal female external genitalia
- Greenish, watery stool in diaper

## MS/Ext

- Weak peripheral pulses
- Muscle tone normal at 5/5 throughout

## Neuro

- Lethargic and sleepy but arousable
- Irritable and crying when awake but no tears noted
- No focal defects noted

## Laboratory Blood Test Results

See Patient Case Table 22.2

| Patient Case Table 22.2 Laboratory Blood Test Results | | | | | |
|---|---|---|---|---|---|
| Na | 137 meq/L | Hb | 13.1 g/dL | WBC | 12,800/mm³ |
| K | 4.4 meq/L | Hct | 40% | • Neutros | 33% |
| Cl | 112 meq/L | Plt | 220,000/mm³ | • Bands | 3% |
| HCO₃ | 11 meq/L | ESR | 18 mm/hr | • Lymphs | 55% |
| BUN | 23 mg/dL | pH | 7.31 | • Monos | 7% |
| Cr | 1.3 mg/dL | PaO₂ | 96 mm Hg | • Basos | 1% |
| Glu, fasting | 95 mg/dL | PaCO₂ | 22 mm Hg | • Eos | 1% |

## UA

Normal except for SG = 1.029

## Stool Examination

(−) leukocytes and bacterial pathogens

---

***Patient Case Question 2.*** The emergency room physician's assessment of the patient's condition was that of *viral gastroenteritis, probably due to rotavirus, with dehydration and metabolic acidosis.* Provide a *minimum of eight* clinical signs and symptoms that support an assessment of viral gastroenteritis.

***Patient Case Question 3.*** Provide a *minimum of fifteen* clinical signs and symptoms that support an assessment of dehydration.

***Patient Case Question 4.*** Provide a *minimum of five* clinical signs and symptoms that support an assessment of metabolic acidosis.

***Patient Case Question 5.*** Is this patient's diarrhea considered *mild* or *severe?*

***Patient Case Question 6.*** Is this patient's diarrhea technically considered *inflammatory* or *non-inflammatory?*

---

# ▬ Clinical Course

J.L. was hospitalized and an intravenous catheter was inserted. Fluid loss from emesis and bowel movements was replaced with intravenous D₅W and electrolytes. No oral fluids were given during the first 24 hours. The infant was also placed in isolation to prevent transmission of possible infectious microbes to other patients or to hospital personnel. J.L. became more active and alert. Her heart rate improved to 120, respirations to 40, blood pressure to 90/58, and urine specific gravity to 1.020. On the second hospital day, oral feedings of Pedialyte and one-fourth strength infant formula were introduced. Intravenous fluids were discontinued after determination that oral intake was sufficient to sustain an adequate fluid volume.

J.L. was discharged from the hospital on the fourth day and her parents were instructed to continue oral feedings. The infant was seen in the pediatric outpatient clinic on the fifth day after her discharge. She was taking infant formula without diarrhea (approximately 25 ounces/24 hours) and had gained a half pound since her discharge. Physical examination findings were within normal limits.

---

***Patient Case Question 7.*** Which of the following factors contributes most prominently to an infant's vulnerability to dehydration?

a. a significantly lower percentage of an infant's total body weight is water when compared with older children and adults

b. an infant's basal metabolic rate is lower than an adult's basal metabolic rate

c. infants normally have a very high rate of water turnover when compared with older children and adults

d. an infant's body weight is composed of a greater proportion of fat than is an adult's body weight

***Patient Case Question 8.*** Which of the following pathophysiologic mechanisms best explains this patient's diarrhea?

a. increased intestinal motility is the result of a neuroendocrine condition

b. an infectious agent in the gastrointestinal tract has probably promoted gastrointestinal secretions while, at the same time, impaired absorption capability

c. both a and b

d. none of the above

***Patient Case Question 9.*** The immediate goal of rapid infusion of intravenous fluids during treatment of dehydration is to replace fluid in which of the following fluid compartments of the body?

a. intracellular

b. intravascular

c. interstitial

d. joint spaces

e. abdominal, pleural, and pericardial cavities

***Patient Case Question 10.*** Vomiting and diarrhea result in hydrogen ion disturbances by causing . . .

a. decreased blood flow and shifting of cells from aerobic metabolism to anaerobic metabolism, which results in the production of lactic acid

b. decreased renal function and decreased excretion of hydrogen ions in the urine

c. a significant bicarbonate loss in diarrheal stools

d. two of the above

e. three of the above

f. none of the above

***Patient Case Question 11.*** Based on the patient's electrolyte levels, which of the following types of dehydration did she have?

a. isonatremic

b. hyponatremic

c. hypernatremic

d. hypokalemic

e. hyperkalemic

***Patient Case Question 12.*** If the patient has a serum osmolality of 280 mmol/kg $H_2O$, a serum sodium concentration of 140 mmol/L, and a serum potassium concentration of 4.0 mmol/L . . .

a. what is the osmotic gap?

b. can the patient have chronic osmotic diarrhea?

# 23

## ESOPHAGEAL VARICES

 *For the Disease Summary for this case study, see the CD-ROM.*

# PATIENT CASE

## ■ History of Present Illness

Mr. P.T. is a 62-year-old accountant who has been admitted to the hospital for treatment of acute gastrointestinal bleeding. The patient had a similar episode five weeks ago. An upper endoscopic exam at that time revealed a bleeding esophageal varix for which he received band ligation therapy. He is well known to the medical community for chronic alcohol abuse. He has had a "drinking problem" throughout most of his adult life. He has lost several jobs for drinking in the workplace or showing up for work drunk. He lost his driver's license for drunk driving, and his drinking has placed a significant strain on his marriage. He and his wife are currently separated. He has tried several self-help programs to stop drinking as well as Alcoholics Anonymous, all with little success.

## ■ Past Medical History

Mr. P.T. has been hospitalized five times during the past 30 months. Most recently, he was discharged seven weeks ago following treatment for bleeding esophageal varices. He has a 44-year history of cigarette smoking (1 pack per day), was diagnosed 5 years ago with alcoholic cirrhosis, and currently drinks an unknown amount of liquor daily. He had been drinking 1–2 six-packs of beer per day for many years.

On previous admissions, he had been treated for acute pancreatitis twice, alcohol withdrawal seizures, ascites, coagulopathy, esophageal varices, peptic ulcer disease, anemia and gastritis, all of which were related to alcohol abuse. Medications at last discharge included:

- Lactulose 30 mL po QD
- Spironolactone 50 mg po QD
- Furosemide 20 mg po QD
- Propranolol 10 mg po TID
- Famotidine 40 mg QD HS

## ■ Current Status

The patient was found unconscious and face down in a pool of bright red, bloody vomitus by his neighbor. He was resuscitated and taken to the hospital by ambulance and admitted to the intensive care unit. Initial vital signs were: BP 90/60, P 112, RR 14, T 98.0°F.

Intravenous infusion with a solution of $D_5W$ and colloid was begun through a central line. Oxygen was started at 3 L/min. Octreotide was administered to help stop the bleeding. A physical examination was performed.

# ■■ Physical Examination and Laboratory Tests

## Skin

- Markedly jaundiced
- (+) spider angiomas on arms
- Normal turgor
- (−) palmar erythema

## HEENT

- Icteric sclera
- PERRLA
- EOMI
- TMs intact
- O/P dry
- No erythema or lesions in O/P

## Neck

- Supple with no nodules
- (−) JVD, thyromegaly, and lymphadenopathy

## Chest

- CTA bilaterally
- Good air exchange bilaterally
- (+) gynecomastia

## Heart

- Tachycardia with normal rhythm
- Normal $S_1$ and $S_2$ with no additional heart sounds
- No murmurs or rubs heard

## Abdomen

- Soft with mild distension and hyperactive bowel sounds
- (+) splenomegaly
- (−) caput medusae
- (−) guarding or rebound tenderness

## Genit/Rect

- External genitalia normal
- Stool heme (+)

## MS/Ext

- Warm with mild (1+) edema
- Pulses symmetric at 2+
- Muscle tone normal
- Full range of motion throughout

## Neuro

- Alert and oriented × 3
- Slow to answer questions
- CNs II–XII intact
- (−) asterixis
- DTRs brisk and equal bilaterally

## ECG

Normal sinus rhythm

***Patient Case Question 1.*** Explain the pathophysiology of each of the following clinical manifestations in this patient.

a. spider angiomas

b. gynecomastia

c. splenomegaly

d. edema

e. jaundice and icteric sclera

***Patient Case Question 2.*** Why has the primary care provider noted the absence of the following unusual clinical manifestations?

a. caput medusae

b. asterixis

## Laboratory Blood Test Results

See Patient Case Table 23.1

### Patient Case Table 23.1 Laboratory Blood Test Results

| | | | | | |
|---|---|---|---|---|---|
| Blood type | B+ | Hematocrit | 28% | PT | 23 sec |
| Sodium | 135 meq/L | White blood cells | 10,100/mm³ | PTT | 54 sec |
| Potassium | 4.6 meq/L | Platelets | 160,000/mm³ | AST | 119 IU/L |
| Chloride | 103 meq/L | Total bilirubin | 10.4 mg/dL | ALT | 94 IU/L |
| Bicarbonate | 22 meq/L | Indirect bilirubin | 9.9 mg/dL | Total protein | 4.9 g/dL |
| BUN | 10 mg/dL | Amylase | 43 IU/L | Albumin | 2.9 g/dL |
| Creatinine | 1.1 mg/dL | $PaO_2$ | 85 mm Hg | Calcium | 8.9 mg/dL |
| Glucose, fasting | 140 mg/dL | $PaCO_2$ | 45 mm Hg | Phosphorus | 2.8 mg/dL |
| Hemoglobin | 9.4 g/dL | pH | 7.38 | HIV | (−) |
| INR | 2.3 | $NH_3$ | 59 μg/dL | | |

***Patient Case Question 3.*** What is the significance of the renal test results?

***Patient Case Question 4.*** What is the significance of the liver enzyme test results?

***Patient Case Question 5.*** What are the *pathophysiology* and *significance* of the total and indirect bilirubin test results?

***Patient Case Question 6.*** Is blood clotting a concern at this time in this patient?

***Patient Case Question 7.*** Why might hemoglobin concentration and hematocrit be abnormal?

***Patient Case Question 8.*** Does this patient have an arterial blood gas problem?

***Patient Case Question 9.*** Give a reasonable explanation for the pathophysiology of the patient's blood glucose concentration.

***Patient Case Question 10.*** What evidence is provided above that this episode is not associated with another attack of alcohol-induced acute pancreatitis?

***Patient Case Question 11.*** What is the purpose of prescribing lactulose for patients with chronic liver disease?

***Patient Case Question 12.*** Why are diuretics like furosemide and spironolactone appropriate for patients with chronic hepatic disease?

## ■ Clinical Course

The patient was further evaluated with upper endoscopy, and the bleeding varices were sclerosed with sodium morrhuate. There were no acute complications of the procedure. The patient recovered satisfactorily in six days and was discharged.

# 24

# GASTRIC CANCER

 *For the Disease Summary for this case study, see the CD-ROM.*

# PATIENT CASE

## History of Present Illness

A.G. is a 62-year-old Latino male who presents to his family PCP complaining of persistent weakness, fatigue, and lack of energy that began approximately three weeks ago. When questioned about abdominal discomfort or pain, the patient noted that he "seemed to get heartburn more often lately despite taking his medication for GERD." He denied vomiting, weight loss, swelling in the abdomen, and early satiety. A CBC was ordered and revealed a red blood cell count of 3.2 million/mm$^3$, hematocrit of 31%, and hemoglobin concentration of 10.1 g/dL. A fecal occult blood test was performed and the stool was positive for blood.

*Patient Case Question 1.* What disorder is suggested by the patient's complete blood count?

## Past Medical History

• Benign prostatic hyperplasia
• Asthma
• Gastroesophageal reflux disease

## Family History

• Mother is alive at age 82 with type 2 diabetes mellitus and hypertension
• Father died at age 59 from acute myocardial infarction
• Patient has two sisters (ages 60 and 64) who are alive and well
• Maternal grandmother died from breast cancer and an aunt passed away from complications secondary to colon cancer

## ■ Social History

The patient is a retired music professor and lives alone since his wife passed away six years ago. He smokes 1½ packs of cigarettes and drinks 3–4 brandy Manhattans daily. He eats a significant amount of hamburger and processed meats, especially wieners. His daily diet does not contain healthy servings of whole grain products, fresh fruits, and vegetables. He does not have a regular exercise program but does "some walking."

## ■ Medications

- Omeprazole 20 mg po QD
- Ipratropium bromide 2 puffs QID
- Triamcinolone MDI 2 puffs QID
- Albuterol MDI 2 puffs PRN
- Terazosin 1 mg HS QD

*Patient Case Question 2.* Which of the drugs listed directly above is the patient taking for benign prostatic hyperplasia?

*Patient Case Question 3.* Which of the drugs listed directly above is the patient taking for asthma?

*Patient Case Question 4.* Which of the drugs listed directly above is the patient taking for gastroesophageal reflux disease?

## ■ Allergies

Aspirin (upset stomach)

## ■ Physical Examination and Laboratory Tests

### General

The patient is a pleasant, overweight Latino male in no apparent distress. He appears to be his stated age.

### Vital Signs

BP 120/95; P 78; RR 15; T 98.5°F; Wt 182 lbs; Ht 5'6½"

*Patient Case Question 5.* Are any of the vital signs above abnormal?

### Skin

- Warm and dry
- No lesions, bruising, or discoloration
- Normal turgor

## Head, Eyes, Ears, Nose, and Throat

- Extra-ocular muscles intact
- (−) nystagmus
- Slightly pale conjunctiva
- Sclera clear
- Normal funduscopic exam without retinopathy
- Auricular canal occluded with wax bilaterally
- Deviated nasal septum without sinus tenderness
- Nose without discharge or congestion
- Oropharynx clear, teeth intact; tongue mid-line and negative for abnormalities; tonsils intact and normal

## Neck

- Supple without masses
- No palpable nodes or auscultated bruits
- Normal thyroid
- (−) jugular vein distension

## Lungs and Thorax

- Clear to auscultation and percussion
- Breath sounds resonant and equal bilaterally
- Good air entry
- No crackles or wheezing

## Heart

- Regular rate and rhythm
- Point of maximal impulse normal at the 5th intercostal space
- Normal $S_1$ and $S_2$
- (−) for murmurs, $S_3$ and $S_4$

## Abdomen

- Soft but tender to palpation
- No masses, swelling, or bruits
- Normal peristaltic activity
- No organomegaly

## Genitalia/Rectum

- Normal male genitalia
- Diffusely enlarged prostate without distinct nodules, consistent with benign prostatic hyperplasia

## Musculoskeletal/Extremities

- Spooning of fingernails (koilonychia)
- (−) cyanosis, clubbing, and edema
- Limited range of motion upper and lower extremities consistent with degenerative joint disease

- Muscle strength and tone 4/5 bilaterally
- Peripheral pulses palpable bilaterally

## Neurological

- Oriented to person, place, and time
- Deep tendon reflexes 2+
- Normal gait
- CNs II–XII intact
- No motor or sensory deficits

## Other

- Serology: (+) for *H. pylori* antibodies
- Peripheral blood smear: hypochromic, microcytic erythrocytes

*Patient Case Question 6.* Identify *five* risk factors for gastric cancer in this patient.

*Patient Case Question 7.* Which type of deficiency is expected by the clinical data presented above?

## Laboratory Blood Test Results

See Patient Case Table 24.1

### Patient Case Table 24.1 Laboratory Blood Test Results

| | | | | | |
|---|---|---|---|---|---|
| Na | 139 meq/L | MCH | 19 pg | Chol | 188 mg/dL |
| K | 4.4 meq/L | MCHC | 26 g/dL | Ca | 9.1 mg/dL |
| Cl | 101 meq/L | WBC | 5,200/mm$^3$ | Iron | 34 µg/dL |
| HCO$_3$ | 22 meq/L | AST | 93 IU/L | TIBC | 720 µg/dL |
| BUN | 14 mg/dL | ALT | 112 IU/L | Transferrin sat | 7% |
| Cr | 0.6 mg/dL | Total bilirubin | 2.1 g/dL | Ferritin | 8 ng/mL |
| Glu, fasting | 104 mg/dL | Total protein | 7.1 g/dL | Vit B12 | 790 pg/mL |
| MCV | 70 fL | Alb | 4.6 g/dL | Folic acid | 340 ng/mL |

*Patient Case Question 8.* Which *ten* laboratory test results from this case study suggest that the patient is iron deficient?

*Patient Case Question 9.* Why was it appropriate to test for vitamin B12 and folic acid levels?

*Patient Case Question 10.* What is suggested by the liver function tests above?

## Specialized Tests

Upper endoscopy revealed a 5 cm × 3 cm mass in the upper stomach near the junction of the esophagus and stomach. A biopsy of suspicious tissue revealed cellular abnormalities consistent with *adenocarcinoma.* An endoscopic ultrasound revealed that the stomach mass had penetrated through the wall of the stomach but had not invaded lymph nodes. A chest x-ray was negative, but an abdominal CT scan was positive for multiple liver lesions. An MRI scan of the brain was negative.

*Patient Case Question 11.* To what stage has this gastric cancer progressed?

*Patient Case Question 12.* Is the 5-year survival probability for this patient greater than or less than 50%?

*Patient Case Question 13.* Would chemotherapy be significantly beneficial for this patient?

# CASE STUDY

# 25

## GASTROESOPHAGEAL REFLUX DISEASE

 *For the Disease Summary for this case study, see the CD-ROM.*

# PATIENT CASE

## ▄▄ Patient's Chief Complaints

"My acid reflux is getting worse and my histamine blocker isn't working anymore. About an hour after a meal, I get a burning pain in the middle of my chest. Sometimes, I have trouble getting food down. It seems to get stuck behind my breastbone. I've never had that problem before. My heartburn is affecting my quality of life again and I want it to stop."

## ▄▄ HPI

W.R. is a 75 yo male with a significant history of GERD. He presents to the family practice clinic today for a routine follow-up visit. The patient reports that during the past three weeks he has experienced increasing episodes of post-prandial heartburn with some regurgitation and dysphagia. He has also begun using antacids daily in addition to histamine-2-receptor blockers for symptom relief. Despite sleeping with three pillows, the patient has also begun to experience frequent nocturnal awakenings from heartburn and regurgitation.

## ▄▄ PMH

- HTN × 15 years
- GERD × 7 years
- Alcoholic cirrhosis × 2 years
- Hiatal hernia

## ▄▄ FH

Non-contributory

## ▄▄ SH

- Patient is widowed and lives alone; daughter lives in same town, checks on him regularly, and takes him grocery shopping every Saturday

- Patient is a retired college basketball coach
- Enjoys cooking, traveling, gourmet dining, and playing poker
- (+) caffeine; 5 cups coffee/day
- (+) EtOH; history of heavy alcohol use; current EtOH consumption reported is 6 beers with shots/week
- (+) smoking; 55 pack-year history; currently smokes ¾ ppd

## Meds

- Verapamil SR 120 mg po QD
- Hydrochlorothiazide 25 mg po QD
- Famotidine 20 mg po Q HS

## All

- Citrus fruits and juices (upset stomach)
- Dogs (itchy eyes, runny nose, sneezing)
- Erythromycin (unknown symptoms)

## ROS

- (−) H/A, dizziness, recent visual changes, tinnitus, vertigo
- (−) SOB, wheezing, cough, PND
- (+) frequent episodes of burning, non-radiating substernal CP
- (+) dysphagia
- (−) sore throat or hoarseness
- (−) N/V, diarrhea, BRBPR or dark/tarry stools
- (−) recent weight change

## PE and Lab Tests

### Gen

The patient is a pleasant, talkative Native American man who is wearing a sports jacket, jeans, and tennis shoes. He looks his stated age and does not appear to be in distress.

### VS

See Patient Case Table 25.1

| Patient Case Table 25.1 Vital Signs | | | | | |
|---|---|---|---|---|---|
| BP | 155/90 | RR | 18 and unlabored | HT | 5′8″ |
| P | 75 and regular | T | 97.9°F | WT | 195 lbs |

### Skin

No rashes or lesions noted

### HEENT

- PERRLA
- EOMI

- (−) arteriolar narrowing and A-V nicking
- Pink, moist mucous membranes
- (−) tonsils
- Oropharynx clear

## Lungs

CTA

## Heart

- Regular rhythm
- (−) additional heart sounds

## Abd

- Normoactive BS
- Soft, NT/ND
- (−) HSM
- (−) bruits

## Genit/Rec

- (−) hemorrhoids
- (−) rectal masses
- Brown stool without occult blood
- Prostate WNL

## Ext

(−) CCE

## Neuro

- A & O for person, time, place
- CNs II–XII intact
- Strength 5/5 upper/lower extremities bilaterally

*Patient Case Question 1.* Which clinical information suggests worsening symptoms of GERD in this patient?

*Patient Case Question 2.* Which symptom(s) indicates the possible severity of the patient's GERD?

*Patient Case Question 3.* Are the patient's symptoms *classic* or *atypical*?

*Patient Case Question 4.* Identify all those factors that may be contributing to the patient's symptoms.

*Patient Case Question 5.* Why is the drug verapamil a potential contributing factor to the patient's symptoms?

*Patient Case Question 6.* What non-pharmacologic therapies or lifestyle modifications might be beneficial in the management of this patient's acid reflux disease?

*Patient Case Question 7.* What pharmacotherapeutic alternatives are available for the treatment of this patient's GERD?

# ■■■ Clinical Course

The patient underwent upper endoscopy, which revealed multiple, circular, confluent erosions of the distal esophagus. There was no evidence of bleeding, ulcerations, stricture, or esophageal metaplasia. The patient was treated with an 8-week course of 30 mg/day lansoprazole and both heartburn and dysphagia resolved. Approximately 10 weeks after PPI therapy was discontinued, the patient reported that his reflux symptoms had returned and that he was again suffering from frequent post-prandial and nocturnal episodes of reflux.

*Patient Case Question 8.* What therapeutic options are now available for this patient?

*Patient Case Question 9.* Based on upper endoscopy test results, what grade of esophagitis can be assigned to this patient's condition?

*For the Disease Summary for this case study,
see the CD-ROM.*

# PATIENT CASE

## ■■ Patient's Chief Complaints

"I've been nauseated again and have thrown up several times since yesterday. I also have a constant aching in my stomach and I feel really bloated again."

## ■■ HPI

J.A. is an 83-year-old man who is a five-day post-status surgical patient for elective repair of an abdominal aortic aneurysm. After nearly nine hours of uncomplicated surgery, the patient was transferred to the surgical intensive care unit. Intravenous methyldopa was used to maintain the patient's systolic blood pressure below 160 mm Hg. He awoke one hour later and was drowsy from the IV morphine sulfate that he was receiving every 90–120 minutes for pain. Vital signs were stable for the next five hours (BP 148/85, P 91, RR 21, Hct 39%) on 40% oxygen by face mask. Then, his abdomen became moderately distended but soft. No bowel sounds were heard during a prolonged period of auscultation. There was no fever or elevated white blood cell count, but there was mild abdominal tenderness with palpation. Plain film radiographs demonstrated a cecal diameter of 10.5 cm (the upper limit of normal cecal size is 9.0 cm) and a diagnosis of acute colonic pseudo-obstruction secondary to surgery was made. Nasogastric and rectal tubes were inserted and low constant suction provided to ensure gastric decompensation. The patient was periodically rolled from side to side and to the prone position in an effort to promote expulsion of colonic gas. Nasogastric output was replaced mL for mL with IV 0.45% saline and 20 meq/L potassium chloride.

On post-operative day 1, repeat abdominal radiographs revealed that cecal diameter remained at 10.5 cm. The patient continued to feel nauseous and vomited twice. Nasogastric output was measured every 4–4½ hours and fluctuated from 50 to 175 mL of green drainage fluid.

*Patient Case Question 1.* Determine the grade of vomiting during the last 24 hours.

On post-operative day 2, analgesia was maintained with 8 mg morphine IM every 4 hours. Abdominal radiographs showed that cecal diameter had increased to 11.5 cm. Two more episodes of vomiting occurred. A single dose of 2 mg neostigmine was given IV and significant colonic decompression occurred within 20 minutes. The patient was monitored for possible neostigmine-induced bradycardia, but no adverse effects developed.

On post-operative day 3, cecal diameter was measured at 9.5 cm, a decrease of 2.0 cm from post-operative day 2. The patient felt considerably less nauseated and had not vomited in the past 12 hours. Nasogastric output had slowed to 60 mL/8 hours. He remained on IV saline and KCl, however, and orders of "nothing by mouth." His abdomen was only mildly distended and soft. Bowel sounds were audible by auscultation in all four quadrants. A decision was made to maintain his tubes in place for one more day.

On post-operative day 4, the patient's tubes were removed and he began taking in a clear liquid diet by mouth in the early morning. By noon, however, he began to complain of increasing abdominal discomfort, feeling bloated and nauseous, and suffered three episodes of vomiting a greenish fluid. Respiration rate was 28/minute, heart rate was 105/minute, and both blood pressure and temperature were normal. Bowel sounds, which had been normoactive upon rising, were now absent. The patient did not respond to neostigmine this time, but responded well to placement of a decompression tube. Within 18 hours, however, symptoms had returned once again.

## ▰▰▰ PMH

- HTN × 20 years
- OA × 18 years
- Type 2 DM
- Hyperlipidemia

## ▰▰▰ PSH

- Right nephrectomy for "benign" renal disease, 23 years ago
- Partial colectomy for polyposis, 14 years ago
- Total right hip replacement for worsening hip pain from OA unresponsive to analgesic treatments, 5 years ago

## ▰▰▰ FH

- Mother and younger sister (both deceased) had "high blood pressure"
- Father died from AMI at age 78
- History of AMI and stroke at young ages in maternal grandparents

## ▰▰▰ SH

- Patient lives with wife of 55 years, is a retired civil engineer (retired at age 65), and enjoys gardening and travel
- No tobacco × 15 years
- No EtOH × 15 years

## ▰▰▰ ROS

- (+) nausea, retching, vomiting, epigastric discomfort, dry mouth, and fatigue
- (−) headache, stiff neck, fever, abdominal pain, diarrhea, melena, urinary frequency/urgency/discomfort, weakness, SOB, numbness/tingling in extremities

# Meds

- Amlodipine 10 mg po Q AM
- Glyburide 10 mg po Q AM, 5 mg po Q PM
- EC ASA 325 mg po QD
- Gemfibrozil 600 mg po BID

*Patient Case Question 2.* How does amlodipine work to relieve hypertension?

*Patient Case Question 3.* How does glyburide work to control blood sugar in type 2 diabetes mellitus?

*Patient Case Question 4.* What are the *two major* contributing factors for nausea and vomiting in this patient?

# All

No known drug or food allergies

# PE and Lab Tests

## Gen

- White male who looks his stated age in moderate distress
- Ill-appearing and slightly lethargic in his hospital bed
- The patient's face is ashen and the eyes are noticeably sunken

## VS

See Patient Case Table 26.1

**Patient Case Table 26.1 Vital Signs**

| BP | 85/60 supine, right arm | RR | 25 and unlabored | HT | 5'7" |
|---|---|---|---|---|---|
| P | 105 and regular | T | 95.3°F | WT | 154 lbs (160 lbs 5 days ago) |

## Skin

- Color: gray
- Temperature: cold
- Turgor: poor, some skin tenting noted
- Feel: dry
- No rash, petechiae, or lesions

## HEENT

- PERRLA
- EOMI
- Fundi benign

- Sclera without icterus
- TMs intact
- Mucous membranes dry

## Neck/LN

- Supple
- Thyroid WNL
- (−) adenopathy, bruits, and JVD

## Lungs/Thorax

- Tachypnea prominent
- Lungs clear to auscultation

## Cardiac

- Sinus tachycardia
- (−) murmurs, rubs, and gallops

## Abd

- Soft and moderately distended with hypoactive BS
- Pain is elicited on light palpation of RLQ
- (−) HSM, rebound tenderness, and masses

## Genit/Rect

- Genital exam not performed
- Normal sphincter tone
- Rectal exam WNL
- No bright red blood or masses visible
- Stool guaiac-negative

## MS/Ext

- Extremities are cold and gray
- Pulses hypoactive at 1+ throughout
- (−) edema and clubbing

## Neuro

- (+) lethargy
- (−) visual abnormalities
- Cranial nerves intact
- DTRs 2+
- Strength is equal bilaterally in all extremities

## Laboratory Blood Test Results

See Patient Case Table 26.2

## Patient Case Table 26.2 Laboratory Blood Test Results

| Na | 147 meq/L | Glu, fasting | 71 mg/dL | Amylase | 31 IU/L |
|---|---|---|---|---|---|
| K | 3.2 meq/L | Mg | 1.8 mg/dL | Hb | 14.6 g/dL |
| Cl | 95 meq/L | $PO_4$ | 2.4 mg/dL | Hct | 41.2% |
| $HCO_3$ | 31 meq/L | Ca | 8.9 mg/dL | Plt | $206 \times 10^3/mm^3$ |
| BUN | 30 mg/dL | T Bilirubin | 0.8 mg/dL | WBC | $3.5 \times 10^3/mm^3$ |
| Cr | 1.2 mg/dL | T Protein | 7.6 g/dL | • PMNs | 58% |
| | | | | • Bands | 0% |
| | | | | • Lymphs | 33% |
| | | | | • Monos | 6% |
| | | | | • Eos | 2% |
| | | | | • Basos | 1% |

*Patient Case Question 5.* List *twelve* clinical manifestations in this patient that are consistent with a diagnosis of *dehydration*.

*Patient Case Question 6.* Has the patient developed *hypokalemia*?

*Patient Case Question 7.* Why can *acute pancreatitis* be ruled out as a cause of nausea and vomiting in this patient?

*Patient Case Question 8.* Perforation of the cecum often occurs when cecal diameter >10 cm. Severe abdominal pain, fever, and leukocytosis are clinical manifestations of perforation. Has the cecum perforated in this patient?

*Patient Case Question 9.* What is believed to be the pathophysiologic mechanism that underlies acute colonic pseudo-obstruction?

*Patient Case Question 10.* Are respiratory and reflex signs *consistent* or *inconsistent with* metabolic alkalosis?

# CASE STUDY

# 27

# PEPTIC ULCER DISEASE

 *For the Disease Summary for this case study, see the CD-ROM.*

# PATIENT CASE

## ■ History of Present Illness

M.S. is a 56-year-old Hispanic male who presents with complaints of a four-week history of gradually increasing upper abdominal pain. He describes the pain as "burning" in nature, localized to the epigastrium, and that previously it had been relieved by drinking milk or Mylanta. The pain is much worse now and milk or antacids do not provide any relief. He scores the pain as a "7" on a scale of 1–10. The patient does not feel the pain radiating into his back and has not noticed any blood in his stools. He denies any nausea, vomiting, weight loss, shortness of breath, neurologic symptoms, or chest pain with exercise. He maintains that his appetite is excellent.

He has been taking 400 mg ibuprofen almost daily for knee pain for the last 18 months. He injured his right knee in a car accident 15 years ago. He also takes daily doses of 81 mg aspirin "for his heart," although this has not been prescribed. He does not take any other pre-scribed or OTC medications. The patient smokes 1½ packs of cigarettes every day and has done so for 5 years since his wife passed away. He does not drink alcohol or use illegal drugs. The patient is allergic to meperidine and develops a skin rash when he is treated with it.

He admits to feeling "stressed out" as he recently lost his job of 20 years as an insurance salesman and has had difficulty finding another. Furthermore, his unemployment compen-sation recently lapsed.

M.S. has been feeling a bit tired lately. He was diagnosed with HTN (stage 1) three years ago and has been managing his elevated BP with diet and regular workouts at the gym. His younger brother also has HTN and both his parents suffered AMIs at a young age. M.S. has a history of gallstones and laparoscopic removal of his gallbladder six years ago. He also has a history of migraine headaches.

*Patient Case Question 1.* Identify *three* factors that may have contributed to a peptic ulcer in this patient.

*Patient Case Question 2.* From your list of factors in Question 1 above that may have contributed to a peptic ulcer in this patient, which factor has likely played the most sig-nificant role?

*Patient Case Question 3.* Why might the healthcare provider have inquired about possi-ble shortness of breath or chest pain with exercise?

# ■■ PE and Lab Tests

The patient is a heavy Hispanic male in mild acute distress. He is rubbing his chest and upper abdomen. Height 5'10", weight 206 lbs, T = 98.8°F po, P = 90 and regular, RR = 18 and unlabored, BP = 156/98 left arm sitting.

***Patient Case Question 4.*** Is this patient *underweight, overweight, obese,* or is his weight *healthy* for his height?

***Patient Case Question 5.*** Why might the PCP order an ECG for this patient?

## HEENT, Neck, Skin

- PERRLA, fundi w/o vascular changes
- Pharynx and nares clear
- Neck supple w/o bruits over carotid arteries
- No thyromegaly or adenopathy
- No JVD
- Skin warm with good turgor and slightly diaphoretic w/o cyanosis
- Yellowed teeth

## Lungs, Heart

- Good lung expansion bilaterally
- Breath sounds clear
- Percussion w/o dullness throughout
- RRR
- No murmurs, gallops, or rubs
- $S_1$ and $S_2$ prominent

## Abdomen, Extremities

- No abdominal bruits, masses, or organomegaly
- Positive bowel sounds present throughout with no distension
- Epigastric tenderness w/palpation but w/o rebound or guarding
- No cyanosis, clubbing, or edema
- Peripheral pulses 2+ throughout

## Rectal Examination

- No hemorrhoids present
- Prostate slightly enlarged but w/o nodules that suggest cancer
- Stool sample submitted for heme testing

## Neurological

- Alert and oriented to time, place, and person, appropriately anxious
- Cranial nerves II to XII intact
- Strength 5/5 bilaterally
- DTRs 2+ and symmetric
- Touch sensation intact
- Gait steady

## Laboratory Test Results

- All blood chemistries including Na, K, Ca, BUN, and Cr normal
- WBC = 7500/mm$^3$ w/NL WBC Diff
- Hct = 37%
- ALT, AST, total bilirubin normal
- Amylase = 90 IU/L
- ECG = normal sinus rhythm w/o evidence of ischemic changes
- Stool heme-positive

*Patient Case Question 6.* What is the significance of the WBC count?

*Patient Case Question 7.* What is the significance of the Hct?

*Patient Case Question 8.* What is the significance of the serum amylase concentration?

*Patient Case Question 9.* Why might tests for ALT and AST be appropriate in this patient?

## ▬ Endoscopy Results

- Normal appearing esophagus
- 1-cm gastric ulcer w/evidence of recent bleeding but no signs of acute hemorrhage in the ulcer crater
- Rapid urease test negative

*Patient Case Question 10.* What is the significance of the urease test result?

*Patient Case Question 11.* What type of management would be appropriate for this patient?

# 28

# ULCERATIVE COLITIS

 *For the Disease Summary for this case study, see the CD-ROM.*

## PATIENT CASE

### ■ HPI

X.P. is a 24-year-old man, who presents to the urgent care clinic with complaints of rectal bleeding and weakness. Five days ago he noticed bright red blood in his stools. Furthermore, daily bowel movements have increased to five or six with significant diarrhea. He states that urges to move his bowels have rapid onset, but there has been no incontinence. He has been weak for approximately 2½ days. He has not traveled outside of the city, been hospitalized, or received antibiotics recently.

**Patient Case Question 1.** What is the relevance of the last sentence directly above?

### ■ PMH

- Chronic sinus infections since age 15
- Ventricular septal defect at birth, surgically repaired at age 1 year

### ■ FH

- Strong positive family history of autoimmune disease on maternal side
- Mother has SLE
- Maternal grandmother (deceased) had Graves disease
- Aunt has myasthenia gravis

**Patient Case Question 2.** What is the significance of the patient's family history?

## ■■■ SH

- College graduate
- Recently discharged after 3 years of active military service in Afghanistan
- Currently employed as user consultant in information technology division at local community college
- Social alcohol use only
- Denies tobacco and IV drug use

## ■■■ ROS

- Negative for lightheadedness and feeling faint with standing
- Negative for nausea, vomiting, visual changes or eye pain, abdominal distension with gas, and joint pain
- Positive for occasional malaise, mild abdominal cramps, loss of appetite, and weight loss of 4 lbs during the past month

## ■■■ Meds

None

## ■■■ All

NKDA

## ■■■ PE and Lab Tests

### Gen

A & O, pleasant, young, white male in NAD; skin color is pale

### VS

BP (sitting, left arm) 120/75, P 93 bpm, RR 20/min, T 99.4°F, SaO$_2$ 95% on RA, Wt 161 lbs (usual weight 165 lbs), Ht 5′10″

*Patient Case Question 3.* What is the significance of the pulse oximetry findings above?

### Skin

- Warm and dry with satisfactory turgor
- Positive for pallor
- No rashes or other lesions

*Patient Case Question 4.* What is a reasonable explanation for pallor in this patient?

## HEENT

- PERRLA
- EOMI
- Negative for uveitis
- Funduscopic exam normal
- TMs intact
- Nose clear and not inflamed
- Moist mucous membranes

---

***Patient Case Question 5.*** What is the significance of the findings described as *satisfactory turgor* and *moist mucous membranes*?

---

## Chest

Lungs CTA & P

## Heart

- RRR
- Normal first and second heart sounds
- No m/r/g or extra heart sounds

## Abd

- BS (+)
- Soft and NT/ND
- No palpable masses
- No HSM
- No bruits

## Rectal

- Somewhat tender
- No hemorrhoids or other lesions
- Heme (+) stool

## MS/Ext

- Equal motor strength at 5/5 in both arms and legs
- Sensation normal
- No CCE
- Peripheral pulses normal

## Neuro

- A & O × 3
- Sensory and motor levels normal
- CNs II–XII intact

- DTRs 2+
- Babinski response negative

---

*Patient Case Question 6.* What constitutes a positive Babinski sign and why is a positive Babinski sign significant?

## Laboratory Blood Test Results

See Patient Case Table 28.1

| Patient Case Table 28.1 Laboratory Blood Test Results | | | | | | | |
|---|---|---|---|---|---|---|---|
| Na$^+$ | 143 meq/L | BUN | 20 mg/dL | Plt | 315,000/mm$^3$ | AST | 33 IU/L |
| K$^+$ | 3.2 meq/L | Cr | 1.1 mg/dL | ESR | 24 mm/hr | ALT | 41 IU/L |
| Cl$^-$ | 108 meq/L | Hb | 10.8 g/dL | CRP | 1.5 mg/dL | T bilirubin | 0.9 mg/dL |
| HCO$_3^-$ | 18 meq/L | Hct | 36% | Ca$^{+2}$ | 8.9 mg/dL | PT | 11.3 sec |
| Glu, fasting | 132 mg/dL | WBC | 9,400/mm$^3$ | PO$_4^{-3}$ | 4.0 mg/dL | Alb | 3.1 g/dL |

---

*Patient Case Question 7.* Identify *eight* abnormal laboratory blood test values and provide a brief pathophysiologic explanation for each of them.

*Patient Case Question 8.* Does the patient have signs of liver disease?

## ■■■ Clinical Course

The patient received 1 L of 0.9% saline with 30 meq KCl IV for 4 hours and was discharged with instructions to return to the urgent care clinic or immediately contact his PCP if symptoms developed again. The patient was referred to the GI clinic.

---

*Patient Case Question 9.* Why was the patient treated with an IV solution?

*Patient Case Question 10.* Why is the concentration of saline that was infused important?

A proctosigmoidoscopy was conducted three days after the patient's discharge from the acute care clinic. Significant pseudopolyp formation could be seen. Biopsies of the colon revealed erosions of the mucosa and ulcerations into the submucosa with mixed acute (i.e., neutrophils) and chronic (lymphocytes and macrophages) inflammatory cells. No dysplastic cells suggesting the development of colon carcinoma were seen. No multinucleated giant cells suggesting Crohn disease were seen. Inflammation and ulceration were limited to the rectum and sigmoid colon only. Crypts of Lieberkühn were intensely inflamed. Marked hemorrhaging of capillaries in the mucosa was also observed.

## ■■■ Pathologist's Dx

Ulcerative colitis

***Patient Case Question 11.*** Based on laboratory tests, physical examination, and the patient's medical history, would disease activity be considered *mild, moderate,* or *severe?* How did you arrive at your answer?

***Patient Case Question 12.*** What is an appropriate initial pharmacotherapeutic approach for this patient?

***Patient Case Question 13.*** If the patient responds unsatisfactorily during three weeks of treatment, what is an appropriate pharmacotherapeutic option?

***Patient Case Question 14.*** Is surgery warranted in this patient?

# VIRAL HEPATITIS

 *For the Disease Summary for this case study, see the CD-ROM.*

# PATIENT CASE

## ■ Patient's Chief Complaints

"I don't really feel seriously sick, but my wife insisted that something is wrong and that I should see a doctor. I've been a bit tired and weak now for nearly three weeks. I've not been working more than usual, my appetite is good, and I'm only 52—so it can't be old age setting in already. Also, and this may be nothing, but I'm a little sore under my right ribcage—not really pain, but it is uncomfortable when I jog."

## ■ HPI

D.H. is a 52 yo white male with no significant past medical history, except for a severe bout of cholecystitis seven years ago that resolved following laparoscopic cholecystectomy. He states that he has been healthy until three weeks ago, when he noticed some fatigue and weakness. He does not recall a past history of liver problems.

## ■ PMH

- MVA in 1996 that required a blood transfusion
- Cholecystitis and cholecystectomy, 7 years ago

## ■ FH

- No known family history of liver disease
- Mother was alcoholic; died 8 years ago in car accident
- Father, age 77, has type 2 DM
- Two younger siblings are alive and well

## ▬ SH

- Divorced, but re-married 3 years ago
- Has 5 children from first marriage (three are still living at home)
- No tobacco use
- Drinks a 6-pack of beer on weekends
- Minimal caffeine consumption
- Has been employed as an information technology consultant at the university in town for the past 11 years
- Has a significant history of IV drug use and cocaine snorting as a young adult but has "been clean now for 15 years"
- Denies any recent international travel
- Exercises daily (jogging and golf in summer, bowling and basketball in winter)
- Denies knowledge of having unprotected sex or living with anyone diagnosed with viral hepatitis

## ▬ ROS

- (+) progressive fatigue and weakness
- (+) slightly elevated liver enzymes during last physical examination 10 months ago; was advised to seek follow-up at the liver clinic—which he failed to do, because he "felt fine"
- (−) yellowing of the skin/sclera; bleeding and bruising; swelling; gynecomastia; decrease in sexual drive; impotence; palmar erythema; spider veins; high blood pressure; rash or other type of skin lesion; itching; loss of appetite; changes in bowel or bladder function; and changes in stool or urine color

## ▬ Meds

None

## ▬ All

No known drug or food allergies

## ▬ PE and Lab Tests

### Gen

- WDWN muscular, white male in NAD
- Wears glasses
- Patient is friendly, soft-spoken, and cooperative and appears to be his stated age
- He appears to be of ideal body weight

### VS

See Patient Case Table 29.1

| Patient Case Table 29.1 Vital Signs | | | | | |
|---|---|---|---|---|---|
| BP | 138/80 | RR | 16 and unlabored | HT | 6 ft-1 in |
| P | 69 and regular | T | 98.3°F | WT | 174 lbs |

## Skin

- Warm and dry with normal color and turgor
- (−) obvious icterus, spider angiomata, palmar erythema, and other types of rash or skin lesions
- (+) large tattoos on both forearms, lower legs, and lower back

## HEENT

- NC/AT
- Pupils equal at 3 mm with normal response to light
- EOMI
- Clear sclera
- (−) nystagmus and conjunctivitis
- Funduscopic exam normal
- TMs WNL bilaterally
- Good dentition
- Oral mucosa pink and moist with no lesions

## Neck/LN

- Neck supple
- (−) cervical, supraclavicular, and axillary lymphadenopathy
- (−) thyromegaly, carotid bruits, masses, and JVD

## Lungs/Chest/Back

- CTA & P bilaterally
- Mild scoliosis noted

## Cardiac

- RRR
- $S_1$ and $S_2$ normal
- (−) $S_3$, $S_4$, rubs, murmurs, and gallops

## Abd

- Soft and non-distended
- Moderate hepatomegaly and tenderness in RUQ with light palpation
- (−) splenomegaly, ascites, masses, and bruits
- (+) BS

## Genit/Rect

- (−) masses, prostate enlargement, hemorrhoids, melena, and testicular atrophy
- Normal anal sphincter tone

## MS/Ext

- (−) CCE
- Peripheral pulses 2+ throughout and without bruits
- Normal ROM

## Neuro

- A & O × 3
- CNs II–XII intact
- DTRs 2+ throughout
- (−) focal deficits
- Toes downgoing
- Sensation, coordination, and gait normal
- Muscle strength 5/5 in all four extremities
- Capillary refill normal at < 2 secs

## Laboratory Blood Test Results

See Patient Case Table 29.2

| Patient Case Table 29.2 Laboratory Blood Test Results | | | | | |
|---|---|---|---|---|---|
| Na | 138 meq/L | PMNs | 51% | Protein, total | 5.6 g/dL |
| K | 3.8 meq/L | Bands | 3% | PT | 12.3 secs |
| Cl | 104 meq/L | Lymphs | 37% | PTT | 29.8 secs |
| HCO$_3$ | 25 meq/L | Monos | 9% | Ca | 8.5 mg/dL |
| BUN | 15 mg/dL | AST | 142 IU/L | Mg | 2.0 mg/dL |
| Cr | 1.0 mg/dL | ALT | 120 IU/L | Phos | 3.9 mg/dL |
| Glu, fasting | 85 mg/dL | Alk Phos | 178 IU/L | Vit D—1,25OH | 51 pg/mL |
| Hb | 14.1 g/dL | Bilirubin, total | 1.5 mg/dL | Vitamin A | 19 mg/dL |
| Hct | 40.7% | Bilirubin, direct | 1.1 mg/dL | Vitamin E | 0.6 mg/dL |
| Plt | 263 × 10³/mm³ | Bilirubin, indirect | 0.4 mg/dL | AFP | 14 ng/mL |
| WBC | 9.9 × 10³/mm³ | Alb | 3.0 g/dL | | |

## Urinalysis

See Patient Case Table 29.3

| Patient Case Table 29.3 Urinalysis | | | | | |
|---|---|---|---|---|---|
| Color | Dark yellow | Protein | (−) | Bacteria | (−) |
| Appearance | Clear | WBC | 1/HPF | Bilirubin | (+) |
| pH | 5.5 | RBC | (−) | Ketones | (−) |
| SG | 1.020 | Nitrite | (−) | Glucose | (−) |

## Serology Testing

See Patient Case Table 29.4

| Patient Case Table 29.4 Serology Testing | | | |
|---|---|---|---|
| (−) | IgG anti-HAV antibody | (+) | HCV RNA = 2.7 million copies/mL |
| (−) | HBsAg | (−) | IgG anti-HDV antibody |
| (−) | IgG anti-HBeAg | (−) | IgG anti-HEV antibody |
| (+) | IgG anti-HCV antibody | HCV Genotype | Type 1 |

## Liver Biopsy

- Lymphocyte aggregates and some macrophages within portal tracts
- Mild periportal fibrosis
- Macrovesicular steatosis
- All pathologic findings consistent with chronic hepatitis

*Patient Case Question 1.* What is an appropriate diagnosis of this patient's condition?

*Patient Case Question 2.* Which *three* tests are most definitive in determining this diagnosis?

*Patient Case Question 3.* Identify this patient's potential risk factors for viral hepatitis.

*Patient Case Question 4.* What is the most likely cause of this patient's viral hepatitis?

*Patient Case Question 5.* Why is a previous blood transfusion not a likely cause of viral hepatitis?

*Patient Case Question 6.* What is the preferred treatment for this patient?

*Patient Case Question 7.* Why were serum concentrations of the vitamins A, D, and E tested?

*Patient Case Question 8.* Why was serum AFP assayed in this patient?

*Patient Case Question 9.* What is the significance of the serum AFP concentration in this patient?

*Patient Case Question 10.* Which patient vital sign—blood pressure, heart rate, temperature, or respiratory rate—would likely be elevated if the patient's liver was not adequately metabolizing cortisol for excretion?

*Patient Case Question 11.* Which two major serum electrolytes may be abnormal if the patient's liver was not adequately metabolizing aldosterone for excretion?

*Patient Case Question 12.* Why is this patient's WBC differential consistent with a diagnosis of viral hepatitis?

*Patient Case Question 13.* Identify *seven* abnormal laboratory blood tests that are consistent with a diagnosis of liver injury and reduced hepatic function.

*Patient Case Question 14.* What is the *single* most significant abnormal finding in the patient's urine and why is this finding consistent with the patient's condition?

*Patient Case Question 15.* Why is it critical that this patient refrain from further use of alcohol?

# RENAL

# DISORDERS

# ACUTE RENAL FAILURE

 *For the Disease Summary for this case study, see the CD-ROM.*

# PATIENT CASE

## ▰ HPI

Mr. J.R. is a 73-year-old man, who was admitted to the hospital with clinical manifestations of gastroenteritis and possible renal failure. The patient's chief complaints are fever, nausea with vomiting and diarrhea for 48 hours, weakness, dizziness, and a bothersome metallic taste in the mouth. The patient is pale and sweaty.

He had been well until two days ago, when he began to experience severe nausea several hours after eating two burritos for supper. The burritos had been ordered from a local fast-food restaurant. The nausea persisted and he vomited twice with some relief. As the evening progressed, he continued to feel "very bad" and took some Pepto-Bismol to help settle his stomach. Soon thereafter, he began to feel achy and warm. His temperature at the time was 100.5°F. He has continued to experience nausea, vomiting, and a fever. He has not been able to tolerate any solid foods or liquids. Since yesterday, he has had 5–6 watery bowel movements. He has not noticed any blood in the stools. His wife brought him to the ER because he was becoming weak and dizzy when he tried to stand up. His wife denies any recent travel, use of antibiotics, laxatives, or excessive caffeine, or that her husband has an eating disorder.

## ▰ PMH

- HTN × 14 years
- Post-AMI × 10 years
- Heart failure × 8 years
- No known renal disease or DM
- Osteoarthritis × 5 years
- DVT at age 61, treated with anticoagulants for 1 year

## ▰ FH

- Father died at age 50 from AMI
- Mother has type 2 DM
- Has two brothers, both living, with no known medical problems
- Has two sons without medical problems

## ■ SH

- Retired pharmacy professor who is living at home with his wife of 34 years
- Denies use of alcohol, tobacco, and illicit drugs
- Has 2 cups of coffee maximum daily

## ■ ROS

Was not performed as patient is acutely ill

## ■ Meds

- Digoxin 0.125 mg po QD
- Furosemide 40 mg po QD
- Enalapril 20 mg po QD (recently added to furosemide to manage HTN)
- OTC acetaminophen 500 mg po PRN

## ■ All

- Sulfa drugs (anaphylaxis)
- Molds (watery eyes and sneezing)

## ■ Physical Examination and Laboratory Tests

### General

The patient is a pale, diaphoretic, elderly Asian male in acute distress. The patient's eyes appear sunken with dark circles around them.

### Arterial Blood Gas Results

See Patient Case Table 30.1

| Patient Case Table 30.1 Arterial Blood Gas Results | | | | | | | |
|---|---|---|---|---|---|---|---|
| pH | 7.35 | $PaO_2$ | 87 mm Hg | $PaCO_2$ | 29 mm Hg | $SaO_2$ | 95% |

*Patient Case Question 1.* Based on the information provided above, which two types of acute renal failure are most likely?

*Patient Case Question 2.* List *four* major risk factors that are likely to be contributing to the patient's kidney failure.

### VS

See Patient Case Table 30.2

| Patient Case Table 30.2 Vital Signs | | | | | |
|---|---|---|---|---|---|
| BP | 92/45 | RR | 30 | WT | 185 lbs |
| P | 115 | T | 101.3°F | HT | 5′11″ |

## Skin

- Pale
- Poor turgor
- Warm to touch
- Patient denies itching

*Patient Case Question 3.* What is the significance of (a) poor skin turgor and (b) an absence of itching?

## HEENT

- PERRLA
- No funduscopic abnormalities
- EOMI
- Conjunctiva pale
- Non-erythematous TMs
- Nose clear w/o exudates or lesions
- Mucous membranes pale and dry
- Tongue rugged
- Slight erythema in throat

## Neck/LN

- Supple
- No JVD or HJR
- No lymphadenopathy or thyromegaly
- No carotid artery bruits

*Patient Case Question 4.* What is the importance of the absence of JVD and HJR?

## Heart

- Normal $S_1$ and $S_2$
- Faint $S_3$
- No murmurs or friction rubs
- Normal sinus rhythm

## Lungs

No crackles bilaterally

*Patient Case Question 5.* What is the significance of the "faint $S_3$" cardiac sound?

*Patient Case Question 6.* What is the significance of the absence of pulmonary crackles?

## Abd

- Diffuse tenderness
- No guarding or rebound

- Soft and non-distended with hyperactive bowel sounds
- No HSM

## Genit/Rect

- Prostate exam normal
- Slightly heme-positive stool in the rectum
- No grossly visible blood

## MS/Ext

- Normal muscle strength bilaterally
- No CCE
- Peripheral pulses weak at 1+ bilaterally
- Patient denies any muscle tenderness

## Neuro

- A & O × 3
- CNs intact
- Motor function—no focal weakness
- Slightly decreased patellar reflex, otherwise normal reflexes
- Normal coordination and gait

**Patient Case Question 7.** What is the significance of the neurological findings in this patient?

## Laboratory Blood Test Results

See Patient Case Table 30.3

| Patient Case Table 30.3 Laboratory Blood Test Results | | | | | | | | | |
|---|---|---|---|---|---|---|---|---|---|
| Na | 144 meq/L | Cr | 2.6 mg/dL | Alb | 4.3 g/dL | PMNs | 29% |
| K | 4.7 meq/L | Glu, random | 155 mg/dL | Hb | 13.9 g/dL | Lymphs | 66% |
| Cl | 111 meq/L | Ca | 9.1 mg/dL | Hct | 48% | Monos | 3% |
| HCO$_3$ | 19 meq/L | Phos | 4.1 mg/dL | Plt | 190,000/mm$^3$ | Eos | 1% |
| BUN | 57 mg/dL | Mg | 2.8 mg/dL | WBC | 11,700/mm$^3$ | Basos | 1% |

**Patient Case Question 8.** Do serum potassium, phosphate, calcium, and magnesium concentrations suggest that intrarenal acute renal failure has developed?

**Patient Case Question 9.** Why might the serum glucose level be abnormal?

**Patient Case Question 10.** Would you expect electrocardiogram abnormalities in this patient? Why or why not?

**Patient Case Question 11.** If acute renal failure progresses to chronic renal failure, hemoglobin and hematocrit may decrease significantly and a peripheral blood smear may indicate a normocytic, normochromic anemia. Suggest two pathophysiologic mechanisms that explain the abnormal hemoglobin level, hematocrit, and peripheral blood smear.

**Patient Case Question 12.** Which laboratory data suggest that the infection is probably viral and not bacterial?

**Patient Case Question 13.** Why is it appropriate that a serum creatinine phosphokinase assay was not ordered?

## UA

- Clear, pale yellow urine
- Microscopy was negative for cells, casts, pigments, and crystals
- SG 1.019
- (–) bacteria
- (–) glucose
- (–) protein
- WBC 1/HPF with no eosinophils
- RBC 1/HPF
- Na concentration = 14 meq/L
- Osmolality = 769 mOsm/kg $H_2O$

*Patient Case Question 14.* Which urinalysis information suggests that acute renal failure in this patient is not the result of glomerular disease?

*Patient Case Question 15.* Do the urinary microscopic analysis, specific gravity, sodium concentration, and osmolality suggest *prerenal* acute renal failure or *intrarenal* acute renal failure associated with acute tubular necrosis?

*Patient Case Question 16.* Calculate the plasma BUN/creatinine ratio and suggest whether the calculated value is consistent with prerenal acute renal failure or acute tubular necrosis.

*Patient Case Question 17.* If the patient's *fractional excretion of sodium* is 0.87%, calculate the patient's urine creatinine concentration.

*Patient Case Question 18.* Why do you expect that an ultrasound study of the patient's urinary tract was not conducted?

*Patient Case Question 19.* Which therapeutic measure should be considered "first and foremost" and may be very beneficial in reversing the signs of acute renal failure?

*Patient Case Question 20.* Would dialysis be appropriate treatment for this patient at this time?

*Patient Case Question 21.* Should sodium polystyrene sulfonate therapy be instituted in this patient?

# CASE STUDY

# 31

# CHRONIC RENAL FAILURE

 *For the Disease Summary for this case study, see the CD-ROM.*

# PATIENT CASE

## ■ History of Present Illness

Mr. M.A. is a 27-year-old white male, who is visiting his primary healthcare provider to discuss recent blood tests. He has been feeling fatigued and weak lately.

## ■ Past Medical History

Three years ago, the patient presented to the emergency room with a six-hour history of coughing up blood. He also complained of difficulty breathing, chills, and chest pain. He had recently suffered a two-week episode of influenza A. Laboratory tests revealed an elevated white blood cell count and iron deficiency anemia. A physical exam revealed moderate hepatosplenomegaly and inspiratory crackles at the base of each lung. He was hospitalized for a thorough clinical workup.

An ELISA test was positive for anti-glomerular basement membrane (GBM) antibodies in the blood, but serum complement levels were within normal limits. Immunofluorescence of the renal biopsy was positive for IgG and complement lining the glomerular membranes. A diagnosis of Goodpasture syndrome was made. The patient was educated about Goodpasture syndrome (that it is a disease in which the immune system attacks the kidneys and lungs) and that a potential serious complication is chronic renal failure.

The patient was immediately placed on methylprednisolone (1 mg/kg/d po divided Q 6–12 hrs) and plasmapheresis was conducted (four plasma exchanges of 1 L each daily for two weeks). After two weeks, the patient's symptoms resolved and serum anti-GBM antibodies were no longer detectable. The patient was maintained for six months on azathioprine (2 mg/kg/d po QD) and 160 mg trimethoprim plus 800 mg sulfamethoxazole 3×/week.

***Patient Case Question 1.*** Which type of immune hypersensitivity reaction causes the destructive renal changes in Goodpasture syndrome—type I, II, III, or IV?

***Patient Case Question 2.*** Why were methylprednisolone and azathioprine given to the patient?

***Patient Case Question 3.*** Why was trimethoprim and sulfamethoxazole prescribed with azathioprine for this patient?

***Patient Case Question 4.*** What is the purpose of plasmapheresis?

During a follow-up visit with a nephrologist in six months, a urinalysis revealed a low-grade proteinuria and hematuria.

***Patient Case Question 5.*** What is the pathophysiology behind the clinical signs of proteinuria and hematuria in this patient?

# Clinical Course

With each patient visit at every six-month interval, proteinuria and hematuria became more severe. Also, increasing BUN and serum creatinine levels indicated that kidney disease was progressing. The patient had one relapse at one year following onset and had been hospitalized and treated again with methylprednisolone, azathioprine, and plasmapheresis.

At the patient's most recent visit with the nephrologist, vital signs were: BP 150/95, P 90, RR 22 and unlabored, T 98.6°F, Ht 5′9″, Wt 170 lb. Serum creatinine test results were compared with previous tests to determine the extent of progression of renal failure. See Patient Case Table 31.1.

### Patient Case Table 31.1 Serum Creatinine Test Results

| Serum Creatinine Measurement | Serum Creatinine Concentration (mg/dL) |
| --- | --- |
| At onset of disease 3 years ago | 1.00 |
| 6 months after onset | 1.18 |
| 1 year after onset | 1.39 |
| 18 months after onset | 1.72 |
| 24 months after onset | 2.38 |
| 30 months after onset | 3.57 |
| 3 days ago | 7.14 |

***Patient Case Question 6.*** Determine the approximate time to end-stage renal disease from this visit.

***Patient Case Question 7.*** Determine the patient's creatinine clearance from tests done three days ago, indicate the stage of chronic renal failure to which the patient has progressed, and identify an action plan.

# Review of Systems

The patient denies any bleeding and bruising, shortness of breath, chest pain with inspiration, anorexia, nausea, vomiting, loss of coordination, unsteady gait, and bone pain. He states, however, that his "skin has been itching some lately. I have been using a lot of lotion on my arms and legs, because sometimes it is really bothersome."

# Physical Examination and Laboratory Tests

The patient is very pale and appears to be in mild acute distress. There is some periorbital edema and mild swelling of his hands. He reports a dull headache for the past four days. "I have been forgetting things a lot lately and I can't seem to concentrate at work anymore."

## Head, Eyes, Ears, Nose, and Throat

- Pupils equal at 3 mm, round, and reactive to light and accommodation
- Extra-ocular muscles intact

- Anti-icteric sclera
- Fundi normal
- Conjunctiva normal
- Tympanic membranes intact and clear
- No exudates or erythema in oropharynx

## Skin

- Very pale, dry with flakiness
- No ecchymoses or purpura

## Neck

- Supple without masses or bruits
- Thyroid normal
- No lymphadenopathy

## Lungs

Mild bibasilar crackles with auscultation

*Patient Case Question 8.* What is a likely cause of the abnormal lung sounds here?

## Heart

- Regular rate and rhythm
- $S_1$ and $S_2$ sounds clear with no additional heart sounds
- No murmurs or rubs

## Abdomen

- Soft, non-tender, and non-distended
- No guarding or rebound with palpation
- No masses, bruits, hepatomegaly, or splenomegaly
- Normal bowel sounds

## Rectal/Genitourinary

- Prostate normal in size with no nodules
- Anal sphincter tone normal
- Stool is guaiac-negative

## Extremities

- Negative for cyanosis or clubbing
- Mild (1+) edema of the hands and feet
- Normal range of motion throughout
- 2+ dorsalis pedis and posterior tibial pulses bilaterally

## Neurological

- Alert and oriented × 3
- No sensory or motor abnormalities

- CNs II–XII intact
- DTRs = 2+ throughout
- Muscle tone 5/5 throughout
- Positive Chvostek sign bilaterally

---

***Patient Case Question 9.*** Describe a positive Chvostek sign and suggest with which abnormal laboratory test below this clinical sign is consistent.

## Laboratory Test Results

See Patient Case Table 31.2

| Patient Case Table 31.2 Laboratory Test Results | | | | | |
|---|---|---|---|---|---|
| Na | 149 meq/L | Plt | 270,000/mm$^3$ | Mg | 3.8 mg/dL |
| K | 5.4 meq/L | RBC | 3.4 million/mm$^3$ | PO$_4$ | 5.9 mg/dL |
| Cl | 116 meq/L | WBC | 9,400/mm$^3$ | PT | 14.2 sec |
| Ca | 6.7 mg/dL | AST | 18 IU/L | PTT | 34 sec |
| HCO$_3$ | 32 meq/L | ALT | 38 IU/L | Protein$_{urine}$ | +++ |
| BUN | 143 mg/dL | Alk Phos | 178 IU/L | Blood$_{urine}$ | +++ |
| Cr | 7.1 mg/dL | Glu, random | 152 mg/dL | pH blood | 7.45 |
| Hb | 9.5 g/dL | T bilirubin | 2.0 mg/dL | Renal ultrasound: significant bilateral atrophy, 8.3 cm each | |
| Hct | 30.7% | Alb | 2.9 g/dL | Chest x-ray: bibasilar shadows | |
| MCV | 80 fL | T protein | 5.0 g/dL | ECG | Normal |

---

***Patient Case Question 10.*** There are *twenty* abnormal laboratory tests above. Identify them and suggest a brief pathophysiologic mechanism for each.

# 32 DIALYSIS AND RENAL TRANSPLANTATION

 *For the Disease Summary for this case study, see the CD-ROM.*

# PATIENT CASE

## ■ Patient's Chief Complaints

"I've had three more kidney infections this past summer. Mentally, I am still very alert. I can still mow the yard with the riding mower, burn the trash, and keep the house clean, but my legs are very weak and I have to strain to walk. I also have an ongoing problem with leg cramps, hand cramps, and stomach cramps, especially when I forget to take my medicine before dialysis."

## ■ History of Present Illness

Mr. M.B. is a 60 yo white male, who presented to the outpatient dialysis center for staff-assisted hemodialysis. He was diagnosed 4½ years ago with a severe case of pyelonephritis that resulted in renal failure. During transport to the hospital, the patient was hypotensive with a blood pressure of 60/44. He was hospitalized for one month, diagnosed with end-stage renal failure, and discharged with total renal function reduced to only 10% of normal. He was started on hemodialysis 41 months ago and currently undergoes dialysis three times each week, during which 2–6 lb excess fluid are removed. He has had recurring episodes of pyelonephritis every 3–4 months for the last three years and three more episodes this past summer in the left kidney that has resulted in total renal function of 1–2%. He is scheduled to have his left kidney removed in the near future to prevent further renal infections and is currently on a waiting list for renal transplantation.

## ■ Past Medical History

- Measles and chickenpox as a child
- "Nervous colitis" diagnosed 35 years ago; new diagnosis of lactose intolerance and irritable bowel syndrome established 4½ years ago
- Diabetes mellitus type 2, 4½ years
- Recurring colds, but none in past 2 years

## ■ Previous Surgeries

- Tonsils and adenoids removed, age 5
- Left inguinal hernia repaired, age 7

- Right inguinal hernia repaired, age 26
- Surgery for fracture of forearm at elbow, age 40
- Kidney stone removed, 4½ years ago
- Chest catheters surgically placed for hemodialysis—41 months, 27 months, and 18 months ago

## History of Previous Trauma

- Head trauma, lost consciousness and fell, age 16
- Minor whiplash injury in motor vehicle accident, age 25

## Family History

- Father had been in good health until he developed kidney cancer and passed away 18 months later at age 77
- Mother, alive at age 81, in good general health and takes no medication other than an occasional acetaminophen
- Sister, age 53, has had DM type 2 for more than 10 years; has lost her toenails and vision is impaired
- Brother, age 46, has had major problem with recreational drug use but quit approximately 6 years ago; currently drinks to excess on weekends but not during the week
- Brother, age 42, has had major problem with recreational drug use and alcohol for 25 years, but quit both approximately 2 years ago
- Sister, who was stillborn when patient was 10 yo
- Has one daughter, age 16, diagnosed with attention deficit disorder at age 4 but condition resolved by age 7; also hospitalized twice with rare type of staphylococcal infection

## Social History

- Divorced nearly 4 years and lives by himself
- Retired approximately 4 years ago; before that he was employed over an 18-year period as a resettlement coordinator, Vietnamese medical and court translator, social worker, and job counselor in Iowa
- Quit social drinking approximately 20 years ago; occasionally will have a small glass of champagne at New Years and on August 5th in commemoration of his father's life
- Has smoked since age 19 and currently smokes 2 ppd
- Has never used recreational drugs
- Has been a church pianist for 47 years
- Enjoys model railroads, vegetable and flower gardening, and the companionship of his miniature dachshund
- Has been too weak to exercise regularly; however, gets some exercise mowing yard, grocery shopping, and cleaning house
- Limits consumption of salt and sugar and totally avoids cola soft drinks, coffee, and pork

## Review of Systems

- (+) dry, itchy skin, especially around ankles; fatigue and weakness; and occasional swelling in feet and lower legs
- (−) for nausea, vomiting, joint pain, headaches, recent chest pain, fevers, confusion, and shortness of breath (unless the weather is very hot)

## Medications

- Pioglitazone, 30 mg po QD
- Ranitidine, 75 mg po QD
- Aspirin, 162 mg po QD

- Multivitamin with lycopene, 1 tablet po QD
- Quinine sulfate, 650 mg po before dialysis
- Levofloxacin, 250 mg po QD after dialysis
- Calcium acetate, 1334 mg po QD after dialysis
- Clonazepam, 0.5 mg po HS after dialysis
- Escitalopram, 10 mg po HS after dialysis

*Patient Case Question 1.* Why is this patient taking pioglitazone?

*Patient Case Question 2.* Why is this patient taking levofloxacin after dialysis?

*Patient Case Question 3.* Why is this patient taking calcium acetate after dialysis?

*Patient Case Question 4.* Why is this patient taking quinine sulfate before dialysis?

# ▰ Allergies

No known drug allergies

# ▰ Physical Examination and Laboratory Tests

## General

The patient is a WDWN white male in NAD who appears his stated age. He is mentally alert and oriented.

## Vital Signs

See Patient Case Table 32.1

| Patient Case Table 32.1 Vital Signs | | | | | |
|---|---|---|---|---|---|
| BP | 125/80, sitting | RR | 15, unlabored | HT | 6′3″ |
| P | 70, regular | T | 98.6°F | WT | 194 lbs. |

## Skin

Dry, scaly skin, especially around the ankles

## Head, Eyes, Ears, Nose, and Throat

- PERRLA
- EOMI
- No A-V nicking, hemorrhages, or exudates
- Clear sclera
- No oral or nasal lesions
- Oropharynx is clear, without exudates
- Mucous membranes moist
- Tongue mid-line

## Neck and Lymph Nodes

- No cervical, supraclavicular, or axillary adenopathy
- Normal thyroid

## Chest and Lungs

CTA & P bilaterally

## Heart

- RRR
- Normal $S_1$ and $S_2$
- (−) for m/r/g

## Abdomen

- Soft, NT, and without HSM
- (–) for bruits

## Musculoskeletal and Extremities

- Mild (1+) bilateral foot/ankle edema
- Normal ROM
- Pulses are normal and equal at 2+
- (−) for clubbing and cyanosis

## Neurological

- A & O × 3
- CNs II–XII intact
- DTRs 2+ in all four extremities
- Strength is 4/5 in upper extremities and 3/5 in lower extremities

***Patient Case Question 5.*** Identify each of this patient's clinical manifestations above that are consistent with end-stage renal failure.

## Laboratory Blood Test Results

See Patient Case Table 32.2

### Patient Case Table 32.2 Laboratory Blood Test Results

| | | | | | |
|---|---|---|---|---|---|
| Na | 142 meq/L | RBC | $3.41 \times 10^6/mm^3$ | Alb | 3.6 g/dL |
| K | 5.3 meq/L | MCV | 81.7 fL | Ca | 8.6 mg/dL |
| Cl | 110 meq/L | MCHC | 33.4 g/dL | Phos | 7.4 mg/dL |
| $HCO_3$ | 20 meq/L | WBC | $6.9 \times 10^3/mm^3$ | Uric acid | 5.5 mg/dL |
| BUN | 120 mg/dL | AST | 16 IU/L | Iron | 90 µg/dL |
| Cr | 9.2 mg/dL | ALT | 21 IU/L | TIBC | 275 µg/dL |
| Glu, fasting | 85 mg/dL | Alk phos | 124 IU/L | Transf sat | 33% |
| Hb | 9.3 g/dL | Total bilirubin | 0.5 mg/dL | Ferritin | 279 ng/mL |
| Hct | 27.9% | Total protein | 6.1 g/dL | PTH | 1835 pg/mL |

***Patient Case Question 6.*** Why does this patient require hemodialysis?

***Patient Case Question 7.*** Describe the pathophysiology that has contributed to this patient's abnormal hemoglobin concentration and hematocrit as shown in Table 32.2.

***Patient Case Question 8.*** With the exception of hemoglobin and hematocrit data, identify all of the abnormal laboratory blood tests in the table above and provide a brief explanation of the pathophysiology associated with *each abnormal blood test.*

*For the Disease Summary for this case study, see the CD-ROM.*

# PATIENT CASE

## ▄▄ Patient's Chief Complaints

"I've been having some dull, aching pain in my left lower back. It's been going on now for 3 days. I think that what's remaining of my own kidney is going bad now."

## ▄▄ HPI

Mr. M.B. is a 58 yo male who developed end-stage renal disease six years ago from post-infectious glomerulonephritis. He received hemodialysis for two years. Then, four years ago, he successfully accepted a kidney transplant from a deceased donor. His health has been fair-to-good since receiving the kidney, although immunosuppressant medications have occasionally caused serious side effects, including hyperglycemia and infections.

## ▄▄ PMH

- H/O ESRD due to post-streptococcal glomerulonephritis that was diagnosed 10 years ago
- 4 years S/P cadaveric renal transplantation, right side
- OA of left knee (had several skiing accidents as an adolescent)
- Mild arthritis involving hands, elbows, and shoulders
- DVT, acute episode 1 year ago
- PUD, diagnosed 4 weeks ago
- Mild recurrent bouts of depression that have not been treated pharmacologically

## ▄▄ FH

- Adopted—no detailed family history available
- Has one daughter (age 38) who is alive and healthy

# SH

- The patient is divorced and lives alone
- He cares for himself but is unable to carry on normal activities (score of 70 on the Karnofsky Performance Status Scale)
- Currently receiving disability benefits
- Retired farmer from the Midwest
- Denies alcohol use but has been a 1 ppd cigarette smoker for 25 years
- Vietnam War veteran
- Hobbies include woodworking and gardening
- Denies non-compliance with his medications
- H/O IVDA in his twenties; none since

# ROS

- OA in left knee limits his mobility and in past 4 months he has not been able to maintain his active walking schedule
- (−) for cachexia
- Denies fatigability, fevers, chills, night sweats, swelling of legs and ankles, blood in urine, cough, hemoptysis, bone pain, nausea, loss of appetite, and jaundice

# Meds

- Tacrolimus 10 mg po Q 12h
- Prednisone 10 mg po QD
- Mycophenolate mofetil 1500 mg po BID
- Misoprostol 400 µg po BID
- Warfarin sodium 7.5 mg po QD
- Ibuprofen 400 mg po PRN

# All

- Food allergy to tofu (hives and wheezing)
- NKDA

# PE and Lab Tests

## Gen

- Cooperative Caucasian male in mild discomfort; pain is 3–4 on a scale of 10
- Patient appears his stated age and is above ideal body weight, but not obese

## VS

See Patient Case Table 33.1

| Patient Case Table 33.1 Vital Signs | | | | | |
|---|---|---|---|---|---|
| BP 125/73 | (sitting, left arm) | RR | 17 and unlabored | HT | 6'2" |
| P | 65 and regular | T | 98.5°F | WT | 220 lbs |

## Skin

- Normal color, hydration, and temperature
- (−) for lesions and bruising

## HEENT

- NC/AT
- (–) periorbital swelling
- PERRLA
- EOMI
- Anicteric sclera
- (−) nystagmus
- Normal funduscopic exam without retinopathy
- TMs non-erythematous and non-bulging
- Deviated nasal septum
- Oropharynx clear

## Neck/LN

- Supple
- Significant bilateral supraclavicular lymphadenopathy
- Normal thyroid
- (−) JVD or bruits

## Back

Significant left CVAT with palpation

## Lungs/Thorax

- Trachea midline
- CTA & P
- Breath sounds equal bilaterally
- (−) for crackles and wheezing

## Heart

- RRR
- Normal $S_1$ and $S_2$
- (−) for m/r/g
- (−) for $S_3$ and $S_4$

## Abd

- Soft with tender, palpable mass in left flank region
- Normal peristalsis
- (−) for bruits and HSM

## Genit/Rect

- (−) for testicular or scrotal enlargement

## MS/Ext

- (−) for C/C/E
- ROM significantly decreased throughout but especially left knee
- Joint enlargement of left knee, changes consistent with DJD
- Pulses 2+ throughout

## Neuro

- A & O × 3
- Deep sensation and visual fields intact
- CNs II–XII intact
- DTRs 2+ throughout
- Normal gait
- Motor level intact
- Muscle strength 5/5 all groups

## Laboratory Blood Test Results

See Patient Case Table 33.2

| Patient Case Table 33.2 Laboratory Blood Test Results | | | | | |
|---|---|---|---|---|---|
| Na | 138 meq/L | Glu, fasting | 71 mg/dL | ALT | 23 IU/L |
| K | 4.1 meq/L | Hb | 11.9 g/dL | Bilirubin | 1.2 mg/dL |
| Cl | 103 meq/L | Hct | 35% | Alk Phos | 54 IU/L |
| $HCO_3$ | 27 meq/L | Plt | $196 \times 10^3/mm^3$ | Ca | 8.9 mg/dL |
| BUN | 19 mg/dL | WBC | $4.1 \times 10^3/mm^3$ | PT | 12.1 sec |
| Cr | 1.1 mg/dL | AST | 25 IU/L | PTT | 27.9 sec |

## UA

- Appearance: yellow and cloudy
- SG 1.016
- pH 6.5
- (−) for glucose, bilirubin, ketones, hemoglobin, protein, nitrite, crystals, casts, bacteria
- WBC: 15/HPF
- RBC: TNTC

## Abdominal Helical CT Scan

- Well-defined, single, irregular, solid 3.5-inch nodule within superior pole of left kidney; signs of invasion into surrounding adipose tissue and through Gerota fascia; left kidney is significantly atrophied from glomerulonephritis
- Right (transplanted) kidney appears normal
- Remainder of CT scan was unremarkable

## Biopsy of Kidney Nodule

Large, pale, polygonal cells that stain poorly with eosin

## Plain X-Rays of Chest

- Right lung: clear
- Left lung: 3 solid, 0.5–1.0-inch lesions in lower lobe consistent with metastatic disease
- Remainder of x-rays were unremarkable

***Patient Case Question 1.*** Is this patient technically considered *overweight* or *obese* or is this patient's weight *normal and healthy*?

***Patient Case Question 2.*** List a minimum of *ten* distinct clinical manifestations in this case study that are consistent with a diagnosis of renal cell carcinoma.

***Patient Case Question 3.*** What are this patient's *two major* risk factors for renal cell carcinoma?

***Patient Case Question 4.*** List any other potential risk factors that may have contributed to renal cell carcinoma in this case.

***Patient Case Question 5.*** Based on the information provided, what is the most likely subtype of renal cell carcinoma in this case?

***Patient Case Question 6.*** Why is this patient taking misoprostol?

***Patient Case Question 7.*** Why is this patient taking warfarin sodium?

***Patient Case Question 8.*** Why is this patient taking tacrolimus?

***Patient Case Question 9.*** To which clinical stage of renal cell carcinoma has the disease advanced?

***Patient Case Question 10.*** What is the probability that this patient will survive 5 years?

***Patient Case Question 11.*** *True or false?* A partial nephrectomy is the best and only treatment required for the patient in this case study.

***Patient Case Question 12.*** What evidence exists that the cancer has metastasized to the liver?

***Patient Case Question 13.*** What evidence exists that the tumor is producing large amounts of renin?

***Patient Case Question 14.*** What evidence exists that the cancer has metastasized to bone?

# 34

# URINARY STONE DISEASE

 *For the Disease Summary for this case study, see the CD-ROM.*

# PATIENT CASE

## ▬ Initial Presentation

H.B. is a 56-year-old, married, white college professor who woke up to severe and intensifying pain in his left flank region this morning. He presented to the emergency room in severe acute distress with significant anxiety, pallor, and diaphoresis. He could not sit still on the ER bed but continued to move around, constantly repositioning himself. Groans from pain were constant. He developed nausea from the pain and vomited twice. The ER nurse gave him promethazine hydrochloride IV for nausea. Since he reported an allergy to meperidine, he was also given morphine IV for pain.

***Patient Case Question 1.*** Describe the pathophysiologic mechanism that caused pallor and diaphoresis in this patient.

***Patient Case Question 2.*** How does promethazine relieve nausea and vomiting?

## ▬ Medical History

- Tonsillectomy for chronic earache and sore throat, age 6
- Non-Hodgkin's T cell-rich B-cell lymphoma, age 48, treated with 6 monthly sessions of CHOP, currently in remission
- IgG immunodeficiency disorder, possibly secondary to lymphoma or chemotherapy, age 52
- Zenker diverticulum, age 52
- Renal stones: ages 35, 43, 52 (all passed spontaneously)

Other than a skin allergy with meperidine, the patient has no other known allergies. He does not smoke or drink. He gets very little exercise and lately has not been compliant with instructions from his PCP to remain hydrated. He is taking rabeprazole daily for acid reflux associated with Zenker diverticulum (ZD). ZD also interferes with his ability to swallow. He is receiving gamma globulin infusions as needed for his immunodeficiency condition, usually once every 5–6 weeks. He is taking one chewable multivitamin tablet daily and one chewable 500-mg vitamin C tablet every day to help boost his immune response.

# ■ Physical Examination and Laboratory Tests

## Vital Signs

T = 98.4°F; BP = 130/86 sitting, right arm; P = 90; RR = 16; Ht = 5'11", Wt = 182 lbs.

## HEENT

- Conjunctiva clear
- Fundi are without lesions
- Nasal mucosa is pink without drainage
- Oral mucous membranes are moist
- Pharynx is clear and pink

## Skin

- Pale, cool, and clammy without lesions or bruises
- Surgical scars from lymph node biopsies on lower abdomen and groin region
- Surgical scars on the back from removal of several sebaceous cysts and biopsy for suspected melanoma (biopsy was negative for cancer)

## Neck

- Supple with no lymphadenopathy or thyromegaly
- 2-cm sebaceous cyst noted in the dorsocervical region
- No bruits auscultated

## Lungs

- Chest expansion is symmetric and full
- Diaphragmatic excursions are equal
- Lung sounds are clear to auscultation

## Heart

- Regular rate and rhythm
- No murmurs, gallops, or rubs

## Abdomen

- Non-distended
- Bowel sounds are present and normoactive
- No hepatomegaly or splenomegaly
- No tenderness or masses
- No bruits auscultated

## Extremities

- Cool
- No edema
- Peripheral pulses full and equal

## Neurological

- Alert and oriented but anxious
- Strength 5/5 in all extremities
- DTR 2+ bilaterally
- Sensory intact to touch

## CT Scan

- 6-mm radiopaque stone in left mid-ureter
- 1-mm radiopaque stone in inferior calyx of right kidney

## Urinalysis

- The patient voided a urine sample in the ER, and microscopic analysis of the specimen revealed significant numbers of RBC and WBC.

## Clinical Course

The stone passed spontaneously within three hours and the patient was released. Stone analysis revealed that the primary component was calcium oxalate. The urologist ordered a blood chemistry panel (see Patient Case Table 34.1) and a 24-hour urine collection test (see Patient Case Table 34.2).

| Patient Case Table 34.1 Laboratory Blood Test Results | | | |
|---|---|---|---|
| $Na^+$ | 140 meq/L | $Cl^+$ | 102 meq/L |
| $K^+$ | 4.3 meq/L | $Mg^{+2}$ | 2.2 mg/dL |
| $Ca^{+2}$ | 10.0 mg/dL | Uric acid | 6.3 mg/dL |
| $PO_4^{-3}$ | 2.7 mg/dL | | |

| Patient Case Table 34.2 24-Hour Urine Collection | | | |
|---|---|---|---|
| Volume | 1,220 mL | pH | 6.3 |
| Calcium | 180 mg | Specific gravity | 1.035 |
| Citrate | 128 mg | Protein, total | 111 mg |

*Patient Case Question 3.* In addition to male gender and Caucasian race, identify *four* more risk factors that have likely contributed to this patient's current urinary stone.

*Patient Case Question 4.* Based on this patient's medical history and all of the laboratory tests, what non-pharmacologic and pharmacologic recommendations might be appropriate?

*Patient Case Question 5.* Which of the clinical findings above are consistent with the fact that the passed stone was not a uric acid stone?

*Patient Case Question 6.* Is allopurinol an appropriate treatment for this patient's recurring nephrolithiasis?

*Patient Case Question 7.* Is penicillamine an appropriate treatment for this patient's recurring renal stones?

*Patient Case Question 8.* Are there any types of kidney stones that can be dissolved with medication?

*Patient Case Question 9.* Rank the following sets of food items as such: 1 = extremely rich in oxalates; 2 = mild to moderately rich in oxalates; 3 = very low oxalate content.

_____ cranberry juice, cooked broccoli, and red, raw raspberries

_____ pecans, baked potatoes, cooked carrots

_____ cooked beet greens, stewed rhubarb, pickled beets

# URINARY TRACT INFECTION

 *For the Disease Summary for this case study, see the CD-ROM.*

## PATIENT CASE

### ▰ HPI

K.N. is a 24 yo woman who presents to the family practice clinic complaining of sudden urgency to urinate, frequent urination, and pain with urination. Symptoms began approximately 48 hours ago. She awoke from sleep with urgency and suprapubic discomfort two nights ago. Her urine now has a strong odor and a cloudy appearance. She has no fever.

> **Patient Case Question 1.** List a minimum of *eight* appropriate questions that you might ask this patient.
>
> **Patient Case Question 2.** What is the significance of this patient's absence of fever?

### ▰ PMH

- UTI 30 months ago, resolved with short course of trimethoprim-sulfamethoxazole (TMP-SMX)
- UTI 14 months ago, TMP-SMX effective
- UTI 8 months ago, treated with TMP-SMX; patient developed urticaria at conclusion of Tx
- H/O iron deficiency anemia
- H/O gonorrhea and chlamydia (2 years ago)

### ▰ FH

Father has DM; remainder of FH is non-contributory

### ▰ SH

- Non-smoker
- Uses marijuana occasionally

- Social EtOH
- Sexually active with multiple partners

# ROS

- Denies any vaginal discharge or bleeding
- Denies chills, nausea, or vomiting
- Reports having some pelvic discomfort and pain during urination

# Meds

- Phenazopyridine OTC 100 mg po PRN
- Ortho-Novum 7/7/7 1 tab po QD
- Ferrous sulfate 300 mg po BID

*Patient Case Question 3.* Why is the patient taking Ortho-Novum?

*Patient Case Question 4.* Why is the patient taking ferrous sulfate?

# All

TMP-SMX, hives with pruritus

# PE and Lab Tests

## Gen

Cooperative woman in mild discomfort

## VS

See Patient Case Table 35.1

| Patient Case Table 35.1 Vital Signs | | | | | | | |
|---|---|---|---|---|---|---|---|
| BP | 100/60 | RR | 15 | WT | 123 lbs |
| P | 74 | T | 98.2°F | HT | 67 in |

## Skin

Dry with decreased turgor; otherwise normal in appearance

## HEENT

- PERRLA
- EOMI
- Fundi benign
- TMs intact
- Mucous membranes dry

## Neck/LN

* Supple with no JVD, bruits, or lymphadenopathy
* Normal thyroid

## Lungs

CTA throughout

## Heart

RRR

## Abd

* Soft with positive BS
* No HSM, bruits, or tenderness

## Back

* No CVAT

## Pelvic

* No vaginal discharge or lesions noted
* LMP 10 days ago
* Mild suprapubic tenderness

## MS/Ext

* Pulses 2+ throughout
* Full ROM
* Strength 5/5 throughout

## Neuro

* A & O $\times$ 3
* CNs II–XII intact
* Patellar reflexes normal at 2+
* Sensory and motor levels intact

## CBC

* WBC 6,400/mm$^3$

## Dipstick Urinalysis

* Color, dark yellow
* Specific gravity 1.035
* pH 5.5
* Protein ($-$)
* Ketones ($-$)
* Bilirubin ($-$)

- Trace blood
- Leukoesterase (+)
- Nitrites (+)
- Urobilinogen (−)

**Patient Case Question 5.** What is the significance of the positive leukoesterase and nitrites findings with the dipstick analysis?

**Patient Case Question 6.** Normal protein, glucose, and ketone concentrations are below the sensitivity of the dipstick. Which disease state causes a significant elevation in all three of these parameters?

**Patient Case Question 7.** List *three* pathophysiologic conditions that may result in a positive bilirubin dipstick test.

**Patient Case Question 8.** What is urobilinogen?

**Patient Case Question 9.** What is one pathophysiologic cause of elevated urobilinogen in the urine?

## Microscopic Examination of Urine

- WBC: TNTC/HPF
- Bacteria: TNTC
- RBC: 3–4/HPF
- Casts: (−)

## Urine Culture

- *E. coli* $>10^5$ cfu/mL

**Patient Case Question 10.** What is your overall assessment of this patient's condition?

**Patient Case Question 11.** What is an appropriate treatment for this patient?

# NEUROLOGICAL DISORDERS

# 36

# ACUTE PYOGENIC MENINGITIS

 *For the Disease Summary for this case study, see the CD-ROM.*

## PATIENT CASE

### ■ Initial History

Mrs. S.N. is a 67-year-old Caucasian female who felt well until approximately one week ago, when she developed an upper respiratory tract infection. She improved slowly but during the past 48 hours has developed a more severe cough with significant production of rust-colored sputum, fever with occasional shaking chills, and muscle aches. Mrs. S.N. was brought to the hospital emergency room by her husband when she woke up this morning mildly confused and complaining of a severe headache.

At the hospital she informs the ER physician (with some difficulty concentrating) that she has had a "bad cold" for about a week, that her "neck feels stiff, sore, and extremely painful when she tilts her head forward," and that "bright lights hurt her eyes." She also tells him that she has had no skin rashes, nausea, or vomiting but has had some "very severe chills." She does not recall any of her recent contacts being ill and she denies any difficulty breathing and chest pain.

***Patient Case Question 1.*** What is the significance of the patient's productive cough with rust-colored sputum?

***Patient Case Question 2.*** List *three* clinical manifestations that strongly suggest that the patient has developed meningitis.

### ■ Past Medical History

Mrs. S.N. denies any past history of head trauma, sinus infection, immunodeficiency disorders, and medications that cause immunosuppression. She has smoked a half-pack of cigarettes each day for the last 45 years, was diagnosed with emphysema five years ago, and had several severe episodes of chronic bronchitis and one episode of pneumonia in the past two years. Her emphysema is being managed with ipratropium bromide delivered with a metered-dose inhaler (2–4 puffs every 6 hours). She has never suffered from episodes of angina or symptoms of heart failure. She has an allergy to peanuts but not to any medications. She is taking no medications other than ipratropium and a conjugated estrogen preparation for menopausal symptoms. The patient was vaccinated for influenza six months ago and pneumococcus when she turned 65.

# ■■■ Physical Examination and Laboratory Tests

The patient is a slight female who is in acute distress with headache and intermittent chills and is constantly coughing. She appears older than her stated age. Her vital signs are as follows: T = 101.5°F; P = 115 and regular; RR = 24 and slightly labored; BP = 160/70 (right arm, sitting); Ht = 5′4″; Wt = 103 lbs.

*Patient Case Question 3.* Explain the abnormalities in the vital signs.

*Patient Case Question 4.* Is the patient technically considered *underweight, overweight, obese,* or does the patient have a *healthy weight based on height?*

## Head, Eyes, Ears, Nose, Throat, and Neck

* Normocephalic with no signs of head injury
* Pupils equal at 3 mm, round, and sluggishly reactive to light
* Difficult to view fundi due to photophobia, but no papilledema observed
* Nares slightly flared, purulent discharge visible
* Pharynx red with purulent post-nasal drainage
* No tonsillar exudates
* Mucous membranes moist
* Neck stiff and painful with flexion
* Neck shows mild anterior cervical lymphadenopathy

*Patient Case Question 5.* Why is it appropriate for the physician to examine the patient for a head injury?

*Patient Case Question 6.* List *two* clinical signs that are consistent with and specific for an upper respiratory tract infection.

*Patient Case Question 7.* Define *papilledema* and explain the significance of a lack of papilledema in this patient.

*Patient Case Question 8.* Explain the pathophysiology behind this patient's lymphadenopathy.

## Lungs

* Significant use of accessory muscles
* Breath sounds markedly decreased in RML and RLL
* Crackles present at right posterior axillary line
* Clear left lung, both upper and lower lobes

## Skin

* Warm, moist, and pale
* No rashes upon careful inspection

## Cardiac

* Distinct $S_1$ and $S_2$ with no murmurs or gallops
* Regular rate and rhythm

## Extremities

- Peripheral pulses full and symmetric in all extremities
- No cyanosis, rashes, or edema
- Mild clubbing

## Abdomen

- Flat, soft, non-distended, with no tenderness to palpation
- Bowel sounds present in all four quadrants are within normal limits
- No masses, bruits, or organomegaly

## Neurological

- Oriented × 3 but conversation is slightly confused
- Level of consciousness assessed at 14 on Glasgow Coma Scale
- Cranial nerves intact, including eye movements
- Strength 5/5 and symmetric throughout
- DTRs 2+ and symmetric
- Gait steady
- Positive Kernig and Brudzinski signs

---

*Patient Case Question 9.* What is the cause of the patient's "significant use of accessory muscles"?

*Patient Case Question 10.* What is the significance of lack of a skin rash?

*Patient Case Question 11.* What has probably caused clubbing in this patient?

*Patient Case Question 12.* Is the patient's rating on the Glasgow Coma Scale *normal* or *abnormal*?

---

## ▬ Clinical Course

Based on the patient's physical examination, a preliminary diagnosis of meningitis is made. Mrs. S.N. was admitted to the hospital for a complete clinical examination. A blood chemistry panel, chest x-rays, and lumbar puncture were ordered (see Patient Case Table 36.1).

| Patient Case Table 36.1 Test Results | | | | | |
|---|---|---|---|---|---|
| Hct | 41% | Chloride | 110 meq/L | CSF WBC | 1,100/mm³ (predominately neutrophils) |
| Hb | 14.8 g/dL | Calcium | 9.3 mg/dL | CSF protein | 125 mg/dL |
| RBC | 5.2 million/mm³ | Bicarbonate | 22 meq/L | CSF glucose | 40 mg/dL |
| WBC | 14,000/mm³ (90% neutrophils) | Glucose, fasting | 123 mg/dL | CSF gram stain: | (+) for encapsulated diplococci |
| Platelets | 280,000/mm³ | BUN<br>Cr | 12 mg/dL<br>1.0 mg/dL | CSF culture: | (+) for *S. pneumoniae* |
| Sodium | 145 meq/L | CSF appearance | cloudy | Sputum gram stain: | (+) for diplococci |
| Potassium | 5.0 meq/L | CSF opening pressure: | 300 mm H₂O | Chest x-rays: RML and RLL shadows consistent with pneumonia; left lung clear but hyperinflated | |

***Patient Case Question 13.*** Identify all *eleven* of the test results directly above that are abnormal.

***Patient Case Question 14.*** Based on all of the available test data in Table 36.1, what is an appropriate neurologic diagnosis for Mrs. S.N.?

***Patient Case Question 15.*** How did this patient's neurologic condition probably develop?

***Patient Case Question 16.*** What is the antibiotic of first choice for this patient and for how long should it be administered?

***Patient Case Question 17.*** What is the antibiotic of choice if the patient does not respond to the first drug of choice (i.e., the microbial agent is resistant to the antibiotic of first choice)?

***Patient Case Question 18.*** Which type of white blood cell predominates in the blood and cerebrospinal fluid of patients with acute bacterial meningitis?

ACUTE VIRAL ENCEPHALITIS

 *For the Disease Summary for this case study, see the CD-ROM.*

## PATIENT CASE

### ■ History of Present Illness

N.C. is an 83 yo male who has made an appointment with his personal internal medicine physician because a mosquito bite has caused the area around his right eye to swell. He received the bite approximately 96 hours ago while camping in Rocky Mountain National Park in Colorado. Periorbital edema has become progressively worse, now to the point where the right eye is swollen shut. The patient also has a mild fever and a mild headache, both of which developed last evening.

### ■ ROS

The patient is alert and oriented. He denies fatigue, body aches, tremors, skin rashes, neck stiffness, muscle weakness, photophobia, and general malaise. His physician suspects that N.C. has developed an arthropod-transmitted infection and refers him to both a neurologist and infectious diseases specialist for immediate follow-up the next morning. He also instructs the patient to take OTC ibuprofen for his fever and headache, to apply ice to the swollen area around the eye to decrease the swelling, and to go directly to the urgent care clinic if his condition worsens.

### ■ VS

- BP 140/95
- P 90 and regular
- RR 16 and unlabored
- T 99.4°F
- HT 5′9″
- WT 165 lbs

*Patient Case Question 1.* What is the pathophysiology of swelling in this case?

*Patient Case Question 2.* Why is the application of ice helpful to relieving swelling in this case?

***Patient Case Question 3.*** Based on the patient's location when he received the mosquito bite, what are several possible diagnoses?

***Patient Case Question 4.*** Based on incubation period only, identify *two* potential types of encephalitis in this patient.

***Patient Case Question 5.*** Are any of the infections that you listed above in your answer to question 3 potentially serious?

# ■ Clinical Course

The next morning N.C. woke up confused and disoriented, with mild tremors. His headache was also much worse. His wife drove him immediately to the urgent care clinic for evaluation.

# ■ PMH

- 18 months S/P cadaveric renal transplantation
- ESRD secondary to DM type 1, diagnosed 10 years ago
- CAD
- COLD × 6 yrs
- Asthma for as long as he can remember
- DM type 1 diagnosed at age 13

# ■ Meds

- Nitroglycerin SR 6.5 mg po Q 8h
- Nitroglycerin 0.4 mg SL PRN
- Theo-Dur 100 mg po BID
- Albuterol MDI 2 puffs QID PRN
- Atrovent MDI 2 puffs BID
- Cyclosporine 250 mg po BID
- Prednisone 10 mg po QD
- Mycophenolate mofetil 1500 mg po BID
- Insulin: NPH insulin 16 units at breakfast and Lispro insulin according to the schedule in Patient Case Table 37.1

## Patient Case Table 37.1 Daily Lispro Insulin Medication Schedule

| Blood glucose (mg/dL) | Units at Breakfast | Units at Lunch | Units at Supper | Units at Bedtime |
|---|---|---|---|---|
| <80 | 4 | – | – | – |
| 81–150 | 5 | – | 8 | – |
| 151–200 | 6 | – | 9 | 1 |
| 201–250 | 7 | 2 | 10 | 2 |
| 251–300 | 8 | 3 | 11 | 3 |
| 301–350 | 9 | 4 | 12 | 4 |
| 351–400 | 10 | 5 | 13 | 5 |
| >400 | 11 | 6 | 14 | 6 |

***Patient Case Question 6.*** Three of the drugs listed above are of particular concern in this patient. Which three drugs should cause concern and why should they cause concern?

## ■ All

- Vancomycin (rash)
- Penicillin (rash, hives, and difficulty breathing)
- Sulfa-containing products (rash)

## ■ PE and Lab Tests

### Gen

The patient is disoriented, pale, is manifesting mild tremors, and appears ill.

### VS

- BP 150/95
- P 105 and regular
- RR 17 and unlabored
- T 100.5°F

### Skin

- Warm and pale
- No rash observed

### HEENT

- PERRLA
- EOM intact
- Fundi reveal old laser scars bilaterally without hemorrhages and occasional hard exudates bilaterally
- Ears and nose unremarkable with no bulging of TMs
- Mucous membranes dry
- Mild non-exudative pharyngitis present
- Wears dentures

### Neck

- Thyroid normal
- Supple with no masses present

### LN

- Cervical and axillary lymph nodes are palpable (approximately 2 cm)
- Femoral lymph nodes are not palpable

### CV

- PMI is normal and not displaced
- $S_1$ and $S_2$ are normal without $S_3$, $S_4$, rubs, or murmurs
- Sinus tachycardia
- Carotid, femoral, and dorsalis pedis pulses are normal at 2+
- No carotid, abdominal, or femoral bruits heard

## Chest

- Lungs are CTA & P with no crackles or wheezes
- There is full excursion of the chest without tenderness

## Abd

- Soft, NT, and without organomegaly or masses
- Bowel sounds are normal

## Rect

- Anus normal
- No masses or hemorrhoids observed
- Stool is heme-negative

## Ext

- No CCE
- Range of motion intact
- Feet are without ulcers, calluses, or other lesions

## Neuro

- Disoriented
- Mild tremor in both hands
- DTRs are 2+ bilaterally for biceps, brachioradialis, quadriceps, and Achilles
- (+) Kernig sign
- (+) Brudzinski sign
- Muscular strength 3/5 throughout
- Slightly decreased sensation to light touch in both feet (consistent with diabetic neuropathy)

*Patient Case Question 7.* Suggest a reasonable explanation for the laser scars in the eyes?

*Patient Case Question 8.* Suggest a reasonable pathophysiologic explanation for the patient's enlarged lymph nodes.

*Patient Case Question 9.* Although not routine practice, why was this patient's feet carefully examined for lesions?

*Patient Case Question 10.* What is suggested by the positive Kernig and Brudzinski signs?

## CBC

Significant lymphopenia

## Lumbar Puncture Results

See Patient Case Table 37.2

**Patient Case Table 37.2 Lumbar Puncture Results**

| CSF lymphocytosis | | Normal glucose | | No CSF RBCs | |
|---|---|---|---|---|---|
| Moderately elevated protein | | Normal lactic acid | | Gram stain | (−) |
| Bacterial culture | (−) | IgM antiviral antibody | (+) | | |

## MRI

Mild diffuse cerebral edema with no intra-cerebral bleeding

## Enzyme Immunoassay with Plaque Reduction Neutralization Test

Positive for West Nile

*Patient Case Question 11.* Based on all the available clinical evidence above, what is a likely diagnosis for this patient's condition?

*Patient Case Question 12.* What is an appropriate treatment approach for this patient?

# 38

# ALZHEIMER DISEASE

 *For the Disease Summary for this case study, see the CD-ROM.*

# PATIENT CASE

## ■ Patient's Chief Complaints

"I got lost in the grocery store and my children think that I need those diapers that old people have to wear."

## ■ HPI

R.M. is an 83-year-old woman who presents to the geriatric care clinic for a routine visit. She is accompanied by her two oldest daughters. The patient was diagnosed with probable Alzheimer disease nine years ago when her children reported short-term memory loss and several cognitive manifestations. They noted that she was constantly misplacing her glasses, hearing aid, and keys and that, on several occasions, had placed familiar household items in illogical places—like the coffee pot in the refrigerator. They also reported that she had taken walks in the neighborhood where she had lived for nearly 45 years and got lost. Neighbors had helped her home on more than one occasion.

It was at about this same time that her children and friends also noticed several changes in her personality. She had become very quiet and passive and seemed to have lost all motivation and interest in everything that she had previously enjoyed, including her flower garden. A complete clinical workup with neuroimaging studies revealed no significant new medical conditions that were causing her neurologic manifestations. However, she scored only 25 out of a possible 30 points on a Folstein Mini-Mental State Examination. She was started on tacrine, but when adverse effects became intolerable (nausea, vomiting, and abdominal pain), her medication was changed to donepezil. Donepezil helped significantly with both memory and mood for several years.

Four years ago, family members noticed another significant change in the patient. Not only had previous manifestations become more severe, she also began developing new features of Alzheimer disease. She started having difficulty with numbers, could no longer balance her checkbook, and even forgot how to play bridge—a game that she had enjoyed for more than 60 years. She also began showing signs of poor judgment—one time leaving the house on a cold, winter morning without a coat and shoes, another time going to the store in her nightgown. Furthermore, there was a small kitchen fire that occurred when she forgot to turn off the stove. Fortunately, her neighbor had come over to check on her and put the fire out. At this time, she was again tested for new systemic disease, but no significant abnormalities were detected other than a mild case of iron deficiency anemia. A CT scan of the brain revealed moderate-to-severe cerebral atrophy in the temporal and parietal lobes bilaterally. Her Folstein Mini-Mental State Examination score had significantly decreased to 18/30. Shortly thereafter, the oldest daughter sold her mother's home and moved her mother in to live with her family. The two oldest daughters shared caregiving responsibilities and the youngest son also contributed significantly to his mother's safety and well-being.

Within the past six weeks, the patient has demonstrated multiple, sudden outbursts of anger. While shopping for groceries earlier this week with her second oldest daughter, the patient became separated, lost, confused, angry, and then violent when store employees and several customers tried to help her. Before she could be calmed, she had thrown several tomatoes at the store manager. She broke into a violent rage again at check-out when the grapes that she was purchasing fell out of the bag onto the floor. Within the last two weeks, she also began having occasional urinary accidents. Caring for their mother is now becoming unmanageable and the children are currently considering admitting their mother into a long-term nursing care facility.

## ■■■ PMH

- HTN × 20 years
- Episode of nephrolithiasis 2 years ago, stone passed without intervention, uric acid was primary component of stone
- Gout × 2 years
- Hypercholesterolemia × 6 months
- Plantar fasciitis of left foot × 3 months
- Occasional constipation

> **Patient Case Question 1.** What is *plantar fasciitis?*

## ■■■ FH

- Both parents are deceased
- Father died from CVA
- Mother developed Alzheimer disease in her 70s
- Brother died from heart disease
- Sister also had Alzheimer disease, died 5 years ago at age 76

## ■■■ SH

- Lives with daughter
- Has been widowed for 14 years (husband died from cancer)
- Does not smoke or drink alcohol

## ■■■ ROS

- No history of trauma or recent infection
- Patient reports occasional bladder incontinence
- No complaints of chest pain, shortness of breath, dizziness, joint pain, foot pain, or bowel incontinence

## ■■■ Medications

- Donepezil 10 mg po Q HS
- Allopurinol 100 mg po QD
- Pravastatin 40 mg po QD
- Lisinopril 20 mg po QD
- Ensure drinks PRN

- Ibuprofen 200 mg q4h PRN
- Docusate sodium 100 mg po BID

 **All**

Co-trimoxazole → rash

---

***Patient Case Question 2.*** Identify this patient's *two* major risk factors for Alzheimer disease.

***Patient Case Question 3.*** Why is the patient taking allopurinol, and why is this medication effective in individuals with this condition?

***Patient Case Question 4.*** Why is the patient taking lisinopril, and why is this medication effective in individuals with this condition?

***Patient Case Question 5.*** Why is the patient taking docusate sodium, and why is this medication effective in individuals with this condition?

## ■■■ PE and Lab Tests

### Gen

- Slightly confused but cooperative elderly woman in NAD
- Becomes less confused with slowly repeated questions and simple explanations
- The patient has a significant tic of the upper lip (2–3 twitches/minute)

### Vital Signs

See Patient Case Table 38.1

| Patient Case Table 38.1 Vital Signs | | | | | |
|---|---|---|---|---|---|
| BP | 140/80 left arm, sitting | RR | 15, unlabored | HT | 5′6″ |
| P | 85, regular | T | 98.8°F | WT | 114 lbs |

### Skin

- Pale and dry with senile lentigines
- Poor turgor
- Multiple minor ecchymoses noted on forearms; no other lesions or abrasions

---

***Patient Case Question 6.*** What are *senile lentigines*?

***Patient Case Question 7.*** What are *ecchymoses*?

### HEENT

- Fundi WNL
- TMs intact
- Dentures present
- Buccal and pharyngeal membranes moist and without lesions or exudate

## Neck/LN

- Neck supple
- No thyromegaly or lymphadenopathy
- Trachea mid-line
- Carotid pulses full and equal bilaterally without bruits
- No JVD

## Chest/Lungs

- Mildly increased chest anteroposterior diameter with mild kyphosis
- Lungs clear to auscultation throughout

## Heart

- RRR
- Normal $S_1$ and $S_2$
- No murmurs or rubs

## Abdomen

- Soft, NT/ND, and symmetric with no apparent masses or hernias
- No scars, lesions, or bruits
- Bowel sounds present
- Tympany to percussion in all quadrants; no masses or organomegaly

## Breasts

No masses, tenderness, discoloration, discharge, or dimpling

## Genitalia

Normal external female genitalia

## MS/Extremities

- No redness, swelling, or cyanosis
- Extremities warm bilaterally
- All peripheral pulses present and equal bilaterally
- No inguinal adenopathy
- With exception of left great toe, which was tender with movement, joints showed full, smooth ROM; no crepitus or tenderness
- Able to maintain flexion and extension against resistance without tenderness

## Neurological

- Pinprick, light touch, vibration intact
- Able to feel key in both hands with eyes closed, but unable to identify it as such
- Rapid alternating movements have deteriorated since the patient's last visit
- DTRs all 2+
- Negative Babinski sign bilaterally
- Gait slightly wide-based and awkward; unable to tandem walk
- No Romberg sign

## Folstein Mini-Mental State Examination

The patient's examination score was 9/30

**Patient Case Question 8.** Have the results of the patient's mini-mental state exam *improved, worsened,* or *remained the same* since her last mental state test?

## Laboratory Blood Test Results (Fasting)

See Patient Case Table 38.2

| Patient Case Table 38.2 Laboratory Blood Test Results (Fasting) | | | | | |
|---|---|---|---|---|---|
| Na | 144 meq/L | ALT | 22 IU/L | HDL | 39 mg/dL |
| K | 4.3 meq/L | Alk Phos | 124 IU/L | LDL | 117 mg/dL |
| Cl | 105 meq/L | T Bilirubin | 1.2 mg/dL | Uric acid | 5.7 mg/dL |
| $HCO_3$ | 29 meq/L | D Bilirubin | 0.4 mg/dL | Vitamin $B_{12}$ | 288 pg/mL |
| Hb | 14.9 g/dL | BUN | 14 mg/dL | Ca | 9.2 mg/dL |
| Hct | 44% | Cr | 1.2 mg/dL | $PO_4$ | 4.5 mg/dL |
| RBC | $4.85 \times 10^6/mm^3$ | Glu | 87 mg/dL | Mg | 2.4 mg/dL |
| Plt | $161 \times 10^3/mm^3$ | Cholesterol | 185 mg/dL | TSH | 3.6 µU/mL |
| WBC | $7.34 \times 10^3/mm^3$ | Trig | 147 mg/dL | $T_4$ | 5.9 µg/dL |
| AST | 28 IU/L | T Protein | 6.5 g/dL | Alb | 4.1 g/dL |

**Patient Case Question 9.** Identify all of the abnormalities associated with this patient's CBC.

**Patient Case Question 10.** Is this patient's renal function *normal* or *abnormal*?

**Patient Case Question 11.** Is this patient's hepatic function *normal* or *abnormal*?

**Patient Case Question 12.** Is this patient's serum lipid profile *normal* or *abnormal*?

**Patient Case Question 13.** Is this patient's thyroid function *normal* or *abnormal*?

**Patient Case Question 14.** Identify any laboratory blood test results in Table 38.2 that might explain the patient's deteriorating neurologic function.

**Patient Case Question 15.** Are there any indications for treating this patient with memantine?

**Patient Case Question 16.** Multi-infarct dementia has to be ruled out as a possible cause of this patient's changes in cognitive function, because this condition presents in a similar manner. Identify *two* risk factors that predispose this patient to multi-infarct dementia.

**Patient Case Question 17.** Does multi-infarct dementia present in the same manner with a CT scan study as does Alzheimer disease?

**Patient Case Question 18.** Clinical depression in an elderly patient is often mistaken for Alzheimer disease. Is there any way to distinguish depression from Alzheimer disease in the geriatric population?

**Patient Case Question 19.** Why might a trial of risperidone be appropriate for this patient?

# CASE STUDY

# 39

# CLUSTER HEADACHE

 *For the Disease Summary for this case study, see the CD-ROM.*

## PATIENT CASE

### ■■■ History of Present Illness

P.T. is a 35-year-old male with a three-year history of cluster headache. He presents to the neurology clinic for follow-up. He states that he has not had any headaches for approximately one year until they returned about six weeks ago. He has recently been through a divorce, lost his mother to cancer, and started a new job. His typical headache "comes out of nowhere" and reaches peak intensity within 10 minutes. The pain is very severe (9 on a pain scale of 1–10), non-throbbing in nature, and is always located on the left side of the head above the eye. In addition, pain extends over into the temple and down into the left cheek. There is always a "runny nose" and a "runny eye" associated with the headaches. Episodes of head pain usually last about 2½ hours, and he has been getting two headaches each day for the last five days. Headaches have been occurring at approximately 9 AM and 9 PM daily. Neither acetaminophen nor ibuprofen is very effective in relieving pain. There are no "flashing lights," sparks, or zig-zags of light associated with the head pain. There has been an occasional bout of nausea but no vomiting.

### ■■■ Past Medical History

- Cluster headaches since age 32, no triggers identified
- Previous clinical evaluation included EEG and head MRI
- No previous signs of PVD, CVA, brain tumor, CNS infection, cerebral aneurysm, or epilepsy
- Drug therapies have included the following:

  Abortive Therapies
  1. Aspirin, acetaminophen, ibuprofen, and Cafergot ineffective
  2. Home self-administration of 100% oxygen very effective

  Prophylactic Therapies
  1. Oral verapamil ineffective as prophylactic agent; causes constipation and dizziness
  2. Oral lithium carbonate moderately effective; causes hand tremor, fatigue, muscle weakness, polydipsia, and polyuria

*Patient Case Question 1.* Why does lithium carbonate cause polydipsia and polyuria as side effects?

# Other Medical Problems

- Scrotal varicocele, 10 years ago, surgically repaired
- Bacterial epididymitis, 8 years ago, cleared with antibiotics
- Anemia of unknown origin, 4 years ago, resolved spontaneously

# Family History

- Mother had history of headaches before her death
- Remainder of family history is unremarkable

# Other Medications

None

# Immunizations

Up-to-date

# Allergies

No known drug allergies

# Social History

- Started new job as baker 5 weeks ago
- Recently divorced
- Father of twin daughters, age 8
- Denies tobacco use and intravenous drug abuse
- Alcohol consumption has increased significantly in past month, up to a 6-pack of beer every night
- Occasional caffeine intake

# Physical Examination and Laboratory Tests

## General Examination

Well-developed, well-nourished, muscular Hispanic male in no acute distress

## Vital Signs

See Patient Case Table 39.1

| Patient Case Table 39.1 Vital Signs | | | |
|---|---|---|---|
| Blood pressure | 132/84 mm Hg | Temperature | 98.3°F |
| Heart rate | 83 beats/minute | Weight | 170 lbs |
| Respiratory rate | 15 respirations/minute | Height | 5'9" |

## Skin

- Intact, warm, and dry
- Normal skin turgor
- No diaphoresis
- No unusual lesions noted

## Head, Eyes, Ears, Nose, and Throat

- Miosis of left pupil with slow response to light
- Ptosis of left upper eyelid prominent
- Negative for conjunctival erythema
- White sclera
- Fundi benign
- Pinnae without lesions
- Auditory canals without lesions or obstruction
- Tympanic membranes clear throughout with no drainage or perforations
- Nasal septum mid-line
- No nasal polyps or bleeding noted
- No nasal discharge
- Oral mucosa clear with no erythema or exudates
- Uvula mid-line

## Neck

- Supple
- No palpable nodes, carotid bruits, or JVD
- Trachea mid-line
- Thyroid without masses or tenderness

## Chest

- Symmetric expansion of rib cage
- Lungs clear to auscultation
- No wheezes, rales, or rhonchi noted

## Heart

- Regular cardiac rate and rhythm
- Normal $S_1$ and $S_2$
- No $S_3$ or $S_4$
- No murmurs, rubs, or gallops

## Abdomen

- Soft and non-tender
- No evidence of ascites
- Spleen is not palpable
- Positive bowel sounds
- No masses or abdominal bruits noted
- Liver size normal

## Genitalia/Rectum

- Normal penis and testicles, healed surgical incision in left scrotum
- Normal rectal exam and rectal tone
- No polyps or hemorrhoids
- Prostate benign
- Negative for hernia
- Guaiac-negative stool

## Musculoskeletal/Extremities

- Skeletal muscle hypertrophy of arms from weight-lifting
- No clubbing, edema, or tenderness
- Radial and femoral pulses palpable bilaterally
- Full range of motion in all extremities
- Upper extremity/lower extremity strength 5/5 with normal tone
- No evidence of thrombophlebitis

## Neurological

- Cranial nerves II–XII intact
- No aphasia
- Negative Romberg response
- Finger-to-nose normal
- Motor: Grip strength strong, bilaterally symmetric
- Deep tendon reflexes (patellar) 2+ and equal
- Sensory: Intact bilaterally
- Babinski response negative bilaterally
- No nystagmus or tremors

## Laboratory Blood Tests

See Patient Case Table 39.2

| Patient Case Table 39.2 Laboratory Blood Test Results | | | | | |
|---|---|---|---|---|---|
| Sodium | 136 meq/L | BUN | 11 mg/dL | Hematocrit | 41% |
| Potassium | 4.8 meq/L | Creatinine | 0.6 mg/dL | Platelets | 403,000/mm$^3$ |
| Chloride | 101 meq/L | Glucose, fasting | 89 mg/dL | WBC | 7,200/mm$^3$ |
| Bicarbonate | 24 meq/L | Hemoglobin | 14.7 g/dL | WBC diff | WNL |

*Patient Case Question 2.* What is an appropriate assessment of the patient's condition?

*Patient Case Question 3.* What are some possible causes/risk factors of this patient's current headache problem?

*Patient Case Question 4.* What is the significance of the primary care provider's observation of "white sclera"?

*Patient Case Question 5.* List *two* clinical signs of cluster headache that were observed during the physical examination.

*Patient Case Question 6.* Do any of the laboratory blood tests indicate a potential cause of headaches in this patient?

*Patient Case Question 7.* What is the significance of the results from the neurologic exam?

*Patient Case Question 8.* Which type of abortive pharmacotherapy might be suggested to the patient in lieu of home oxygen treatment?

*Patient Case Question 9.* Which type of prophylactic pharmacotherapy might be suggested to the patient?

*Patient Case Question 10.* Define the term *ascites*.

*Patient Case Question 11.* Define the term *nystagmus*.

*Patient Case Question 12.* List *seven* distinguishing features that suggest that the patient has been having cluster headaches and not migraines.

# 40 COMPLEX PARTIAL SEIZURE

 *For the Disease Summary for this case study, see the CD-ROM.*

# PATIENT CASE

## ■ Patient's Chief Complaints

"I think that I'm having partial seizures. I'm not sure what is causing them, but, at my age, statistics suggest that it may be bad news."

## ■ History of Present Illness

Dr. D.K. is a 59 yo physician who visits his brother, also a physician, while vacationing one summer in San Diego. "Jeannie (i.e., D.K.'s spouse) has told me that the clinical manifestations were subtle at first but have become more disturbing of late. The last time that I had an episode I would have fallen down a flight of stairs if she hadn't caught hold of me. She tells me that during one of these things, I don't respond to anything but I do not lose consciousness either. She says that I just stare off into space and fidget with my tie or the buttons on my shirt. I don't respond to my surroundings and don't seem to know what is going on at all, that I'm not in the present. It has been going on now for about three weeks and the episodes last three or four minutes every time. At first it was every three days; now, it's every other day. When I come out of it, I'm extremely confused and unable to speak clearly for some time. I try to talk but, apparently, my words are incoherent. I remember very little about the attacks. I do remember several things, however—especially, the taste of what seems like soap in my mouth immediately before I black out and some mild stomach discomfort. And when I do become aware again, I feel a distinct sense of loss of time . . . and sometimes I'm so exhausted that I need a nap. I guess that, if there is any good news at all, it is that I haven't had a grand mal yet. . . . but it could be just around the corner."

Dr. K's brother strongly encourages him to see a neurologist as soon as possible and volunteers to refer him to a good specialist and make an appointment.

## ■ Past Medical History

- Malignant melanoma on lower back removed 14 years ago
- Two colonic polyps removed 7 years ago during colonoscopy
- Diverticulosis × 4 years
- Occasional back pain
- Tension headaches

## ■ Family History

- No family history of seizure disorder, cancer, or cardiovascular disease
- Mother died from MVA at age 69
- No information available for father
- One brother, age 54, is alive and well

## ■ Social History

- Married for 39 years, lives with his wife who is a nurse, and has 2 daughters who are in good physical health
- Family practice physician who attended medical school in New York; also teaches "Introduction to Clinical Medicine" and acts as preceptor to first-year medical students
- Has a positive history of alcohol use but states that "he hasn't had a drop in 20 years"
- Non-smoker
- (–) IVDA
- Works out 3–5 times per week at the gym and jogs most mornings
- Eats healthy and is conscientious of calories, fats, and sugars

## ■ Review of Systems

- Recently has noticed a decrease in stamina and tires easily
- (–) for head injury, increase in frequency or change in nature of headaches, nausea, vomiting, visual or other sensory changes, irritability, hemiparesis, TIA, tingling or numbness, HIV disease, history of febrile seizures, problems with balance, and identifiable triggers of attacks
- Patient's interview details and his overall score on the Quality of Life in Epilepsy Questionnaire (QOLIE-31, see *Appendix G*) show that seizures are beginning to impact significantly on his quality of life; however, his overall scores on energy/fatigue, pain, and social support domains are high in comparison with a cohort of other patients with recurrent seizure activity.

## ■ Medications

- Multiple vitamin 1 tablet po QD
- Denies any herbal products
- Occasional acetaminophen for headaches and back pain

## ■ Allergies

- NKDA
- Dogs → itchy eyes and sneezing

## ■ Physical Examination and Laboratory Tests

### General

- WDWN, pleasant white male in NAD
- Patient is cooperative, oriented, and appears to be his stated age, but seems tired

### Vital Signs

See Patient Case Table 40.1

| Patient Case Table 40.1 Vital Signs | | | | | |
|---|---|---|---|---|---|
| BP | 138/80 (sitting, right arm) | RR | 14 and unlabored | HT | 5'10½" |
| P | 60 and regular | T | 98.8°F | WT | 174 lbs |

## Skin

- Warm, soft, dry, and non-jaundiced
- (–) for rashes, bruises, and other lesions
- Hair quality, distribution, and texture unremarkable

## Head, Eyes, Ears, Nose, and Throat

- NC/AT
- PERRLA
- EOMI without nystagmus
- Optic disc margins appropriately sharp
- Wears eyeglasses
- TMs pearly gray, revealing good cone of light bilaterally
- Nasal mucous membranes moist
- (–) for erythema of pharynx and oral ulcers

## Neck/Lymph Nodes

- Neck supple without stiffness
- (–) for adenopathy, bruits, JVD, and thyromegaly

## Chest

- Normal breath sounds
- Good air entry

## Cardiac

- RRR
- (–) for murmurs, rubs, and gallops

## Abdomen

- Soft, NT/ND
- (+) BS
- (−) for masses, organomegaly, and guarding

## Genitalia/Rectum

- Genitalia normal
- Circumcised male
- Rectal exam not performed

## Musculoskeletal/Extremities

- (–) for adenopathy, lesions, rashes, joint swelling, and tenderness
- Good ROM throughout
- (–) for edema, clubbing, and cyanosis
- Peripheral pulses 2+ throughout

## Neurological

- CNs II–XII intact
- DTRs exaggerated at 3+ throughout
- A & O to person, place, and time
- No focal abnormalities
- Normal strength and tone
- Plantar flexion WNL

## Laboratory Blood Test Results (Fasting)

See Patient Case Table 40.2

| Patient Case Table 40.2 Laboratory Blood Test Results (Fasting) | | | | | |
|---|---|---|---|---|---|
| Na | 138 meq/L | Hb | 14.2 g/dL | Alb | 3.9 g/dL |
| K | 3.9 meq/L | Hct | 40.7% | PT | 14.3 sec |
| Cl | 103 meq/L | Plt | $417 \times 10^3/mm^3$ | PTT | 31.8 sec |
| $HCO_3$ | 26 meq/L | WBC | $6.2 \times 10^3/mm^3$ | AST | 28 IU/L |
| BUN | 13 mg/dL | Ca | 8.3 mg/dL | ALT | 44 IU/L |
| Cr | 1.0 mg/dL | Mg | 2.3 mg/dL | Bilirubin, total | 1.1 mg/dL |
| Glu | 92 mg/dL | Phos | 2.7 mg/dL | Alk Phos | 68 IU/L |

## CT Scan

- 1.5-inch irregular mass in left temporal lobe
- No herniation of brain tissue noted

## Electroencephalogram

WNL but 72 hours since last attack

## Biopsy of Left Temporal Lobe Lesion

- Highly vascular and anaplastic neoplasm with histologic features consistent with poorly differentiated astrocytoma (*glioblastoma multiforme*)
- Clinical course of this type of brain cancer is usually rapidly progressive with poor prognosis; metastasis is rare; total surgical removal is usually not possible; radiation and chemotherapy may prolong survival

*Patient Case Question 1.* Identify a minimum of *ten* distinct patient complaints that are consistent with a diagnosis of complex partial seizure activity.

*Patient Case Question 2.* Can motor automatisms in this case study be considered *simple* or *complex*?

*Patient Case Question 3.* Identify any risk factors that predispose this patient to recurrent complex partial seizures.

*Patient Case Question 4.* What is the cause of complex partial seizure activity in this patient?

*Patient Case Question 5.* Does this patient's condition satisfy the technical definition of epilepsy?

*Patient Case Question 6.* Is this patient a good candidate for long-term treatment with an anti-seizure medication, such as phenytoin or carbamazepine?

***Patient Case Question 7.*** Does this patient's condition satisfy the technical definition of idiopathic epilepsy?

***Patient Case Question 8.*** Does this patient have any signs of renal dysfunction at this time?

***Patient Case Question 9.*** Does this patient have any signs of hepatic dysfunction at this time?

***Patient Case Question 10.*** Does this patient have any signs of pulmonary or cardiovascular dysfunction at this time?

***Patient Case Question 11.*** Identify as many possible other abnormal exam or test results that you did not previously list in Question 1 above.

***Patient Case Question 12.*** Do brain tumors have to be malignant/cancerous to cause epilepsy?

***Patient Case Question 13.*** If this patient had reported that TIAs were accompanying seizure activity, what might have been a possible cause of recurrent complex partial seizures?

# 41

## GENERALIZED TONIC-CLONIC SEIZURE

 *For the Disease Summary for this case study, see the CD-ROM.*

## PATIENT CASE

### ■ Patient's Chief Clinical Manifestations

Provided by patient's football coach: "His arms and legs were as rigid as lead pipes, his eyes were rolling, and he was shaking all over. It was horrible! I've never seen one in person before, but I think that he had a convulsion."

### ■ History of Present Illness

C.S. is a 17-year-old boy, who was brought to the emergency room by his high school football coach and two teammates. The patient had been practicing for Friday night's high school football game when clinical manifestations developed suddenly. It had been a very hot afternoon and all of the players were sweating profusely. When the offensive line positioned itself to run a final play from scrimmage for the afternoon, the patient fell to the ground and appeared to lose consciousness. His body stiffened with arms and legs extended. He suddenly let out a shrill cry and appeared to stop breathing for about 15 seconds. The coach removed his football helmet just before C.S. went into a series of violent, rhythmic, muscle contractions accompanied by hyperventilation. His eyes were rolling and his face became grossly contorted. Suddenly, the jerking movements began to ease up and progressively became less intense until they stopped all together. He then took a deep breath and the incident seemed to be over. The entire episode lasted approximately 3–4 minutes. C.S. woke up confused with no recall of the attack. However, he complained of a headache and extremely sore muscles.

The patient had complained to his mother that morning before school of a "lightheaded feeling," and she had strongly suggested that he consider skipping practice today. He dismissed the symptoms with, "I'll be fine" and "It will pass." Just before he left for practice, his mother asked him how he was feeling. He reported that he "was feeling fine and ready for a good practice."

In the emergency room, 45 minutes after the incident, the patient still could not remember the episode and reported that his first memory was that of finding himself flat on the ground with all of his teammates standing around him and Coach saying, "Are you okay, Big Man?"

### ■ Past Medical History

* The patient's birth followed a normal pregnancy with good prenatal care
* Developmental milestones were all WNL
* No previous history of seizure activity

- To his recall, he has not had any recent infections (confirmed by mother)
- He has a history of one concussion while playing football 2 years ago
- Diagnosed with mild hypertension at age 15 for which he has been under the care of a physician, and taking a low dose of a mild diuretic

## ▰▰ Family History

- Younger brother (age 12) was diagnosed with epilepsy (primarily complex partial seizures) at age 3
- Older sister (age 18) and father are alive and in good health
- Mother has osteoarthritis, which she treats with OTC NSAIDs PRN
- No other information on family history was obtained

## ▰▰ Social History

- Denies drinking alcohol or taking any illegal recreational substances
- Reports doing well at school and at home with "no unusual stress in his life at this time"
- Denies tobacco use
- Plays offensive tackle for high school football team; was awarded "Offensive Lineman of the Year" honors in the conference last season
- Enjoys "fixing up his car" and "hanging out with friends"

## ▰▰ Review of Systems

- Reports feeling "weak and sleepy"
- There was no nausea, vomiting, bladder incontinence, or bowel incontinence during or after the incident

## ▰▰ Medications

Hydrochlorothiazide 12.5 mg po QD

## ▰▰ Allergies

**NKDA**

*Patient Case Question 1.* Identify *two* potential and significant contributing factors to this patient's seizure.

*Patient Case Question 2.* Identify a minimum of *twelve* clinical manifestations in this patient that are consistent with a diagnosis of grand mal seizure.

## ▰▰ Physical Examination and Laboratory Tests

### General Appearance

- Patient is a large, well-developed but obese white teenage male who is alert but tired
- He is in NAD
- He is wearing a football uniform that is moist from diaphoresis

## Vital Signs

See Patient Case Table 41.1

| Patient Case Table 41.1 Vital Signs | | | | | |
|---|---|---|---|---|---|
| BP | 125/79, right arm, sitting | RR | 15, regular, unlabored | HT | 6'3" |
| P | 80, regular | T | 98.4°F | WT | 252 lbs |

## Skin

- Warm, moist, and pale
- Face is flushed
- No lesions or abrasions

## HEENT

- Atraumatic
- Pupils round and equal at 3 mm, responsive to light
- Conjunctiva pink but dry
- Visual acuity 20/20 bilaterally
- Fundi with sharp disks and no abnormalities
- Nasal mucosa pink but dry and without lesions or discharge
- Bite wounds on right lateral tongue and inside right cheek
- Tongue dry and rugged
- Pharynx dry with no exudate or erythema

## Neck/Lymph Nodes

- Neck supple
- Negative for thyromegaly, lymphadenopathy, JVD, and carotid bruits

## Chest/Lungs

- Lungs CTA throughout all lobes with no crackles
- Normal diaphragmatic position and excursion
- Chest expansion full and symmetric

***Patient Case Question 3.*** What is the importance of the chest/lung exam results?

## Heart

- Apical pulse normal at 4th intercostal space, mid-clavicular line
- Regular rate and rhythm
- Normal $S_1$ and $S_2$ with no additional cardiac sounds
- Negative for murmurs, gallops, and rubs

## Abdomen

- Soft, obese, and non-tender
- Liver percussion normal at 2 cm below right costal margin
- Negative for HSM, masses, and bruits
- BS present and normoactive

## Genitalia/Rectum

Deferred

## Musculoskeletal/Extremities

- Brisk capillary refill at 2 seconds
- Negative for edema, cyanosis, or clubbing
- Peripheral pulses 2+ and symmetric throughout
- Muscular hypertrophy of the upper extremities secondary to weight-lifting
- Full ROM

## Neurologic

- Oriented but slightly sleepy
- Cranial nerves II–XII intact
- Muscular tone and strength 5/5 throughout
- DTRs 2+ and symmetric
- Sensory intact to touch
- No motor deficits noted
- Able to perform rapid alternating movements smoothly and without error
- Negative for Babinski sign
- Cerebellar function and gait normal

## Laboratory Blood Test Results

See Patient Case Table 41.2

| Patient Case Table 41.2 Laboratory Blood Test Results | | | | | | |
|---|---|---|---|---|---|---|
| Na | 127 meq/L | Ca | 9.8 mg/dL | WBC | | $7.6 \times 10^3/mm^3$ |
| K | 4.5 meq/L | Mg | 2.3 mg/dL | DIFF<br>• Neutros<br>• Lymphs<br>• Monos<br>• Eos<br>• Basos | | 65%<br>26%<br>5%<br>3%<br>1% |
| Cl | 96 meq/L | $PO_4$ | 2.5 mg/dL | AST | | 12 IU/L |
| $HCO_3$ | 28 meq/L | Hb | 15.0 g/dL | ALT | | 16 IU/L |
| BUN | 16 mg/dL | Hct | 48% | Bilirubin, total | | 0.6 mg/dL |
| Cr | 1.0 mg/dL | MCV | 92.5 fL | Alb | | 4.3 g/dL |
| Glu, fasting | 100 mg/dL | Plt | $191 \times 10^3/mm^3$ | Protein, total | | 6.7 g/dL |

***Patient Case Question 4.*** Identify *the single most critical laboratory result* in Table 41.2 that may have contributed to the patient's seizure.

***Patient Case Question 5.*** Provide a reasonable explanation for the abnormal laboratory finding that you identified in Question 4 above.

## Head MRI Scan

Normal

## EEG

- Showed generalized background slowing
- No focal changes or epileptiform activity present
- Photic stimulation failed to induce changes in pattern

## ■ Clinical Course

While in the emergency room, the patient became progressively irritable and anxious and experienced a second seizure with sudden loss of consciousness and a generalized tonic convulsion that was closely followed by alternating clonic convulsions. The event lasted for approximately 3 minutes. The patient slept for 15 minutes after the seizure and awakened confused. He was treated with intravenous fosphenytoin to provide long-term seizure control, and his electrocardiogram was monitored for cardiac rhythm abnormalities (which are potential side effects when phenytoin is rapidly administered).

A second physical examination revealed a regular heart rate of 115, a regular and unlabored respiration rate of 20, and a blood pressure of 140/85. His lungs were clear to auscultation. His skin was diaphoretic, warm, and not cyanotic. The patient was sleepy and oriented to name only. A focused neurologic exam was essentially normal. Blood was drawn within 20 minutes after termination of the clonic phase of the seizure and submitted for a serum prolactin determination. The prolactin level was 462 ng/mL.

The patient was admitted to the hospital, monitored closely throughout the night, and continued on fosphenytoin. He did well with no further seizures. He continued to feel weak and tired but had no other adverse effects. He was discharged on the morning of the third day and referred to a specialist for further treatment.

*Patient Case Question 6.* Based on what you have learned in this case study, would you say that this patient's seizures were *provoked* or *unprovoked?*

*Patient Case Question 7.* What is the significance of the patient's serum prolactin test?

*Patient Case Question 8.* What do you consider the *most appropriate initial treatment trial* for control of further seizure activity in this patient?

*Patient Case Question 9.* Are the terms *seizure* and *convulsion* synonymous?

# 42

# INTRACRANIAL NEOPLASM

 *For the Disease Summary for this case study, see the CD-ROM.*

# PATIENT CASE

## ■ Chief Complaints

Provided by patient's spouse: "My husband was okay until about 4 months ago in Arizona when he began having trouble driving. He also couldn't recall where he put things and, soon after that, couldn't remember our friends' names. He became more withdrawn and not very talkative. Eventually we figured out that he could not understand what other people were saying. Then he began having problems walking and that progressed rapidly and confined him to a wheelchair. He has also complained of back pain and was scheduled for a prostate biopsy because of a large prostate and high PSA. However, we had to cancel, because R. came down with the flu. He is also having major problems with bowel and bladder control. He makes no effort to go to the bathroom and poops and pees in bed. He has recently developed some annoying repetitive habits—rubbing and picking at his face and eyebrows, scratching himself, and wiping his nose with the back of his hand. It is probably Alzheimer's."

## ■ HPI

Mr. R.L. is 78-year-old African American male who was referred to the neurology clinic. His initial symptoms consisted of progressive problems with memory, followed by gait problems, and finally incontinence. This presentation suggests a process involving the frontal and temporal lobes of the brain. The patient has also shown evidence of a loss of inhibitions, which might also reflect abnormal frontal lobe function. There is no recent history of fever, chills, or loss of appetite.

## ■ PMH

* Recent diagnosis of thrombophlebitis in lower extremities
* Recent diagnosis of depression
* History of visual hallucinations

## ■ Past Surgical History

* Surgical correction of abnormality in nasal septum, 24 years ago
* Surgical repair of inguinal hernia, 20 years ago
* Bilateral blepharoplasty for ptosis, 8 years ago

## FH

- Mother died from respiratory complications but was diagnosed with mental illness 7 years prior to her death
- Father committed suicide by gunshot wound at age 23
- One brother died from testicular cancer at age 26

## SH

- No history of smoking, alcohol abuse, or IVDA
- History of eating cow brains 10 years ago

## PE and Lab Tests

### Gen

The patient is sitting in a wheelchair and appears to be in NAD. His appearance is disheveled and he presents with a mask-like facies (characteristic of Parkinson disease). He appears to be moderately overweight.

### VS

See Patient Case Table 42.1

| Patient Case Table 42.1 Vital Signs | | | | | |
|---|---|---|---|---|---|
| BP | 135/75 sitting | RR | 17 | HT | 6'2" |
| HR | 83 regular | T | 98.0°F | WT | 211 lbs |

### Neck

Supple and negative for thyromegaly, carotid bruits, and lymphadenopathy

### Chest

Clear to auscultation

### Cardiac

Normal heart sounds

### MS/Ext

2+ pitting edema with petechiae in RLE and LLE

### Neurologic Exam Results

See Patient Case Table 42.2

## Patient Case Table 42.2 Neurologic Exam Results

**Mental Status**

- Awake, alert, and responsive
- Mini-mental status exam = 12/30
- Patient did not know month, city, or president
- Unable to recall three objects
- Could not spell "body" backwards
- Unable to draw a stick-man or clock or follow a 3-step command
- Refused to write his name

**Cranial Nerve Function**

| | |
|---|---|
| • II | Unable to assess visual fields as patient was uncooperative |
| | Pupils were 3 mm bilaterally and reactive |
| | Optic discs were negative for papilledema |
| • III, IV, VI | Patient followed finger in all directions of gaze |
| | Positive for nystagmus |
| • V | Difficult to test |
| | Patient responded equally to pinpricks on the face bilaterally |
| | Corneal reflexes were symmetric and WNL |
| • VII–XI | Symmetric responses |
| | Gag response WNL |
| • XII | Normal appearance of tongue, mid-line position, no functional defects |

**Motor Exam**

- Normal muscle bulk but tone is increased
- Muscle strength appeared to be 4/5 in all muscle groups in upper extremities
- Strength in lower extremities was not assessed as patient was uncooperative
- Patient could stand only with bilateral support

**Reflexes**

- Symmetric in upper and lower extremities with hyperreflexia at 3+/4 in biceps, triceps, brachioradialis, and knees
- Ankle reflexes could not be assessed
- Plantar reflexes were downgoing bilaterally

**Sensory Exam**

- The patient responded equally to painful stimuli in all four limbs

**Cerebellar Function**

- Inability to judge distances bilaterally in upper extremities when reaching for objects
- Negative for swaying of the head and trunk when sitting

**Evaluation of Gait and Sense of Position**

- Extremely unsteady
- Could stand only with bilateral support and took only two steps with great difficulty
- Could not evaluate for Romberg sign

## Laboratory Blood Test Results

See Patient Case Table 42.3

## Patient Case Table 42.3 Laboratory Blood Test Results

| | | | | | |
|---|---|---|---|---|---|
| Na | 142 meq/L | Hct | 48% | LDH | 99 IU/L |
| K | 3.9 meq/L | Plt | $229 \times 10^3/mm^3$ | Alk Phos | 88 IU/L |
| Cl | 101 meq/L | WBC | $8.6 \times 10^3/mm^3$ | ALT | 28 IU/L |
| $HCO_3$ | 23 meq/L | Ca | 9.7 mg/dL | AST | 35 IU/L |
| BUN | 16 mg/dL | Mg | 2.5 mg/dL | Bilirubin, total | 0.6 mg/dL |
| Cr | 0.9 mg/dL | Phos | 4.2 mg/dL | TSH | 4.8 µU/mL |
| Glu, fasting | 88 mg/dL | Alb | 3.7 g/dL | Vitamin $B_{12}$ | 144 pg/mL |
| Hb | 15.5 g/dL | Protein, total | 6.7 g/dL | HIV | Negative |

## CT Scan

- Large mass in both frontal lobes crossing the corpus callosum and consistent with "butterfly tumor," greater on the right, with some calcification, suggests astrocytoma
- No enhancement of mass with contrast media, ruling out lymphoma, central nervous system infection, and white matter inflammatory disorder

## Biopsy

- Stereotactic needle biopsy of tissue acquired from right frontal lobe
- Hypercellularity, angiogenesis, pleomorphism, and necrosis consistent with glioblastoma multiforme

## ■■■ Clinical Course

Following biopsy, the patient demonstrated a significant decrease in level of consciousness and developed left-sided hemiparesis. He also developed a deep vein thrombus in the left leg. Because the patient was post-operative, IV heparin could not be given. After considering the prognosis carefully, the family chose not to opt for treatment. The patient remained stable and plans were made to transfer him to a hospice facility close to his spouse.

*Patient Case Question 1.* The patient was initially believed to have Jacob-Creutzfeldt disease. Why?

*Patient Case Question 2.* What evidence is available that helps rule out a central nervous system infection as the cause of this patient's disability?

*Patient Case Question 3.* Why was serum TSH checked?

*Patient Case Question 4.* Why was serum vitamin $B_{12}$ checked?

*Patient Case Question 5.* Why was the patient tested for HIV?

*Patient Case Question 6.* Does any of the laboratory data suggest that this intracranial neoplasm has metastasized outside of the central nervous system?

*Patient Case Question 7.* Does the patient have any known risk factors for the development of a brain tumor?

*Patient Case Question 8.* What evidence suggests that intracranial pressure was not significantly elevated?

## ■■■ Patient Mini-Case 1

See Patient Case Table 42.4

### Patient Case Table 42.4 Patient Mini-Case 1

**Patient History**

- 52-year-old female smoker
- History of hypertension and diabetes mellitus—type 2
- Health began deteriorating 18 months ago
- Morning headaches that would regress with time
- Began having hearing problems on left side 9 months ago
- Constantly had to turn right side of head to hear
- Recent intermittent loss of sensation on left side of face
- Could not feel her husband's hand on her face
- Taking hydrochlorothiazide and captopril for hypertension
- Taking glyburide and metformin for diabetes
- Has no known allergies

**Physical Examination**

- Slight drooping of left side of mouth and left lower eyelid
- Incomplete closure of left eyelid with touch to cornea
- Reduced pain and sensation of light touch on left side
- Funduscopic exam revealed bilateral papilledema

*Patient Case Question 9.* What does *headache* and *papilledema* suggest in the patient in mini-case 1?

# Patient Mini-Case 2

See Patient Case Table 42.5

## Patient Case Table 42.5 Patient Mini-Case 2

**Patient History**

- 37-year-old male, non-smoker
- 20-month history of loss in initiative, depression, and rejection of personal relationships
- Progressive loss of drive to win all the big deals at work
- 4-month history of headache that did not respond to over-the-counter agents
- Progressive increase in lethargy during past several months
- Uncontrollable right arm convulsion for approximately 2 minutes occurred 2 days ago
- Last evening right arm shook violently and right side of face began twitching while watching TV
- Patient presents without fever, loss of appetite, or fatigue

**Physical Examination**

- Bilateral papilledema
- Increased deep tendon reflexes of right bicep and triceps
- Positive Babinski sign of right foot
- Reduced leg strength on right side

*Patient Case Question 10.* Should a patient with a first-time seizure receive an immediate imaging test of the brain?

*Patient Case Question 11.* With reference to the patient's personality changes in mini-case 2, in which anatomic region of the brain is the intracranial neoplasm located?

*Patient Case Question 12.* How should the symptoms be treated for the patient in mini-case 2?

*Patient Case Question 13.* What test could have been done in the absence of neuroimaging in mini-case 2?

# Patient Mini-Case 3

See Patient Case Table 42.6

## Patient Case Table 42.6 Patient Mini-Case 3

**Patient History**

- 2-year-old male
- 3-week history of excessive crying and no interaction with children at daycare
- Began pointing to his head often
- Recently began vomiting daily
- Began wobbling even though he learned to walk 6 months ago
- This morning patient was vomiting and hitting himself in the head

**Physical Examination**

- Bilateral papilledema
- Abnormal gait

*Patient Case Question 14.* In mini-case study 3, why was the child hitting his head?

*Patient Case Question 15.* Why is *brain cancer* not synonymous with *intracranial neoplasm*?

*Patient Case Question 16.* Why are some anti-cancer drugs incapable of crossing the blood–brain barrier and gaining access to an intracranial neoplasm?

*For the Disease Summary for this case study,*
*see the CD-ROM.*

# PATIENT CASE

## ■■■ Initial History

N.B. presents to her primary care provider at the clinic with a "pounding and throbbing" headache, the third of its kind within the past month. The patient is a 41-year-old white female who appears slightly overweight and shows some signs of acute distress. She is a single mother of three sons (ages 2–6), a recent divorcee, has a part-time job at Walmart, and is taking nursing school classes in the evening. She describes her head pain as being localized to the right temple, increasing to peak intensity within one hour, and having a pain score of 9/10. She also complains of neck pain. There is no pain in the orbit or cheek and she denies lacrimation and rhinorrhea. The bright lights in the clinic bother her and she feels nauseous and dizzy but has not vomited. She denies sensitivity to sound. Previous similar headaches have lasted about six hours, have not been responsive to any type of OTC medication, and do not appear to be associated with menses. She was previously diagnosed with migraine headaches at 9 years of age. She adds that she feels "totally exhausted" when the headaches finally subside and often falls into a deep and long sleep afterwards. She denies any symptoms prior to the onset of head pain (such as "bright flashes of light"). She has no known allergies, does not use alcohol or tobacco products, and denies the use of illegal drugs. She sleeps only about five hours every night and has rather poor eating habits. She eats "more chocolate than she should" and drinks 3–4 caffeinated soft drinks each day.

N.B. has been recently diagnosed with major depressive disorder and Zenker diverticulum (localized dilation or outpouching of the esophagus that causes difficulty swallowing). Her medications include rabeprazole for heartburn associated with Zenker diverticulum and phenelzine sulfate for depression. Her mother and younger sister also suffer from migraine headaches.

*Patient Case Question 1.* Is it more likely that the patient is having *classic* or *common* migraines and how did you arrive at your answer?

*Patient Case Question 2.* List *four* potential precipitating factors or contributing factors for migraine in this patient.

# ■ PE and Lab Tests

## Vital Signs

- BP = 135/90 (sitting), 140/95 (lying), 2 minutes apart
- P = 90 and regular
- RR = 14 and unlabored
- T = 98.5° F (oral)
- Wt = 165 lbs
- Ht = 5'6"

***Patient Case Question 3.*** What can be said about the patient's blood pressure?

***Patient Case Question 4.*** Is this patient technically considered *underweight*, *overweight*, *obese*, or is this patient's weight *healthy*?

# ■ HEENT, Neck, and Skin

- No bruises, lacerations, masses, or deformities on head
- Scalp is tender
- Pupils 3 mm and reactive to light
- Funduscopy without lesions
- Ears—cerumen in left ear canal
- Positive for neck soreness, but no adenopathy, thyromegaly, or bruits
- Skin is warm, dry, and pink

***Patient Case Question 5.*** Are the patient's pupils and pupillary response *normal* or *abnormal*?

## Lungs, Chest

- Lungs clear to auscultation
- Resonant to percussion

## Abdomen

- Soft and slightly protuberant
- Not tender to palpation
- No organomegaly or masses
- No aortic, iliac, or renal bruits

## Extremities

- Pulses equal and full
- No edema
- Cardiac NSR

## Neurologic

- Oriented and alert
- Cranial nerves II–XII intact

- Sensory intact to pinprick and light touch
- DTRs = 2+

## Blood Chemistry Panel

- $Na^+$ = 144 meq/L
- $K^+$ = 3.7 meq/L
- $Ca^{+2}$ = 8.5 mg/dL
- $Mg^{+2}$ = 0.9 mg/dL
- $PO_4^{-3}$ = 2.7 mg/dL
- $HCO_3^-$ = 30 meq/L
- $Cl^-$ = 110 meq/L

*Patient Case Question 6.* Identify the *single* abnormal finding in the blood chemistry panel above and explain its possible association with the patient's migraine headaches.

*Patient Case Question 7.* Why might prophylactic pharmacologic therapy be appropriate for this patient?

*Patient Case Question 8.* Name *one* drug that the primary care provider may prescribe initially for prophylactic treatment of migraines in this patient.

*Patient Case Question 9.* Identify *five* features of the patient's headache that help exclude cluster headache as a potential diagnosis.

# 44

# MULTIPLE SCLEROSIS

 *For the Disease Summary for this case study, see the CD-ROM.*

## PATIENT CASE

### Patient's Chief Complaints and History of Present Illness

Mrs. H.J. is a 40-year-old woman with an 18-year history of multiple sclerosis. Her chief complaints today are numbness on the left side of her face and tongue, progressive weakness in her right leg, and constipation. "My balance is getting lousy when I walk," she states. "Sometimes I veer like an old drunken sailor." She has not had a bowel movement in three days. She denies pain during straining episodes. Over-the-counter laxatives have been ineffective. She developed a "bad cold" two weeks ago and these symptoms began occurring at the same time as she was recovering from the illness.

### Past Medical History

- First attack of apparent MS at age 22: Patient had been in excellent health and suddenly lost sensation in tip of index finger of right hand, spread to all fingers of right hand, up into right arm and neck, right arm and neck muscles became weak; symptoms resolved
- Second attack of apparent MS at age 25: Vision in left eye became distorted, colors faded (especially red), vision became blurry with vigorous exercise, eyesight recovered after several weeks
- Third attack of MS at age 28: Weakness in left leg and foot, patient had to be extremely cautious with each step, bringing the entire leg up with the knee bent and extending the leg outward with an exaggerated movement, diagnosis of MS confirmed
- Fourth attack of MS at age 32: Severe constipation with stomach cramps, resolved
- Fifth attack of MS at age 36: Sensations of "electrical buzzing" in her body whenever she lowered her head; right hand became severely numb during the course of 24 hours, soon followed by sensation of numbness in the right hip; the next day, patient developed a sensation of "spinning," became extremely nauseous with severe vomiting, lost sense of balance and had to hold onto objects to remain vertical; left foot became numb and muscles in both legs and left arm became weak; developed mild incontinence; began losing sight in right eye
- Sixth attack of MS at age 38: Complete loss of balance, could not stand, vertigo and muscle weakness, period of vomiting; developed limp after walking a short distance; chronic fatigue; muscle cramps frequent; none of the symptoms seemed to remit

- Mild recurrent bouts of depression often associated with relapses of MS
- Negative for chlamydial infections or syphilis
- Negative for seizures

# ■■■ Family History

The patient is of Belgian descent. She was born and raised in northeastern Wisconsin. She has no siblings. Both parents are alive and well. There is no family history of neurologic disease.

---

***Patient Case Question 1.*** Identify *four* risk factors in this patient that are consistent with multiple sclerosis.

***Patient Case Question 2.*** What probably precipitated this most recent attack of multiple sclerosis?

---

# ■■■ Social History

The patient is married and employed as a special procedures nurse at the hospital. She and her husband have one son (age 20, in college). She denies smoking and intravenous drug use. Patient drinks 1 cup of coffee every morning and has 3–4 glasses of wine each week with dinner. She is involved in a strictly monogamous relationship with her husband of 22 years. Patient enjoys music and reading. She plays cello. She gave up tennis years ago due to weakness and loss of coordination in her arms and legs.

# ■■■ Medications

Ibuprofen 400 mg po PRN for occasional headache

# ■■■ Allergies

No known drug allergies

# ■■■ Review of Systems

- Progressive weakness in arms and legs
- Reports feeling "run down"
- Recent past difficulty with incontinence
- Subjective feeling of extreme weakness in hot weather
- Reports lower abdominal fullness
- Denies any current swallowing or speech problems

# ■■■ Physical Examination and Laboratory Tests

## General

The patient is a middle-aged white woman who appears to be her stated age. She does not appear to be in acute distress. The patient's gait is slow and deliberate, but she is able to walk without assistance. Her affect is sad and she is tearful throughout the examination. She states that she is very concerned about the progression of her disease.

## Vital Signs

See Patient Case Table 44.1

| Patient Case Table 44.1 Vital Signs | | | | | |
|---|---|---|---|---|---|
| BP | 115/70 | RR | 13 and unlabored | WT | 121 lbs |
| P | 74 and regular | T | 97.2°F | HT | 5′5″ |

**Patient Case Question 3.** Should any of the patient's vital signs be a cause for concern?

## Skin

- Warm and dry with normal turgor and color
- No rashes or lesions noted

## Head, Eyes, Ears, Nose, and Throat

- Pupils equal at 3 mm, round, reactive to light and accommodation
- Funduscopic exam normal
- Nystagmus is present
- Slight dysfunction of extra-ocular muscles bilaterally
- External auricular canals clear
- Tympanic membranes intact
- Oropharynx well hydrated without erythema

## Neck/Lymph Nodes

Supple without adenopathy or thyromegaly

## Heart

- Regular rate and rhythm
- $S_1$ and $S_2$ normal with no additional cardiac sounds
- No gallops, murmurs, or friction rubs

## Lungs

Clear to auscultation throughout

## Abdomen

- No tenderness or guarding
- No masses or bruits
- Hypoactive bowel sounds
- (−) organomegaly
- (+) slight distension

# Rectal

- Diminished anal reflex
- Heme-negative stool
- Large amount of stool in rectal vault
- No fissures, hemorrhoids, or strictures

**Patient Case Question 4.** Does the rectal examination provide any information that the patient's constipation is a result of multiple sclerosis?

# Musculoskeletal/Extremities

- Normal range of motion
- Peripheral pulses 2+ throughout

# Neurologic

- Alert, oriented, and cooperative
- Mild subjective sense of auditory distortion despite intact auditory acuity
- Cranial nerves II–XII intact
- Motor strength 4/5 upper extremities and left leg, 3/5 in right leg
- Motor tone is spastic throughout
- Deep tendon reflexes 3+ throughout
- Sensory exam reveals significant reductions in light touch and pinprick bilaterally
- Coordination testing reveals moderate-to-severe unsteadiness with walking
- Positive Romberg sign

**Patient Case Question 5.** Briefly explain how a Romberg maneuver is done and what it may reveal.

**Patient Case Question 6.** Is a positive Romberg sign *good* or *bad?*

# Laboratory Blood Test Results

See Patient Case Table 44.2

| Patient Case Table 44.2 Laboratory Blood Test Results | | | | | |
|---|---|---|---|---|---|
| Na | 143 meq/L | Hb | 14.2 g/dL | AST | 12 IU/L |
| K | 4.0 meq/L | WBC | 6,900/mm$^3$ | ALT | 39 IU/L |
| Cl | 109 meq/L | Plt | 292,000/mm$^3$ | Alk phos | 67 IU/L |
| HCO$_3$ | 23 meq/L | BUN | 11 mg/dL | Total bilirubin | 0.6 mg/dL |
| Ca | 9.2 mg/dL | Cr | 0.8 mg/dL | Alb | 3.9 g/dL |
| Hct | 38% | Glu, fasting | 109 mg/dL | Total protein | 6.8 g/dL |

**Patient Case Question 7.** Identify all of the abnormal blood chemistry test results in Table 44.2 and provide a reasonable explanation for each abnormal test result.

## Spinal Tap

- CSF clear and colorless
- (+) mild lymphocytosis
- (+) elevated IgG concentration
- (+) elevated myelin basic protein level
- Glucose: 60 mg/dL
- Protein: 60 mg/dL

*Patient Case Question 8.* Are the patient's cerebrospinal fluid glucose and protein levels *normal, abnormally high,* or *abnormally low*?

*Patient Case Question 9.* Why is lymphocytosis in the CSF consistent with an attack of multiple sclerosis?

## MRI Scanning of Brain and Spinal Cord

Multiple plaques in the perivascular white matter, cerebellum, and spinal cord. Plaque sizes have uniformly increased in size since MRI 3 years ago. New plaques observed since last MRI.

*Patient Case Question 10.* Before a definitive diagnosis of multiple sclerosis is made, healthcare providers will often conduct various tests on patients. Briefly explain the rationale for each of the following tests.

a. serum vitamin B12 concentration

b. serum folate concentration

c. erythrocyte sedimentation rate

d. antinuclear antibody (ANA) test

e. serology for Lyme disease

e. VDRL test

*For the Disease Summary for this case study, see the CD-ROM.*

# PATIENT CASE

## Chief Complaint

Provided by caregiver: "His medicine for Parkinson's doesn't seem to be working as well anymore."

## HPI

E.A. is a 68 yo man who presents with his caregiver to the neurology clinic for his routine three-month evaluation. He feels that he still has some "good days," but there seem to be more "bad days" now. His medications do not seem to be as effective as they have been in the past. He complains that he often awakens in the morning with a painful cramp in his left foot. He also complains of "feeling more wooden" recently. His tremors have become less pronounced during the last three weeks. His appetite has decreased and he states that he is "just not interested in food." He eats three small meals daily: ½ bowl oatmeal, ½ banana, and orange juice in the morning; ½ sandwich, cup of soup, and serving of melon medley for lunch; and small portions of meat, potatoes, and vegetables and slice of whole grain bread for supper, which he rarely finishes. His caregiver states that he is not interested in wood-carving anymore and that he appears depressed much of the day "until the kids come home from school." He is always happy to see the children, even smiles when they visit with him. During the day, he will often sit in his chair staring at the television for hours, often not moving. Last week, he fell sideways out of his chair when reaching for a peanut that fell onto the floor, but he was not injured. He has to be reminded to blink his eyes once in a while, and the caregiver will often tap his brow lightly to initiate and maintain a blink response. The family will often play cribbage with him and are very patient as E. slowly lays down his cards and pegs his points. Non-disabling dyskinesia secondary to therapy occurs less than 25% of the day and becomes most prominent in the evening when he is tired.

## PMH

- DM type 2 × 23 years
- Three amputations of the RLE—at the ankle 15 years ago, at the knee 9 years ago, at the hip 7 years ago
- PD × 11 years

- GERD × 2 years
- Hyperlipidemia × 2 years

## FH

- Father died from HTN-related cerebral hemorrhage at age 64
- Mother died from renal failure secondary to DM at age 73
- One brother alive and well
- No children

## SH

- (−) for alcohol, tobacco, and illicit drug abuse; 2 cups caffeinated coffee each morning
- Retired farmer of 31 years
- Married for 42 years, wife passed away 3 years ago
- Relocated after his wife's death and now living with family of four in Wyoming; mother/wife of family is LPN and caregiver in the home
- E. has his own room in the house
- Enjoys playing board games and cribbage with his family
- Family has constructed a ramp in front of the house for wheelchair accessibility

## ROS

The patient has no complaints other than those noted in the HPI. He denies nausea, vomiting, sweating, heartburn, tearing, paresthesias, blurry vision, constipation, and dizziness. He also reports no problems at this time with chewing, swallowing, and urination. He is sleeping "OK" at night and often takes a short afternoon nap.

*Patient Case Question 1.* Which of the following clinical manifestations (that are also listed in the ROS directly above) are more likely caused by diabetes than by Parkinson disease?

a. excessive sweating and tearing

b. problems with chewing and swallowing

c. paresthesias and blurry vision

d. all of the above

e. none of the above

## Meds

- Omeprazole 20 mg po QD × 2 years
- Glyburide 6 mg po QD × 1 year
- Carbidopa/levodopa 25/100 1 tablet @8:30 AM, 12:30 PM, 4:30 PM, and 8:30 PM (started 2 years ago with multiple dose changes since that time)
- Pergolide 1 mg po TID × 6 years
- Simvastatin 20 mg po HS × 1 year
- Metformin 850 mg po BID × 8 months

*Patient Case Question 2.* For which condition is this patient receiving omeprazole?

*Patient Case Question 3.* For which condition is this patient receiving glyburide?

*Patient Case Question 4.* For which condition is this patient receiving simvastatin?

*Patient Case Question 5.* For which condition is this patient receiving metformin?

# All

PCN (hives and edema of the face and tongue)

# PE and Lab Tests

## Gen

The patient is an elderly, overweight white male in NAD who appears his stated age. He is well groomed, cleanly shaven, and his overall personal hygiene seems to be very good. He is sitting in a wheelchair and appears interested and cognizant of all that is going on around him. He speaks in a soft, monotone voice.

## Vital Signs

See Patient Case Table 45.1

| Patient Case Table 45.1 Vital Signs | | | | | |
|---|---|---|---|---|---|
| BP | 130/80 | RR | 14 | HT | 5'9" |
| P | 73 | T | 98.4°F | WT | 205 lb |

*Patient Case Question 6.* Is this patient technically considered *underweight, overweight, obese,* or is this patient's weight *normal and healthy*?

## Skin

- Normal turgor
- Erythema and dry, white scales on forehead and in nasal folds
- Mild dandruff of scalp, within and behind the ears
- No bruises noted

## HEENT

- Speaks only in short, simple phrases
- Mask-like facial expression
- Eye blinking, approximately 1/minute
- PERRLA
- EOMI
- R & L funduscopic exam without retinopathy
- TMs intact
- Nares clear
- Oropharynx without redness, exudate, or lesions
- Mucous membranes moist
- Wears dentures

## Neck/LN

- Flexion of the head and neck prominent
- No masses, bruits, or JVD
- Normal thyroid

## Lungs/Thorax

- CTA & P
- No crackles or wheezes
- Localized kyphosis with an exaggerated lordosis of the lumbar spine

## Heart

NSR without murmurs

## Abd

- Soft, NT, and ND
- Liver and spleen not palpable
- No palpable masses
- (+) BS

## Genit/Rec

- Prostate moderately enlarged but no nodules palpated
- No rectal polyps or hemorrhoids

## MS/Ext

- Resting tremor, bilateral, L > R
- Rigidity
- Poor postural stability
- Poor fine motor coordination
- Peripheral pulses moderately subnormal
- DTRs 2+
- Muscle strength 4/5 throughout
- Left foot with normal sensation and vibration

## Neuro

CNs intact
Unified Parkinson Disease Rating Scale (during an on-period for the patient)
See Patient Case Table 45.2

## Schwab and England Activities of Daily Living

20%—can do nothing alone, can help slightly with some chores, severe invalid

## Hoehn and Yahr Staging of Parkinson Disease

Stage 4—severe symptoms, rigidity, and bradykinesia, no longer able to live alone (cachexia not yet present)

## Patient Case Table 45.2 Unified Parkinson Disease Rating Scale

(Adapted with permission from Fahn S, Elton R, and members of the UPDRS Development Committee. In: Recent Developments in Parkinson's Disease, Volume 2 (Fahn S, Marsden CD, Caine DB, and Goldstein M, eds). Floram Park, NJ: Macmillan Health Care Information, 1987:153–163, 293–304.)

| | |
|---|---|
| **I. Mentation, Behavior, and Mood: 11/16 (0 no disability—16 total disability)** | |
| **3/4** | Severe memory loss with disorientation to time and often place, severe impairment managing complex problems |
| **3/4** | Frequent hallucinations or delusions without insight, interference with daily activities (Claims that he saw "skiers on the roof of the house next door" recently) |
| **2/4** | Duration of depressive episodes, often greater than 1 week |
| **3/4** | Loss of initiative or disinterest in day-to-day activities |
| **II. Activities of Daily Living: 25/43 (0 no disability—43 total disability)** | |
| **3/4** | Speech affected, asked to repeat |
| **1/3** | Slight but noticeable increase in salivation, has minimal drooling |
| **1/4** | Swallowing, rare choking |
| **2/4** | Handwriting small but legible |
| **3/4** | Food must be cut, but can feed self |
| **3/4** | Considerable help required with dressing but can do some things alone |
| **3/4** | Requires assistance for washing, brushing teeth, going to bathroom |
| **3/4** | Can initiate turning in bed/adjusting bed covers but cannot initiate/adjust alone |
| **1/4** | Rare falls unrelated to freezing |
| | Freezing when walking: cannot evaluate |
| | Walking: cannot evaluate |
| **2/4** | Moderate tremor, bothersome to patient |
| **3/4** | Frequent painful sensation (LLE) |
| **III. Motor Exam: 52/92 (0 no disability—92 total disability)** | |
| **2/4** | Speech monotone, slurred but understandable, moderately impaired |
| **4/4** | Masked or fixed face, lips parted ¼ inch or more with complete loss of expression |
| **0/4** | Tremor at rest, face, absent |
| **2/4** | Tremor at rest, RUE, mild and present most of time |
| **3/4** | Tremor at rest, LUE, moderate and present most of time |
| | Tremor at rest, RLE, cannot evaluate |
| **0/4** | Tremor at rest, LLE, absent |
| **0/4** | Tremor with action, RUE, absent |
| **0/4** | Tremor with action, LUE, absent |
| **2/4** | Rigidity, neck, mild/moderate |
| **4/4** | Rigidity, RUE, severe |
| **3/4** | Rigidity, LUE, marked, full ROM |
| | Rigidity, RLE, cannot evaluate |
| **3/4** | Rigidity, LLE, marked, full ROM |
| **3/4** | Finger taps, right, severely impaired, frequent hesitations and arrests |
| **2/4** | Finger taps, left, moderately impaired, definite and early fatiguing, may have occasional arrests |
| **4/4** | Open-close hand rapidly, right, can barely perform |
| **2/4** | Open-close hand rapidly, left, moderately impaired, definite and early fatiguing, may have occasional arrests |
| **3/4** | Pronate-supinate hand, right, severely impaired, frequent hesitations and arrests |
| **2/4** | Pronate-supinate hand, left, moderately impaired, definite and early fatiguing, may have occasional arrests |
| | Leg agility, heel tap, right, cannot evaluate |
| **3/4** | Leg agility, heel tap, left, severely impaired, frequent hesitations and arrests |
| **2/4** | Arising from chair, pushes self up from arms |
| **2/4** | Posture, definitely abnormal, moderately stooped, may lean to one side |
| | Gait, cannot evaluate |
| **2/4** | Postural stability, would fall if not caught |
| **4/4** | Body bradykinesia, marked slowness/poverty/amplitude |

*Patient Case Question 7.* Does the disease in this patient seem to be more advanced on the left or right side of the body?

## Laboratory Blood Test Results

See Patient Case Table 45.3

### Patient Case Table 45.3 Laboratory Blood Test Results

| | | | | | |
|---|---|---|---|---|---|
| Na | 139 meq/L | Glu (random) | 289 mg/dL | Bilirubin | 1.0 mg/dL |
| K | 5.1 meq/L | Ca | 9.8 mg/dL | Cholesterol | 238 mg/dL |
| Cl | 102 meq/L | Phos | 3.3 mg/dL | LDL | 168 mg/dL |
| $HCO_3$ | 22 meq/L | AST | 19 IU/L | HDL | 42 mg/dL |
| BUN | 19 mg/dL | ALT | 13 IU/L | Triglycerides | 170 mg/dL |
| Cr | 1.2 mg/dL | Alk Phos | 43 IU/L | $HbA_{1c}$ | 8.2% |

## Urinalysis

- (−) protein
- (−) microalbuminuria

*Patient Case Question 8.* Renal failure is a major complication of diabetes mellitus and a common cause of death among people with diabetes. Does this patient have any signs of renal dysfunction secondary to diabetes at this time and, if so, what are these signs?

*Patient Case Question 9.* Evaluate control of this patient's hyperlipidemia.

*Patient Case Question 10.* Which laboratory tests indicate that this patient's diabetes could be better controlled?

*Patient Case Question 11.* Identify this patient's single major risk factor for Parkinson disease.

*Patient Case Question 12.* Identify this patient's cardinal signs of Parkinson disease.

*Patient Case Question 13.* Does this patient satisfy the minimum criteria for a definitive diagnosis of Parkinson disease?

# PSYCHIATRIC DISORDERS

# CASE STUDY

# 46

## ATTENTION DEFICIT/HYPERACTIVITY DISORDER

 *For the Disease Summary for this case study, see the CD-ROM.*

## PATIENT CASE

### ▅▅ Mother's Chief Complaints

"I'm at the end of my rope and I don't know what to do anymore. My son won't behave or listen at school and he most certainly will not listen to me at home. He always seems to be in motion and can't sit still for even 5 minutes. He likes watching cartoons on TV but gets bored with them in a matter of minutes. His first grade teacher tells me that he can't sit still at school, that he is constantly squirming in his seat, and that sometimes he will get up during the middle of a class and roam around the room looking at different things. She has also told me that he is problematic when he has to wait for things that he wants—like in the lunch line—and he is always grabbing things away from other children. She is always reminding him not to interrupt when others are speaking and to wait until she finishes asking a question before he begins his answer. I have to do that, too, at home."

### ▅▅ HPI

S.P. is a 6-year-old boy who presents to the pediatric clinic with his mother, Ms. A.T. She states that her son has shown hyperactive and inattentive behaviors now for almost one year, but "everything seems to be getting worse." Teachers complain that he does not listen to them, does not follow instructions like the other children, is easily bored during activities, and has difficulty both waiting his turn and engaging in playground games for any significant length of time. The boy's behavior has been so disruptive that no daycare centers will accept him. This is a major concern, because Ms. A.T. is a single parent and must work to support her child and herself.

### ▅▅ PMH

- Mother had taken her son to a pediatrician about 4 months ago and complained of similar problems, but the pediatrician had dismissed her complaints by telling her that she "needed to set more boundaries for her child both at home and at school"
- Pregnancy and delivery with S.P. were normal
- Vaccinations are current
- No prior surgeries, serious medical problems, or established psychiatric illnesses

# ■■■ FH

- Mother does not know of father's whereabouts as he disappeared soon after learning that she was pregnant at age 17
- Both maternal grandfather and maternal uncle have history of hyperactivity as children
- Mother denies drug, tobacco, and alcohol abuse during pregnancy

# ■■■ SH

- Lives with mother in ghetto section of inner city
- Mother is a single parent with no other children

# ■■■ ROS

Occasional GI upset and colds, otherwise non-contributory

# ■■■ Meds

None

# ■■■ All

NKDA

# ■■■ Limited PE and Lab Tests

## Gen

The patient is a healthy-appearing, well-nourished boy. He is moving constantly, fidgeting with both his hands and feet, is easily distracted by minor noises, and interrupts the pediatrician and his mother repeatedly.

## VS

See Patient Case Table 46.1

| Patient Case Table 46.1 Vital Signs | | | | | |
|---|---|---|---|---|---|
| BP | 112/70 | RR | 15 | HT | 3'9" |
| P | 65 | T | 98.2°F | WT | 50 lbs |

## Hearing

WNL

## Vision

WNL

***Patient Case Question 1.*** Are any of the boy's vital signs a major cause for concern?

***Patient Case Question 2.*** What is the patient's single most critical risk factor that is consistent with ADHD?

## Skin

- Skin warm and dry with no discoloration
- Normal hair and nails

## HEENT

- PERRLA
- TMs intact
- Nose clear
- Throat without erythema
- Mucous membranes normal

## Neck/LN

Neck supple without obvious nodal enlargement or thyromegaly

## Heart

RRR with no m/r/g

## Lungs

Clear, normal breath sounds

## Genit

Normal external male genitalia with circumcised penis

## Abd

Soft and non-tender with normal bowel sounds and no palpable viscera or masses

## MS/Ext

- (–) CCE
- ROM intact
- Good peripheral pulses bilaterally

## Neuro

- A & O
- CNs II–XII intact
- DTRs 3+ throughout
- Sensory and motor function intact and gait normal

## Laboratory Blood Test Results

See Patient Case Table 46.2

| Patient Case Table 46.2 Laboratory Blood Test Results | | | | | |
|---|---|---|---|---|---|
| Hb | 15.1 g/dL | Plt | 290,000/mm³ | TSH | 3.8 µU/mL |
| Hct | 43% | BUN | 11 mg/dL | $T_4$, total | 6.8 µg/dL |
| WBC | 7,250/mm³ | Cr | 0.7 mg/dL | Glu, fasting | 75 mg/dL |

***Patient Case Question 3.*** An overactive thyroid gland can mimic many of the clinical manifestations of ADHD. Can hyperthyroid disease be ruled out as a cause of hyperactivity in this child? Why or why not?

***Patient Case Question 4.*** Is this patient's CBC *normal* or *abnormal*?

***Patient Case Question 5.*** What is the significance of this patient's BUN and Cr concentrations?

***Patient Case Question 6.*** Does this patient satisfy all of the criteria that are required for a diagnosis of ADHD?

***Patient Case Question 7.*** Is this patient *predominantly hyperactive, predominantly inattentive,* does he show signs of *combined inattention and hyperactivity,* or are the minimal diagnostic criteria for ADHD lacking?

***Patient Case Question 8.*** Which of the following is the most appropriate therapy for this patient?

a. Ritalin hydrochloride, 5 mg before breakfast and lunch

b. Ritalin hydrochloride, 20 mg before each meal

c. Cylert, 37.5 mg as a single dose every morning

d. Adderall, 5 mg once daily + psychotherapy

e. Tofranil, 25 mg twice daily + psychotherapy

# CASE STUDY

## 47

## BIPOLAR DISORDER

 *For the Disease Summary for this case study, see the CD-ROM.*

## PATIENT CASE

### ■■■ Chief Complaints

Provided by an older sister: "Our mother died three weeks ago and we lost our father several months ago. I think that my sister was depressed and just wanted to be with them."

### ■■■ HPI

B.J. is a 31-year-old female who was brought to the hospital by ambulance. She was found slumped over in her car in front of the funeral home where memorial services for both her father and mother had been recently held. There were two empty bottles of sleeping pills on the seat beside her, a Bible opened to the 23rd Psalm, and a note that read: *I am going to be with mom and dad. It is just too sad being here anymore without them. I love you all and you will be in my prayers. Your sister, B.* When she was found by the director of the funeral home, her hair was oily and unkempt and she smelled as if she had not bathed in a long time. She was simply dressed in a dirty, orange tee shirt, jeans, and tennis shoes.

### ■■■ PMH

Episodes of depression first occurred when the patient was a junior in high school and led to psychiatric admissions at 15 and 19 years of age. She met her first husband in the psychiatric ward of the hospital at age 19 following a suicide attempt. The patient was treated with antidepressants and psychotherapy and discharged on both occasions after approximately 5 weeks.

### ■■■ Interview with Patient's Older Sister

"The kids in our family have had a hard life. Our parents were both alcoholics and I remember that, when we were little, they would go to a bar almost every night and leave us in the car for several hours. There were 8 of us. Later on, it got so bad that the state took all of us away and placed us in foster homes or Catholic girls' homes. Some of the foster homes were absolutely horrible! We were beaten on many occasions and some of the girls were sexually abused.

My sister has been in several detoxification centers for alcohol abuse, as have many of us kids. She's on her second marriage now and I hope that it works out for her and the girls. She has three daughters now and they really need their mother.

She was diagnosed with bipolar disorder about 6 years ago. I remember that her divorce was finalized, she had just gotten married for the second time, was beginning a new job that she really liked and seemed to be getting it all together for the first time. But, after she had her third baby, she went into a terrible depression. She saw a 'head doctor' for about 3 months and he finally decided to put her on an antidepressant—Paxil, I think. Well, after about 3 weeks, she really got weird. She told me that movie stars were talking to her whenever she went to the movies. Her speech became impossible to understand and it seemed like her mind and mouth were moving at the speed of light. She would stay up all night and just pace about the house. At first, the doctors thought that she had a thyroid condition, but it turned out to be BD. Sometimes she would call me at three in the morning to talk. When I told her that I couldn't talk anymore, because I had to go to work in the morning, she became sarcastic, hostile, and would hang up on me. Then, she would call back, apologize, and start talking . . . . no, it was more like rambling again. She would go on and on in sentences that seemed would never end. She preached to me about everything from politics to religion to our bad parents . . . . to sex!

All of us tried to convince her that she needed help, but she believed that she was absolutely fine. 'You all are just jealous, because I'm finally happy and feeling good about myself,' she would tell me in this annoying, loud, sing-songy voice. She would also go on shopping sprees for 2–3 days at a time and max out all of her credit cards. We tried to tell her that this was dangerous behavior, but she would not have any of it. When she finally crashed, we took her to the hospital and that's when they diagnosed her with bipolar. She's been on lithium ever since and it has helped until now. Our father had been sick for a while, but our mother's death took us all by surprise. She went downhill so fast. B. just could not cope with it. I know that she hadn't been eating at all, because she was losing weight. She was also smoking and drinking more than usual."

## FH

* Strong history of mental illness—paternal grandmother suffered from depression; two maternal aunts diagnosed with bipolar disorder
* Both parents have died—her father from pancreatic cancer that had metastasized to bone and her mother from heart failure
* Both parents had a long history of alcohol abuse
* Father was previously diagnosed with pancreatitis and then diabetes mellitus for which he had been taking insulin
* Mother had been relatively well (except for a "smoker's cough") with few serious medical problems until her husband's death; some said that she "died from a broken heart"
* Patient has 3 living brothers, 3 living sisters, and 3 daughters
* One brother died from AMI at age 34; another brother died at age 6 months from "water on the brain"

## SH

* Divorced and remarried
* Has worked primarily as a nurse's aide and, more recently, as a health insurance claims adjuster
* Is religious and goes to church regularly
* Has smoked 1 ppd for nearly 15 years
* Has history of alcohol abuse with several Driving While Intoxicated violations
* History of IVDA but has not used for more than 10 years

## Meds

* Lithium 600 mg po Q AM and 600 mg po Q HS
* Sumatriptan 50–200 mg po PRN

## ■ All

ASA → swelling of face

## ■ ROS

Migraine headaches, 2–3/month, (–) for aura but (+) for nausea, vomiting, and photophobia

## ■ PE and Lab Tests

Performed three hours after regaining consciousness

### Gen

The patient is a tired-looking, white female in NAD. She is very pale and there are "dark rings" under her eyes.

### VS

See Patient Case Table 47.1

| Patient Case Table 47.1 Vital Signs | | | | | |
|---|---|---|---|---|---|
| BP | 110/72 (supine) | RR | 16 and unlabored | HT/WT | 5′6″/135 lbs |
| P | 81 and regular | T | 98.6°F | SaO$_2$ | 97% on room air |

*Patient Case Question 1.* Are any of the patient's vital signs significantly abnormal?

*Patient Case Question 2.* Why has the patient been taking sumatriptan as needed?

*Patient Case Question 3.* Identify this patient's *two* most significant risk factors for bipolar disorder.

*Patient Case Question 4.* Identify *two* additional potential contributing factors to bipolar disorder in this patient.

### Skin

• Comedones on forehead, nose, and chin with several cystic lesions on chin (consistent with acne)
• Normal turgor
• Soft, intact, warm, dry, and very pale
• No evidence of rash, ecchymoses, petechiae, or cyanosis

### Head

Normocephalic and atraumatic

### Eyes

• PERRLA
• EOMI
• Funduscopy revealed normal, clear disc margins without lesions
• (–) nystagmus

## Ears

TMs intact

## Nose

(–) discharge or congestion

## Throat

- (–) exudates or erythema
- Dry mucous membranes

## Neck

- Supple
- No enlarged nodes, thyromegaly, bruits, or jugular venous distension

## Heart

- RRR
- $S_1$ and $S_2$ normal without additional cardiac sounds
- (–) murmurs, rubs, or gallops

## Lungs

CTA & P bilaterally

## Abd

- (+) BS
- (–) pain or tenderness
- Soft and non-distended
- (–) hepatomegaly, splenomegaly, masses, or bruits

## Breasts

Exam deferred

## Genit/Rect

Exam deferred

## MS/Ext

- Full ROM
- Distal pulses normal at 2+ bilaterally
- (–) edema, cyanosis, or clubbing
- No joint swelling or tenderness

## Neuro

- Slightly lethargic but oriented to person, place, and time
- Deep tendon reflexes full and symmetric
- Babinski negative bilaterally

- Normal strength throughout
- Tone normal
- Sensation intact
- CNs II–XII intact
- Speech: no dysarthria, rate normal
- Gross and fine motor coordination are normal
- Cerebellar: finger-to-nose and heel-to-shin WNL
- Good sitting and standing balance
- Able to toe and tandem walk without difficulty
- Gait normal in speed and step length
- Able to perform serial 7s and can abstract
- Short- and long-term memories intact

## Laboratory Blood Test Results

See Patient Case Table 47.2

### Patient Case Table 47.2 Laboratory Blood Test Results

| | | | | | |
|---|---|---|---|---|---|
| Na | 139 meq/L | MCV | 90.2 fL | Bilirubin, total | 0.7 mg/dL |
| K | 3.7 meq/L | MCH | 31 pg | Alb | 2.9 g/dL |
| Cl | 108 meq/L | MCHC | 34.4 g/dL | Protein, total | 4.8 g/dL |
| HCO$_3$ | 23 meq/L | Plt | 150,000/mm$^3$ | Ca | 8.7 mg/dL |
| BUN | 10 mg/dL | WBC | 9,400/mm$^3$ | Mg | 2.0 mg/dL |
| Cr | 0.7 mg/dL | Diff | | Lithium | 0.08 meq/L |
| | | • Neutros | 65% | Steady-state serum lithium | |
| | | • Lymphs | 25% | concentrations should | |
| | | • Monos | 7% | always be maintained at a | |
| | | • Eos | 2% | concentration of | |
| | | • Basos | 1% | 0.6–1.2 meq/L. | |
| Glu, fasting | 102 mg/dL | AST | 33 IU/L | Phos | 3.2 mg/dL |
| Hb | 12.2 g/dL | ALT | 20 IU/L | TSH | 4.1 µU/mL |
| Hct | 36.8% | Alk Phos | 59 IU/L | Cortisol @ 8AM | 9.3 µg/dL |
| RBC | 4.73 × 10$^6$/mm$^3$ | GGT | 82 IU/L | Vitamin B12 | 203 pg/mL |

## Urinalysis

See Patient Case Table 47.3

### Patient Case Table 47.3 Urinalysis

| | | | |
|---|---|---|---|
| Color | *Yellow* | SG | *1.021* |
| Appearance | *Cloudy* | Blood | *Negative* |
| Glucose | *Negative* | pH | *6.3* |
| Bilirubin | *Negative* | Protein | *Negative* |
| Ketones | *Negative* | Nitrites | *Negative* |

**Patient Case Question 5.** Does this patient have any signs of abnormal renal function?

**Patient Case Question 6.** Does this patient have any signs of abnormal hepatic function?

***Patient Case Question 7.*** Identify this patient's *three* most significant abnormal blood laboratory test results and propose a reasonable explanation for these results.

***Patient Case Question 8.*** What is suggested by the patient's serum TSH, cortisol, and vitamin B12 concentrations?

***Patient Case Question 9.*** List a minimum of *eight* clinical manifestations observed in this patient that were helpful toward an initial diagnosis of bipolar disorder.

***Patient Case Question 10.*** Identify all signs of brain damage that may have occurred from the patient's most recent suicide attempt.

***Patient Case Question 11.*** Does the patient in this case study require *inpatient* treatment or is *outpatient* therapy totally appropriate?

***Patient Case Question 12.*** Do you think that the prognosis for this patient is *favorable* or *less than favorable*? Explain your answer.

# 48

# GENERALIZED ANXIETY DISORDER

 *For the Disease Summary for this case study, see the CD-ROM.*

## PATIENT CASE

### ▬ HPI

L.K. is a 23 yo woman who was evaluated by the student health service physician for complaints of "worrying all the time about everybody and everything" and "waking up at 3 AM every morning and not being able to go back to sleep." In addition to being a full-time student, she works 20 hours every week as a waitress to pay for her education and living expenses. She states that she has had difficulty concentrating on her studies and her "grades have not been good lately." She constantly worries about school, grades, meeting her financial responsibilities, and her parents—who are both healthy and happily married. Her worries have been present for as long as she can remember, but they seem to have increased in both frequency and intensity during the past four months. She is preoccupied by her worries most days of the week and now she is worried that she may have developed a mental illness. The physician decides to refer her to one of the clinic psychiatrists.

### ▬ PMH

L.K. has been treated previously with medications for anxiety (paroxetine and sertraline), but she complained of sexual problems and stopped taking them after only two months of usage.

Three years ago, she checked herself into the detoxification unit of a local hospital for alcohol abuse. She attends AA meetings regularly and has not had any alcohol since detoxification.

Her medical records show that she has been a constantly anxious patient who has worried incessantly since early adolescence.

### ▬ FH

Mother had an extended episode of depression when her parents were both killed in a small plane accident 8 years ago. Father has some traits of OCD and a history of alcohol abuse. She has two brothers with no major psychological or medical problems.

### ▬ SH

- Student in third year of nursing school
- Smokes 3–6 cigarettes/day

- Drinks up to a half-dozen cups of coffee/day
- No alcohol use
- Denies use of illicit drugs
- Denies use of OTC medications or herbal formulations

## Psychiatric Evaluation Notes: ■ Patient Comments

- "Hard to remember a time when I wasn't worrying about something."
- "I always seem to be anticipating disaster."
- "Sometimes, simply the thought of getting through the day makes me nervous."
- "I wish that I could shake all of my concerns, but I just can't seem to manage. I always have these nagging feelings of worry or anxiety."
- "I have a difficult time relaxing, I don't get any satisfying sleep anymore, and I'm tired all day long. I've also been very grouchy lately . . . or so my boyfriend tells me."
- "I have been missing some work days lately and I'm afraid that I might get fired."
- "I don't think my health is very good anymore."
- "Yes, I usually am aware that my anxiety is more intense than the situation warrants. Sometimes I'm worried and I can't identify the source."
- "Last week, I was giving a presentation in my public speaking course and my mind suddenly went blank. That has never happened to me before."
- "Yes, I do feel insecure sometimes and I often interpret people's intentions as negative."
- "What do I worry about? Work, school, tests, grades, money, health, safety, even my car breaking down. If you can name it, I will worry about it."
- "Sometimes, in social situations, I start to sweat and get a lump in my throat."
- "Yes, I've tried heroin and cocaine, but I've not used them since high school."
- "I get a little bit down on myself once in a while but, no, I have never given a thought to ending my life. I can get through this."

## ■ ROS

- (+) for "jumpiness," an occasional "smothering sensation" when she turns out the lights in her apartment at night, and a strange tingling sensation in her hands
- Denies any trembling, twitching, suicidal thoughts or attempts, muscle tension, headaches, hot flashes, problems with sexual function including menstruation, chest pain, rapid breathing, lightheadedness, shortness of breath, nausea, diarrhea, palpitations, pruritus, urinary frequency, and epigastric pain

## ■ Meds

Ortho-Novum 7/7/7 1 tablet po QD

## ■ All

NKDA

## ■ PE and Lab Tests

### Gen

Alert, pleasant, attractive, and well-dressed, cooperative female patient in no apparent distress

## VS

See Patient Case Table 48.1

| Patient Case Table 48.1 Vital Signs | | | | | |
|---|---|---|---|---|---|
| BP | 145/92 | RR | 18 | Ht | 65 in |
| P | 80 | T | 98.4°F | Wt | 122 lbs |

***Patient Case Question 1.*** Are any of the patient's vital signs abnormal?

## Skin

Warm and dry with no discoloration or lesions

## HEENT

- PERRLA
- Fundi benign
- Ears, nose, and throat clear
- TMs intact

## Neck/LN

Supple and without enlarged nodes, thyromegaly, JVD, or carotid bruits

## Lungs

Clear to A & P

## Breasts

Normal without lumps, discoloration, or dimpling

## Heart

NSR with no m/r/g or extra cardiac sounds

## Abd

Soft and nontender with (+) BS

## Neuro

- A & O × 3
- DTRs 3+ throughout
- (–) for Romberg sign
- CNs II–XII intact
- Normal gait
- Light touch and vibration intact

## Laboratory Blood Test Results

See Patient Case Table 48.2

| Patient Case Table 48.2 Laboratory Blood Test Results | | | | | | | | |
|------|-----------|--------|-----------|-------------|-----------|------|-----------|
| Na | 138 meq/L | HCO₃ | 28 meq/L | Glu, fasting | 100 mg/dL | TSH | 1.9 µU/mL |
| K | 4.2 meq/L | BUN | 17 mg/dL | Hb | 13.9 g/dL | T₄ | 5.4 µg/dL |
| Cl | 105 meq/L | Cr | 0.9 mg/dL | Hct | 38% | Cortisol, 8am | 10 µg/dL |

**Patient Case Question 2.** Why was it appropriate to test for thyroid function and what were the results of those tests?

**Patient Case Question 3.** Why was it appropriate to obtain a morning serum cortisol concentration and what was the result of that test?

## UA

- Toxicology screen (–)
- Urinary catecholamines normal

## EEG

Normal

**Patient Case Question 4.** Why was it appropriate to test for urinary catecholamines?

## ■ Assessment

Generalized anxiety disorder

**Patient Case Question 5.** Does this patient have at least three of the six required clinical manifestations that must accompany worry and anxiety before a diagnosis of GAD can be rendered?

**Patient Case Question 6.** What specific lifestyle changes might be made to reduce this patient's nervous feelings?

**Patient Case Question 7.** Why is an EEG an appropriate test for this patient?

## ■ Clinical Course

The patient was referred to a cognitive and behavioral psychologist for treatment of GAD. Her psychiatrist also decided to start her on a trial of venlafaxine. After five weeks of behavioral and psychotherapy and excellent compliance with her new medication, L.K. noticed that her anxiety had diminished significantly and she was better able to cope with anxious thoughts. She is also sleeping better at night, feels more rested in the morning, and able to concentrate on her studies, and wants to continue seeing her therapist. She has suffered no significant adverse effects from her medication.

**Patient Case Question 8.** Would you characterize this patient's generalized anxiety disorder as being *acute* or *chronic*?

# CASE STUDY

# 49

# MAJOR DEPRESSIVE DISORDER

 *For the Disease Summary for this case study, see the CD-ROM.*

# PATIENT CASE

## ■ Patient's Chief Complaints

"I don't know how much longer I can go on like this. I've been down in the dumps for years and it isn't getting any better. I've lost everyone who has ever meant anything to me. I've disappointed my son to the point that he'll never forgive me. I've asked God to help me through this, but it seems that He isn't listening. Now my wife is telling me that I have Alzheimer's. Nothing is fun and I don't believe that life is worth living anymore."

## ■ History of Present Illness

Mr. H.B. is a 75 yo white male who presents to the clinic with the above complaints. He lost his first wife to a stroke 19 years ago after 27 years of a "wonderful marriage." The patient emphatically states that she was the "love of his life" and can never be replaced. "I realize now more than ever what a good woman she was." He remarried 2 years after her death. His second and current wife was a former co-worker. "I was lonely and I probably married again too soon," he admits.

He explains that his current wife has been a very difficult person with which to live. It all began about a year after their marriage when she insisted that he put up a privacy fence between their house and the neighbor's house. The patient had been a close friend to his neighbors for more than 25 years and knew that putting up a fence would cause discord. Soon thereafter, his current wife insisted that the patient no longer visit his elderly father-in-law or sister-in-law from his first marriage even though they had been friends for nearly 50 years. "When you married me, you divorced that whole family," she had said. Then, on one occasion and while the patient was at work, she would not allow his son, his son's wife, and their newborn baby into the house to visit. The patient began to feel that he was distancing himself from family and friends that he had known and loved for many years. He tried to resolve issues between his son and wife, but his wife was closed to any suggestions.

The patient began to feel guilty, very much alone, and extremely sad. He began attending church more than usual—on weeknights in addition to Sunday mornings—just to get out of the house. This went on for years. At one time, he visited with the pastor of his church and related his unhappiness. Although his pastor was a Catholic priest, he suggested that H. consider a divorce for the benefit of his health. When he confronted his wife with the topic of divorce, however, she burst into tears and told him that she would change and be a better wife to him. She changed—for about 6 months—and then reverted to her former means of manipulation.

Recently, the patient's wife insisted that they sell the house in which the patient had lived for 46 years and move into an apartment. He totally rejected the idea. "We agreed when we got married that we would live there. If she wants me out of that house, she'll have to carry me out herself," he stated with defiance. When the patient considered divorce as an option for a second time, he dismissed it quickly, because he was a devout Catholic and believed that he would be condemned for that decision. He also decided that "he had made his bed and now must sleep in it" and continued in his sadness and despair.

The patient notes that his memory and ability to make simple decisions have been deteriorating significantly during the last several months. His wife has told him that he has become so forgetful that he probably has Alzheimer disease and should see a doctor. "I've been eating all right and I try to get some exercise every day, but I wake up often now during the night and am usually up for good by 5 o'clock every morning—then I feel tired by 9 AM and throughout the day. I am becoming increasingly depressed. I am ready now to give up the fight and be with K. (his first wife). I know that she is waiting for me."

## ■■■ Past Medical History

The patient has been relatively healthy throughout his 75 years. He has had all of the usual childhood illnesses, but has no current non-psychiatric adult illnesses and takes no medications. At age 54, he was diagnosed by neurologists with a rare eye disorder characterized by poor peripheral vision. The doctors had attributed this condition to trauma that he suffered during the 1941 attack at Pearl Harbor where he had been stationed as an army cook. He sustained temporary deafness for six months due to the noise of the bombings. He has had no other incidents of trauma during his lifetime.

He has never been treated for any psychiatric illnesses, although he reports a 15-year history of many periods of intense sadness, loneliness, and guilt that have lasted weeks to months. He has not had any surgeries performed and there has been no significant travel history. The patient has no dietary restrictions and, although he has no strict exercise program, he walks every day to maintain a healthy weight. His last tetanus booster was six years ago.

## ■■■ Family History

- Father, died from colon cancer at age 67
- Mother, died from influenza epidemic at age 24 (when patient was 2 years old)
- No known family history of depression or other mental illness
- No biological siblings; one half-brother

## ■■■ Social History

- High school graduate
- Married to high school sweetheart for 27 years, then widowed
- Currently married to second wife for 17 years
- Retired; 25-year career as a baker; when the company moved to another part of the state, patient took a job in maintenance where he met his second wife
- Attends Catholic mass regularly and has always been very religious
- Drinks 1–2 beers several times a week, but denies drinking to intoxication
- Has never smoked or used illegal substances
- Rarely drinks coffee anymore as it causes GI distress; often drinks hot tea
- He has never driven a motor vehicle due to poor peripheral vision

## ■■■ Review of Systems

- Feels tired much of the time
- No complaints of headache, body aches, dizziness, fainting spells, tinnitus, ear pain, ear discharge, nasal congestion, diarrhea, constipation, change in appetite, skin abnormalities, or genitourinary symptoms

- Often feels stiff and tense in neck and shoulders
- Denies periods of extreme elation or irritability that alternate with periods of sadness
- Denies being depressed more during winter than other seasons

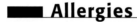 ## Medications

None

## Allergies

None

## Physical Examination and Laboratory Tests

### General

The patient appears tired but in no apparent distress. His face and arms are well tanned. His weight seems to be healthy. He has male pattern baldness and wears bifocals. His hair is cut short and he is clean-shaven and appropriately dressed. Speech is appropriately paced and content is normal.

### Vital Signs

See Patient Case Table 49.1

| Patient Case Table 49.1 Vital Signs | | | | | |
|---|---|---|---|---|---|
| BP | 118/73 | RR | 16 | HT | 5ft-11 in |
| P | 83 | T | 98.8°F | WT | 174 lbs |

### Skin

Skin, hair, and nails unremarkable

### HEENT

- PERRLA
- EOMI without nystagmus
- Fundus exam: discs sharp with no retinopathy
- Negative for nasal discharge or polyps
- TMs gray and shiny bilaterally
- Minor accumulation of cerumen bilaterally
- Significant dental repair for caries

### Neck/Lymph Nodes

Neck supple without adenopathy or thyromegaly

### Chest/Lungs

- Negative for tachypnea or SOB
- Chest CTA and resonant throughout

## Heart

RRR without murmur

## Abdomen

* Soft, NT, and ND
* Positive bowel sounds
* No organomegaly
* No bruits

## Genitalia/Rectum

Deferred

## Musculoskeletal/Extremities

Unremarkable

## Neurologic

* CNs II–XII intact
* Finger-to-nose testing normal
* Motor: normal grip strength, bilaterally symmetric
* DTRs 2+ and equal
* Sensory: intact bilaterally

## Mental Status

* No homicidal thoughts, hallucinations, paranoia, or delusions
* Suicidal thoughts are a major concern. The patient has a 22-caliber rifle in the home and has considered using it to end his life.

## Laboratory Blood Test Results

See Patient Case Table 49.2

| Patient Case Table 49.2 Laboratory Blood Test Results | | | | | |
|---|---|---|---|---|---|
| Na | 138 meq/L | PSA | 4.9 ng/mL | GGT | 38 IU/L |
| K | 4.2 meq/L | Hb | 14.3 g/dL | T bilirubin | 0.8 mg/dL |
| Cl | 102 meq/L | Hct | 41.4% | T protein | 7.0 g/dL |
| $HCO_3$ | 27 meq/L | MCV | 92 fL | Alb | 4.4 g/dL |
| BUN | 11 mg/dL | MCH | 29 pg | $T_4$ | 8.6 µg/dL |
| Cr | 0.9 mg/dL | Plt | $250 \times 10^3/mm^3$ | TSH | 2.8 µU/mL |
| Glu, fasting | 106 mg/dL | WBC | $7.3 \times 10^3/mm^3$ | Cortisol 8AM | 7.8 µg/dL |
| Ca | 9.5 mg/dL | AST | 34 IU/L | Vitamin B12 | 98 pg/mL |
| Mg | 1.8 mg/dL | ALT | 42 IU/L | Folic acid | 333 ng/mL |

## Urinalysis

See Patient Case Table 49.3

### Patient Case Table 49.3 Urinalysis

| Color | Pale yellow | Glucose | Negative | Bacteria | Negative |
|---|---|---|---|---|---|
| Appearance | Clear | Ketones | Negative | Epithelial cells | Negative |
| pH | 5.8 | Bilirubin | Negative | WBC | 1/HPF |
| SG | 1.016 | Protein | Negative | RBC | 0/HPF |

*Patient Case Question 1.* Identify *three* major risk factors that have possibly contributed to depression in this patient.

*Patient Case Question 2.* Does this patient satisfy all of the diagnostic criteria for major depressive disorder?

*Patient Case Question 3.* Should hospitalization be considered for this patient or should outpatient treatment be adequate?

*Patient Case Question 4.* Identify a minimum of *twelve* clinical manifestations that are consistent with major depression in this patient.

*Patient Case Question 5.* Is bipolar depression a reasonable alternative diagnosis in this patient?

*Patient Case Question 6.* Does thyroid disease appear to be a potential contributing cause of depression in this patient?

*Patient Case Question 7.* Does an iron deficiency state appear to be a potential contributing cause of depression in this patient?

*Patient Case Question 8.* Does a vitamin B12 or folate deficiency state appear to be a potential contributing cause of depression in this patient?

*Patient Case Question 9.* Does Cushing syndrome or Addison disease appear to be a potential contributing cause of depression in this patient?

*Patient Case Question 10.* Does the patient have any abnormal urinalysis findings?

*Patient Case Question 11.* Which of the following four therapies is the most appropriate initial treatment for this patient?

a. psychotherapy + fluoxetine, 20 mg by mouth daily

b. psychotherapy + amitriptyline, 500 mg by mouth daily

c. psychotherapy + phenelzine, 3 mg by mouth 3 times daily

d. phototherapy, 60 minutes in the morning + psychotherapy

*Patient Case Question 12.* Provide a reasonable justification for determination of serum γ-glutamyltranspeptidase (GGT) in this patient.

# CASE STUDY

## 50

# SCHIZOPHRENIA

 *For the Disease Summary for this case study, see the CD-ROM.*

## PATIENT CASE

### ■ Patient's Chief Complaints

"You are all morons! I want to go home. There's nothing wrong with me and I shouldn't be here. Don't you see that there are alien doctors at this hospital and they are helping to take over if we don't do something to stop them?"

### ■ History of Present Illness

This is the first admission for P.P., a 37-year-old woman who was brought to the state psychiatric hospital by the police. The patient is apparently homeless. The precipitating event that caused her admission to the hospital was an attack on a police officer under a city bridge. The patient had stolen food from a nearby grocery store, has been delusional, and claims that she needs to store food for later when the aliens come in large numbers and the "War between the Worlds" begins. She also believes that she has been repeatedly raped by alien men on the street, that the water supply to the city has already been poisoned by Martians, and that she has been receiving messages through the city's overhead electrical wires that more aliens are coming and to prepare for a war. She believes that aliens have been doing plastic surgery and making themselves look like her. "I've seen aliens who look exactly like me under the bridge where I live." She claims that four years ago she had been abducted by aliens and they had performed brain surgery on her and inserted a computer chip in her brain that allowed her to hear voices whenever she passed under electrical wires and transformers.

Her speech is rambling, she is oddly dressed, and her hair is greasy and unwashed. She is wearing a red bandana on her head, a pink shawl over her shoulders, a man's yellow striped shirt, a blue-and-white spotted skirt, and sandals. She claims that the red bandana will help protect her from the aliens, because "aliens are afraid of red." She keeps repeating an invented phrase that sounds like "Ohm U Et Nostra," which she also claims will help her to ward off aliens.

The patient claims to be the Assistant Secretary of State for the United States, who is trying to negotiate with the aliens to prevent a war. "I am a powerful person, so you should be sure to treat me with total respect."

### ■ Past Psychiatric History

The patient has no prior hospital admission record for mental illness, but has a short history of meeting with a psychologist five years ago for depression related to the death of her son in a hurricane. She denies the use of street drugs or any type of substance abuse and her medical records confirm this. She smokes cigarettes "when I can find them or trade for them."

## Past Medical History

- The patient has no previous official documentation of having been raped
- Arthroscopy of right knee 8 years ago, complicated 10 days later by an invasive streptococcal infection for which she received 3 weeks of intravenous vancomycin therapy
- Intermediate-grade T cell-rich B-cell lymphoma diagnosed 7 years ago, treated with 6 cycles of CHOP with excellent response and remission
- Seroconverted to PPD+ 6 years ago, treated for 12 months with isoniazid

*Patient Case Question 1.* Identify the *four* cancer chemotherapeutic drugs that are administered in CHOP therapy.

*Patient Case Question 2.* To which microbe has the patient been exposed if she tests positive for PPD?

*Patient Case Question 3.* If a person tests positive for PPD, does this suggest active disease?

## Family Psychiatric History

- Records show that her mother was diagnosed at about the same age (age 36) with a schizophrenic illness.
- Maternal grandfather was "placed in an insane asylum for hysteria."

## Medications

OTC ibuprofen 400 mg for headache as needed, not daily

## Allergies

- "Mycins" (upset stomach)
- Bactrim (rash)

## Social History

- Divorced with a daughter; son is deceased
- Heterosexual
- Homeless (She reports that "my family disowned me years ago")
- Employment history unknown, but she reports that she has "had difficulty keeping a job in the past"

## Mental Status Examination

The patient appears alert and in no acute distress. However, her speech is incoherent and rambling with many persecutory and some grandiose delusions. Illogical and disconnected thoughts are common. She tends to pass rapidly from one subject to another without pause or focus on one topic. There is no evidence of auditory hallucinations at this time and she denies visual and other types of hallucinations. She also denies any thoughts of suicide or homicide, but she verbalizes in great detail about aliens taking over the world. She has pronounced delusional and disorganized speech symptoms with paranoid ideation prominent. All aspects of her memory (immediate, recent, and remote) appear to be fair-to-good. Looseness of associations is present. Cognition and concentration are marginal. Intellectual function is within normal limits. Insight (with anosognosia) and judgment are markedly impaired. She says that she has no pleasure in her life anymore and has very few social contacts "that she can really and truly trust."

# Review of Systems

- Denies loss of appetite or recent weight loss
- Reports that she has occasional headaches due to surgery performed by the aliens
- Otherwise negative

# Physical Examination and Laboratory Tests

## General

The patient is a thin, Hispanic female who is very talkative and appears older than her stated age. She is unkempt, disheveled, and is not wearing any makeup.

## Vital Signs

See Patient Case Table 50.1

| Patient Case Table 50.1 Vital Signs | | | | | |
|---|---|---|---|---|---|
| BP | 143/84 | RR | 16 | HT | 5ft-4 in |
| P | 82 | T | 97.7°F | WT | 109 lbs |

## Head, Eyes, Ears, Nose, and Throat

- Normocephalic and atraumatic
- Pupils equal at 3 mm, round, responsive to light and accommodation
- Extra-ocular muscles intact
- (–) nystagmus
- Funduscopy: discs sharp, no retinopathy
- No nasal discharge or nasal polyps
- Tympanic membranes gray and shiny bilaterally; minor accumulation of cerumen
- Mucous membranes moist
- Throat clear without exudates or lesions

*Patient Case Question 4.* Is funduscopy a test of the head, eyes, ears, nose, or throat?

## Skin

- Warm and dry
- Color and turgor WNL
- No lesions

## Neck and Lymph Nodes

- Supple without thyromegaly or jugular venous distension
- Cervical, axillary, inguinal, and femoral lymph nodes are non-palpable

## Cardiovascular

- Normal sinus rhythm without murmur
- $S_1$ and $S_2$ normal
- No rubs or gallops
- Point of maximal impulse is normal and non-displaced
- Carotid and femoral pulses are normal
- There are no carotid or femoral bruits

## Chest/Lungs

- Frequent sighing during examination
- No tachypnea or shortness of breath
- Lungs clear to auscultation
- There is full excursion of the chest without tenderness

## Abdomen

- Soft, non-tender, and not distended
- Normal bowel sounds
- No organomegaly, bruits, palpable viscera, or masses

## Breasts

No masses, discoloration, discharge, or tenderness

## Extremities

- Full range of motion
- Peripheral pulses 2+ throughout
- Prominent saphenous vein visible bilaterally with multiple varicosities

## Neurologic

- No localizing signs
- CNs II–XII intact
- Negative Romberg
- Toes downgoing
- Finger-to-nose normal
- Motor—5/5 grip strength bilaterally
- DTRs 2+ bilaterally for biceps, brachioradialis, quadriceps, and Achilles
- Normal gait
- Feet are sensitive to light touch, pinprick, and vibration

## Laboratory Test Results

See Patient Case Table 50.2

## Patient Case Table 50.2 Laboratory Blood Test Results

| | | | | | |
|---|---|---|---|---|---|
| Na | 140 meq/L | • Neutros | 67% | Alb | 4.5 g/dL |
| K | 4.0 meq/L | • Lymphs | 25% | Total protein | 7.0 g/dL |
| Cl | 102 meq/L | • Monos | 7% | Ca | 9.9 mg/dL |
| $HCO_3$ | 22 meq/L | • Eos | 1% | $PO_4$ | 3.2 mg/dL |
| BUN | 14 mg/dL | • Basos | 0% | TSH | 2.33 μU/mL |
| Cr | 0.8 mg/dL | Plt | 264,000/mm³ | Cholesterol | 152 mg/dL |
| Glu (PPBG) | 134 mg/dL | AST | 21 IU/L | LDL | 109 mg/dL |
| Hb | 14.6 g/dL | ALT | 15 IU/L | HDL | 50 mg/dL |
| Hct | 42% | Alk Phos | 45 IU/L | Trig | 100 mg/dL |
| RBC | 4.2 million/mm³ | Mg | 2.7 mg/dL | Urine drug screen | Neg |
| WBC | 6,000/mm³ | Total bilirubin | 0.9 mg/dL | Pregnancy test | Neg |

## Urinalysis

See Patient Case Table 50.3

## Patient Case Table 50.3 Urinalysis

| | | | | | |
|---|---|---|---|---|---|
| Color | Light Yellow | Specific Gravity | 1.017 | Leukocyte Esterase | Neg |
| Appearance | Clear | Blood | Neg | WBC | 0/HPF |
| Glucose | Neg | pH | 5.8 | RBC | 1/HPF |
| Bilirubin | Neg | Protein | Neg | Bacteria | Neg |
| Ketones | Neg | Nitrites | Neg | | |

*Patient Case Question 5.* Endocrine disorders, such as thyroid disease, may mimic some of the clinical manifestations of schizophrenia. Why can thyroid disease be ruled out in this patient?

*Patient Case Question 6.* Identify *all* abnormal blood laboratory tests and urinalysis findings in this patient.

*Patient Case Question 7.* The patient has reported the presence of *ten* different delusions in this case study. Identify *eight* of them.

*Patient Case Question 8.* Identify the *single* hallucination in this case study.

*Patient Case Question 9.* Identify the *eleven* remaining clinical manifestations (other than delusions and hallucinations) that are consistent with a diagnosis of schizophrenia.

*Patient Case Question 10.* Identify the *single* risk factor that predisposes this patient to schizophrenia.

*Patient Case Question 11.* Does this patient manifest only positive symptoms, only negative symptoms, or both positive and negative symptoms of schizophrenia?

*Patient Case Question 12.* Why might olanzapine be a more appropriate antipsychotic agent than haloperidol for this patient?

*Patient Case Question 13.* Based on this patient's specific set of symptoms, which subtype of schizophrenia is most likely?

# NEUROENDOCRINE DISORDERS

# 51 ADDISON DISEASE

 *For the Disease Summary for this case study, see the CD-ROM.*

## PATIENT CASE

### ■■■ Patient's Chief Complaints

"I've been feeling weaker and more tired over the past 4 months, but it has taken a more severe turn for the worst since last week. I haven't been able to enjoy any outdoor activities with my family but, for some strange reason, I've been getting an unusual tan."

### ■■■ HPI

C.K. is a 48 yo white woman who presents to her sister's primary care provider with loss of appetite, progressive fatigue, and mild nausea for the past five days. C.K. and her husband are visiting her sister in Wyoming for two weeks, but she has not felt well enough to bicycle, hike, or climb for the past week. Her sister has insisted that she see a healthcare professional.

### ■■■ PMH

- Appendicitis treated surgically, 10 years ago
- Seroconverted to PPD (+) 6 years ago; treated for 12 months with INH
- Pernicious anemia × 5 years
- Hypercholesterolemia × 1 year; controlled with diet and exercise

### ■■■ FH

- No family history of cancer
- Father died from cardiac arrest at age 65
- Mother currently resides in a nursing home as a consequence of CVA; also has rheumatoid arthritis
- Has two sisters (ages 46 and 45) with Hashimoto thyroiditis and one sister (age 52) with Graves disease
- Has one brother (age 53) who is alive and well

*Patient Case Question 1.* What is the major significance of this patient's family history?

# ■ SH

- Born and raised in Dallas, TX
- Owns and manages a bed-and-breakfast motel with her husband in Anchorage, AK
- Husband underwent triple bypass surgery and was diagnosed with Addison disease last year
- Drinks wine with dinner occasionally and socially
- Denies tobacco use and IVDU
- Loves traveling, camping, hiking, biking, and climbing
- Walks on a treadmill three times/week and is trying to follow a dietician-designed, low-cholesterol diet

# ■ Meds

Cyanocobalamin, 200 µg IM on the 15th of every month (her personal physician back home has recently increased the dosage)

*Patient Case Question 2.* Why is this patient taking cyanocobalamin?

*Patient Case Question 3.* Why is oral cyanocobalamin not an option for her condition?

# ■ All

- ASA → swelling of face
- TMP-SMX → bright red rash that covered her torso and face, reportedly with fever

# ■ ROS

- (−) for fever, chills, shortness of breath, night sweats, and cough
- (+) for weight loss of 6 pounds in the last month
- (+) for salt cravings before nausea developed
- (+) for several bouts of dizziness, one fainting spell in last 6 months
- (+) for few aches and pains
- (−) for recent changes in vision
- (−) for changes in menstrual cycle
- (+) for prominent tanning of the skin, although she denies significant exposure to the sun

# ■ PE and Lab Tests

## Gen

Tired-looking, tanned Caucasian woman in NAD who appears to be her stated age

## VS

See Patient Case Table 51.1

| Patient Case Table 51.1 Vital Signs | | | |
|---|---|---|---|
| BP | 95/75, P 83/min sitting, right arm | T | 98.0°F |
| BP | 80/60, P 110/min standing, right arm | HT | 5 ft–6½ in |
| RR | 14/min | WT | 124 lbs |

*Patient Case Question 4.* Explain the significance of the varying blood pressure and heart rate readings with change in position by the patient.

## Skin

- Intact, warm, and very dry
- Subnormal turgor
- Pigmented skin creases on palms of hands and knuckles
- Generalized tanned appearance, even at sites not exposed to the sun
- Sparse axillary hair

## HEENT

- PERRLA
- EOMI
- Normal funduscopic exam
- TMs intact
- Dry mucous membranes

## Neck

- Supple with normal thyroid and no masses
- Shotty lymphadenopathy

## Lungs

Clear, normal vesicular and bronchial lung sounds to A & P

## Breasts

- Equal in size without nodularity, masses, or tenderness
- Very dark areolae
- Hyperpigmentation prominent along brassiere lines

## Cardiac

- RRR
- No m/r/g

## Abd

- Soft and NT
- (−) HSM
- (+) BS

## GU

- Normal external female genitalia
- LMP 2 weeks ago
- Normal pelvic exam without tenderness or masses

## MS/Ext

- No CCE
- Normal ROM
- Pigmented skin creases on elbows
- Pedal pulses moderately weak at 1+
- Muscle strength 5/5 throughout

## Neuro

- A & O × 3
- Bilateral deep tendon reflexes intact at 2+
- Normal gait
- CNs II–XII intact

## Laboratory Blood Test Results (Fasting, Drawn at 8:20 AM)

See Patient Case Table 51.2

| Patient Case Table 51.2 Laboratory Blood Test Results | | | | | |
|---|---|---|---|---|---|
| Na | 126 meq/L | Hct | 33.2% | Alk Phos | 115 IU/L |
| K | 5.2 meq/L | RBC | 4.1 million/mm³ | Bilirubin | 1.2 mg/dL |
| Cl | 97 meq/L | MCV | 85 fL | Protein | 8.0 g/dL |
| HCO₃ | 30 meq/L | Plt | 410,000/mm³ | Albumin | 4.7 g/dL |
| BUN | 20 mg/dL | WBC | 6,800/mm³ | Cholesterol | 202 mg/dL |
| Cr | 1.2 mg/dL | • Neutros | 49% | Triglycerides | 159 mg/dL |
| Glu | 55 mg/dL | • Lymphs | 36% | Fe | 89 µg/dL |
| Ca | 8.8 mg/dL | • Monos | 7% | TSH | 3.2 µU/mL |
| Phos | 2.9 mg/dL | • Eos | 7% | Free T₄ | 16 pmol/L |
| Mg | 2.9 mg/dL | • Basos | 1% | Cortisol | 2.0 µg/dL |
| Uric acid | 3.6 mg/dL | AST | 33 IU/L | ACTH | 947 pg/mL |
| Hb | 11.4 g/dL | ALT | 50 IU/L | Vitamin B₁₂ | 700 pg/mL |

## UA

- Clear and yellow
- SG 1.016
- pH 6.45
- (−) blood

## Imaging

Abdominal CT scan revealed moderate bilateral atrophy of the adrenal glands

## Rapid ACTH Stimulation Test

See Patient Case Table 51.3

| Patient Case Table 51.3  Rapid ACTH Stimulation Test | | |
|---|---|---|
| Condition | Cortisol Assay | Aldosterone Assay |
| Pre-cosyntropin | 2.0 µg/dL | 3.8 ng/dL |
| 30 min post-cosyntropin | 1.9 µg/dL | 3.8 ng/dL |

## Antibody Testing

- (+) 21-hydroxylase
- (−) 17-hydroxylase
- (−) C-P450

## Peripheral Blood Smear

Normochromic, normocytic erythrocytes

---

*Patient Case Question 5.* What is the *single* greatest risk factor for Addison disease in this patient?

*Patient Case Question 6.* What is the most likely cause of Addison disease in this patient?

*Patient Case Question 7.* Why can tuberculosis be ruled out as a cause of Addison disease in this patient?

*Patient Case Question 8.* Which *two* test results are most suggestive of the *cause* of Addison disease in this patient?

*Patient Case Question 9.* Would supplementation with fludrocortisone be appropriate in this patient?

*Patient Case Question 10.* Does this patient have any signs of hypothyroidism, a disorder that is commonly associated with Addison disease?

*Patient Case Question 11.* There are 19 clinical signs and symptoms in this case study that are consistent with Addison disease. Identify *15* of them.

*Patient Case Question 12.* Which *single* test result is diagnostic for Addison disease in this patient?

*Patient Case Question 13.* Which *three* test results support the assessment that the patient's anemia is not the result of iron deficiency?

*Patient Case Question 14.* Which *two* test results support the assessment that the patient's anemia is not the result of vitamin B12 deficiency?

*Patient Case Question 15.* Why is *shotty lymphadenopathy* consistent with a diagnosis of Addison disease in this patient?

# 52 CUSHING SYNDROME

 *For the Disease Summary for this case study, see the CD-ROM.*

# PATIENT CASE

## ■ Current Status

M.K. is a 35-year-old Caucasian woman who presents to her PCP complaining of a dull but persistent headache, a significant weight gain over the past six weeks, significant facial hair growth, menstrual abnormalities, and both an excessive thirst and appetite. She also feels very depressed, does not have much energy, and has stopped performing all the activities that she had previously enjoyed (tennis, bridge, and shopping for new clothes). M.K. is married, has an adolescent son (age 16) and daughter (age 13) and has been in relatively good health throughout her life. She is the third oldest of four children. One of her brothers was diagnosed with type 1 diabetes mellitus at age 11 and was recently evaluated for hypertension. Her two sisters are in good health. Her father is a cancer survivor of childhood leukemia and her mother has a history of rheumatoid arthritis and breast cancer.

The patient does not smoke and only consumes alcohol in moderation at social functions. She has several allergies (ragweed and cat dander) and is not taking any medications other than a daily multivitamin tablet and ibuprofen (as needed) for headache.

## ■ Physical Examination and Laboratory Tests

The patient is an alert but anxious, moderately overweight white female with a noticeably round, full face. T = 98.3°F orally; P = 85 beats/min and regular; RR = 14 breaths/min and unlabored; BP = 185/105 mm Hg left arm, sitting; Ht = 5′0″; Wt = 141 lbs.

*Patient Case Question 1.* Of the vital signs listed above, which of them has to be of most concern to the patient's PCP?

*Patient Case Question 2.* Assuming that the patient has hypercortisolism, briefly explain the pathophysiology of the abnormal vital sign noted in Question 1.

*Patient Case Question 3.* Is this patient technically *underweight, overweight, obese,* or is her weight considered *healthy and normal*?

*Patient Case Question 4.* Assuming that M.K. has hypercortisolism, what are two possible causes of this patient's persistent, dull head pain?

> ***Patient Case Question 5.*** What is the significance in the patient's report that she is not taking any medications other than a daily multivitamin pill and ibuprofen?

## HEENT, Skin, Neck

- Head exam normal except for significant facial hair growth
- Fundi without lesions, PERRLA
- Nares, tympanic membranes, and pharynx clear
- Skin appears hyperpigmented and thin with some bruising on the arms and hands
- Gingiva show localized areas of hyperpigmentation
- Neck supple
- No bruits
- Fat deposits in dorsocervical region
- Thyroid non-palpable
- No palpable cervical, supraclavicular, infraclavicular, or axillary adenopathy

## Lungs, Cardiac

Exams unremarkable

## Abdomen

- Protuberant with striae and minimal bruising
- Bowel sounds heard in all four quadrants
- No abdominal bruits, masses, tenderness, or organomegaly

## Breast Exam

- Symmetric breasts
- No signs of dimpling, discoloration, or nipple discharge
- Two small, mobile, cystic nodules palpable in the UOQ of right breast suggest benign condition, probably fibrocystic change
- Mammogram pending

## Extremities

- No edema
- Both upper and lower extremities show areas of hyperpigmentation
- Pulses full in both feet
- Muscular atrophy significant in all four limbs

## Neurologic

- Alert and oriented
- Cranial nerves II–XII intact (including excellent visual acuity)
- Strength 3/5 throughout
- Sensory to light touch, proprioception, and vibration normal
- DTRs +2 and symmetric
- Gait within normal limits

## Laboratory Test Results

See Patient Case Table 52.1

| **Patient Case Table 52.1 Laboratory Test Results** | | | |
|---|---|---|---|
| Serum Na⁺ | 145 meq/L | Urinary free cortisol | 190 µg/24 hrs |
| Serum K⁺ | 3.1 meq/L | pH arterial, whole blood | 7.46 |
| Serum Cl⁻ | 105 meq/L | Serum testosterone | 160 ng/dL |
| Serum glucose, fasting | 170 mg/dL | Hct | 41% |
| Plasma ACTH | 290 pg/mL | RBC | $5.9 \times 10^6/mm^3$ |
| Serum cortisol, 8 AM | 73 µg/dL | WBC differential: 75% neutrophils, 15% lymphocytes, 7% monocytes/macrophages, 2% eosinophils, 1% basophils | |

**Patient Case Question 6.** Identify the *nine* abnormal laboratory test results in Table 52.1.

**Patient Case Question 7.** Why is serum glucose elevated?

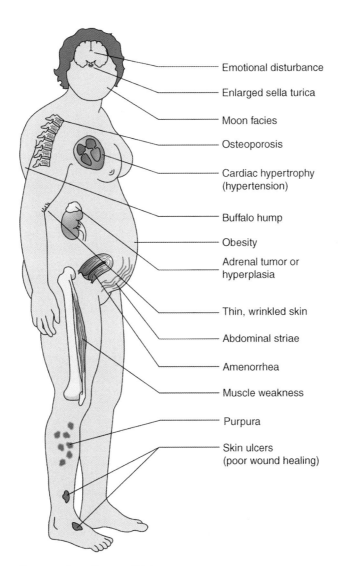

Emotional disturbance

Enlarged sella turica

Moon facies

Osteoporosis

Cardiac hypertrophy
(hypertension)

Buffalo hump

Obesity

Adrenal tumor or
hyperplasia

Thin, wrinkled skin

Abdominal striae

Amenorrhea

Muscle weakness

Purpura

Skin ulcers
(poor wound healing)

PATIENT CASE FIGURE 52.1

Illustration showing the potential clinical manifestations of Cushing syndrome. (Reprinted with permission from Rubin E, Farber JL. Pathology, 3rd ed. Philadelphia: Lippincott Williams & Wilkins, 1999.)

*Patient Case Question 8.* Explain the pathophysiology that underlies *polydipsia* in this patient.

*Patient Case Question 9.* Do laboratory test results suggest that hypercortisolism in M.K. is ACTH-dependent or ACTH-independent?

*Patient Case Question 10.* What is the significance of the serum $K^+$ concentration and the pH of the arterial blood?

*Patient Case Question 11.* Note that *hyperpigmentation of the skin and gingiva* was a physical finding in this patient. Is this clinical manifestation more characteristic of ACTH-dependent or ACTH-independent Cushing syndrome?

*Patient Case Question 12.* Which imaging techniques might be critical to establishing a specific cause of hypercortisolism in this patient?

*Patient Case Question 13.* What type of menstrual abnormality would be suspected in this patient and which abnormal laboratory test result is consistent with this type of abnormality?

*Patient Case Question 14.* What is the treatment of choice for curing hypercortisolism in this patient?

*Patient Case Question 15.* Patient Case Figure 52.1 shows that an *enlarged sella turcica* is a potential clinical manifestation of Cushing syndrome/disease. Explain the association.

*Patient Case Question 16.* Why is *cardiac hypertrophy* shown as a clinical manifestation of Cushing syndrome in Patient Case Figure 52.1?

# 53   DIABETES MELLITUS, TYPE 1

 *For the Disease Summary for this case study, see the CD-ROM.*

# PATIENT CASE

## ■■ Patient's Chief Complaints

"I have been throwing up since yesterday, I have a stomach ache, and I feel very weak."

## ■■ HPI

S.C. has been an active 13-year-old until recently. She has enjoyed relatively good health except for an occasional cold or episode of influenza. She has never been hospitalized. She has an older brother (age 17) with type 1 diabetes diagnosed at age 10.

A few months ago, Mrs. C noticed that her daughter seemed pale and less active than usual. S.C. stated that she had been feeling tired and was seriously thinking about quitting the volleyball team. It seemed that she was always hungry and thirsty and she was constantly eating snacks. Despite both an increase in food and fluid intake, she lost weight. Her clothing began to feel "too big" for her. She also noticed that she was going to the bathroom much more often than previously. Furthermore, she often became irritable and had difficulty concentrating on her homework. Mrs. C became alarmed by all of the changes that she was suddenly observing in her daughter and took S.C. to the family physician. S.C. was diagnosed with type 1 diabetes mellitus. S.C. and her parents were taught proper insulin administration, blood glucose testing, urine testing, foot care, and menu planning. The patient was started on a daily schedule of insulin.

> **Patient Case Question 1.** "Some people I know with diabetes can take pills," says S.C. "Why can't I take pills instead of having to take insulin?" she asks. What is an appropriate response to her question?

Last night before supper, the patient took her usual dose of insulin, lispro, for a blood glucose concentration of 193 mg/dL. She began feeling nauseated right before retiring to bed and she woke up with a stomach ache around midnight and began vomiting. Her blood glucose at that time was 397 mg/dL. Her mother asked her to try sipping diet ginger ale and eating a few crackers, but she was unable to keep anything down. She vomited several more times and then began breathing very heavily. It was at this time that Mrs. C suspected ketoacidosis and took her daughter to the hospital emergency room.

S.C. denies fever or chills. However, she confirms mild diarrhea for the past 36 hours. Furthermore, several of her classmates had been recently ill with flu-like stomach symptoms. She denies cough, sore throat, and painful urination.

*Patient Case Question 2.* What is the single greatest risk factor for type 1 diabetes mellitus that this patient has?

*Patient Case Question 3.* What causes heavy breathing in a patient with type 1 diabetes mellitus?

*Patient Case Question 4.* What is this heavy breathing called?

*Patient Case Question 5.* Why is it appropriate for the physician to inquire about fever, chills, diarrhea, cough, sore throat, and painful urination?

## Meds

- Insulin lispro according to a sliding scale
- NPH insulin at breakfast and bedtime
- Additional insulin lispro if urinary ketones are elevated

## FH

- Both mother and father live in the household and are well
- One older brother, age 17, with type 1 DM
- Two younger sisters, ages 9 and 11, without health problems
- Maternal grandmother died at age 50 from renal complications of type 1 DM

## SH

- "B" student in school
- Member of volleyball team and school band

## ROS

- HEENT: Denies blurry vision, dizziness, head trauma, ear pain, tinnitus, dysphagia, and odynophagia
- CV: No complaints of chest pain, orthopnea, or peripheral edema
- RESP: Denies coughing, wheezing, or dyspnea
- GI: Vomiting with nausea, abdominal pain, mild diarrhea, and food-fluid intolerance as noted above
- GU: Had polyuria (large volumes every 2 hours) last evening but has not urinated since waking up. No complaints of dysuria or hematuria.
- OB-GYN: Started menstruating 13 months ago. Menses flows for 5 days and is regular every 28 days. Not sexually active and denies any vaginal discharge, pain, or pruritus.
- NEURO: Denies weakness in the arms and legs. No complaints of headache, paresthesias, dysesthesias, or anesthesias.
- DERM: No history of rash or other skin lesions and no diaphoresis
- ENDO: Denies heat or cold intolerance

*Patient Case Question 6.* Distinguish between *paresthesias, dysesthesias,* and *anesthesias.*

*Patient Case Question 7.* Describe the pathophysiology of paresthesias, dysesthesias, and anesthesias.

*Patient Case Question 8.* Which types of endocrine disorders are characterized by heat and cold intolerance?

# ▪ PE and Lab Tests

## Gen

- Thin white girl who looks ill
- Deep respirations
- Smell of acetone on her breath
- Alert and oriented

## VS

See Patient Case Table 53.1

| Patient Case Table 53.1 Vital Signs | | | | | |
|---|---|---|---|---|---|
| BP | 90/65 supine | RR | 28 | HT | 5 ft |
| P | 126 | T | 99.5°F | WT | 87 lbs |

*Patient Case Question 9.* Is this patient technically *underweight, overweight, obese,* or is this patient's weight *healthy and normal*?

## Skin

- Pale and dry without lesions
- Moderately decreased turgor

## HEENT

- NC/AT
- PERRLA
- EOM intact
- Fundi normal
- Mucous membranes dry
- Pharynx erythematous without tonsillar exudates
- Ears unremarkable

## Neck

No thyromegaly or masses

## LN

No cervical, axillary, or femoral lymphadenopathy

## CV

- PMI normal and non-displaced
- $S_1$ and $S_2$ normal without $S_3$, $S_4$, murmurs, or rubs
- RRR
- Carotid, femoral, and dorsalis pedis pulses are weak bilaterally
- No carotid, abdominal, or femoral bruits heard

---

***Patient Case Question 10.*** Identify *three* signs that suggest this patient is dehydrated.

---

## Chest

- Lungs are CTA & P
- There is full excursion of the chest without tenderness

## Abd

- Soft and NT without organomegaly or masses
- Bowel sounds are subnormal

## Rect

- Anus is normal
- No masses or hemorrhoids noted
- Stool is heme occult (−)

## Ext

- There is no pretibial edema
- Feet are without ulcers, calluses, or other lesions

## Neuro

- DTRs bilaterally are 2+ for the biceps, brachioradialis, quadriceps, and Achilles
- Plantars are downgoing bilaterally
- Vibratory perception is normal
- Muscle strength is 5/5 throughout

---

***Patient Case Question 11.*** Are "downgoing plantars" a normal or abnormal neurologic response?

---

## Laboratory Blood Test Results

See Patient Case Table 53.2

---

***Patient Case Question 12.*** Identify *four* laboratory test results that are consistent with a diagnosis of diabetic ketoacidosis.

## Patient Case Table 53.2 Laboratory Blood Test Results

| | | | | | |
|---|---|---|---|---|---|
| Na | 127 meq/L | Glu, fasting | 554 mg/dL | MCHC | 33 g/dL |
| K | 6.1 meq/L | Acetone | 3+ | WBC | 11,500/mm³ |
| Cl | 98 meq/L | Hb | 13.1 g/dL | • Neutros | 40% |
| HCO₃ | 15 meq/L | Hct | 48% | • Bands | 11% |
| Anion gap | 20.1 meq/L | RBC | 5.3 million/mm³ | • Lymphs | 45% |
| BUN | 23 mg/dL | Plt | 358,000/mm³ | • Monos | 4% |
| Cr | 1.5 mg/dL | MCV | 90 fL | ESR | 18 mm/hr |

*Patient Case Question 13.* How was *anion gap* determined in this patient?

*Patient Case Question 14.* Identify *three* laboratory test results that are consistent with a diagnosis of dehydration.

*Patient Case Question 15.* What has probably caused this patient's abnormal plasma sodium and chloride concentrations?

*Patient Case Question 16.* Why is this patient's serum potassium concentration abnormal?

## ABG (on Room Air)

pH 7.23, $PaO_2$ 107 mm Hg, $PaCO_2$ 20 mm Hg, $O_2$ saturation 97%

*Patient Case Question 17.* Why is this patient's blood pH abnormal?

*Patient Case Question 18.* Explain the pathophysiology of this patient's low $PaCO_2$.

## UA

- SG 1.018
- pH 5.5
- Glucose 3+
- Protein (−)
- Ketones 3+

## Chest X-Ray

Normal

## ECG

Sinus tachycardia

*Patient Case Question 19.* What is the single major precipitating factor for this patient's ketoacidosis?

*Patient Case Question 20.* Provide *seven* clinical manifestations for your answer to Question 19 above.

*Patient Case Question 21.* How is ketoacidosis most effectively managed?

# CASE STUDY

# 54

## DIABETES MELLITUS, TYPE 2

 *For the Disease Summary for this case study, see the CD-ROM.*

# PATIENT CASE

## ■ Patient's Chief Complaints

"My left foot feels weak and numb. I have a hard time pointing my toes up."

## ■ History of Present Illness

C.B. is a significantly overweight, 48-year-old woman from the Winnebago Indian tribe who had high blood sugar and cholesterol levels three years ago but did not follow up with a clinical diagnostic work-up. She had participated in the state's annual health screening program and noticed that her fasting blood sugar was 141 and her cholesterol was 225. However, she felt "perfectly fine at the time" and could not afford any more medications. Except for a number of "female infections," she has felt fine until recently.

Today, she presents to the Indian Hospital general practitioner complaining that her left foot has been weak and numb for nearly three weeks and that the foot is difficult to flex. She denies any other weakness or numbness at this time. However, she reports that she has been very thirsty lately and gets up more often at night to urinate. She has attributed these symptoms to the extremely warm weather and drinking more water to keep hydrated. She has gained a total of 65 pounds since her last pregnancy 14 years ago, 15 pounds in the last 6 months alone.

## ■ Past Medical History

- Seasonal allergic rhinitis (since her early 20s)
- Breast biopsy positive for fibroadenoma at age 30
- Gestational diabetes with fourth child 14 years ago
- Morning sickness with all four pregnancies
- HTN × 10 years
- Moderate-to-severe osteoarthritis involving hands and knees × 4 years
- Multiple yeast infections during the past 3 years that she has self-treated with OTC antifungal creams and salt baths
- Occasional constipation

## ■ Past Surgical History

C-section 14 years ago

## ■ OB-GYN History

- Menarche at age 12
- Menopause, natural, at age 46½; despite problematic hot flashes, she has chosen not to initiate HRT
- First child at age 17, last child at age 34, $G_4P_4A_0$, all babies were healthy, 4th child weighed 10 lbs 6½ oz at birth
- Last Pap smear 4 years ago

## ■ Family History

- Type 2 DM present in younger sister and maternal grandmother; both were diagnosed in their late 40s; maternal grandmother died from kidney failure while waiting for a kidney transplant; sister is taking "pills and shots"
- Father had emphysema
- Two older siblings are alive and apparently well
- All four children are healthy

## ■ Social History

- Married 29 years with 4 children; husband is a migrant farm worker
- Family of 5 lives in a 2-bedroom trailer
- Patient works full-time as a seamstress in a small, family-owned business
- Smokes 2 ppd (since age 14) and drinks 2 beers most evenings
- Has "never used illegal drugs of any kind"
- Rarely exercises and admits to trying various fad diets for weight loss but with little success; has given up trying to lose weight and now eats a diet rich in fats and refined sugars

## ■ Review of Systems

### General

Admits to recent onset of fatigue

### HEENT

Has awakened on several occasions with blurred vision and dizziness or lightheadedness upon standing; denies vertigo, head trauma, ear pain, ringing sensations in the ears, difficulty swallowing, and pain with swallowing

### Cardiac

Denies chest pain, palpitations, and difficulty breathing while lying down

### Lungs

Denies cough, shortness of breath, and wheezing

## GI

Denies nausea, vomiting, abdominal bloating or pain, diarrhea, or food intolerance, but admits to occasional episodes of constipation

## GU

Has experienced increased frequency and volumes of urination, but denies pain during urination, blood in the urine, or urinary incontinence

## Ext

Denies leg cramps or swelling in the ankles and feet; has never experienced weakness, tingling, or numbness in arms or legs prior to this episode

## OB-GYN

Menses stopped 2 years ago; is not sexually active but denies sexual dysfunction; also denies any vaginal discharge, pain, or itching

## Neuro

Has never had a seizure and denies recent headaches

## Derm

No history of chronic rash or excessive sweating

## End

Denies a history of goiter and has not experienced heat or cold intolerance

## ■■■ Allergies

Sulfa drugs → confusion

## ■■■ Medications

- Lisinopril 20 mg po QD
- Acetaminophen 500 mg with hydrocodone bitartrate 5 mg 1 tablet po Q HS and Q 4h PRN
- Naproxen 500 mg po BID (for mild-to-moderate osteoarthritis × 3½ years)
- Omeprazole 20 mg po QD
- Docusate sodium 100 mg po TID
- Loratadine 10 mg po QD PRN

*Patient Case Question 1.* Why is this patient taking lisinopril?

*Patient Case Question 2.* Why is this patient taking acetaminophen with hydrocodone?

*Patient Case Question 3.* Why is this patient taking omeprazole?

*Patient Case Question 4.* Why is this patient taking docusate sodium?

*Patient Case Question 5.* Why is this patient taking loratadine?

# ■ Physical Examination and Laboratory Tests

## General

- Significantly overweight Native American woman who appears slightly nervous
- The patient is alert, oriented, and uses appropriate words
- She does not appear to be acutely distressed and looks her stated age

## Vital Signs

See Patient Case Table 54.1

| Patient Case Table 54.1 Vital Signs | | | |
|---|---:|---|---:|
| BP | 165/100 without orthostatic changes | T | 98.0°F |
| P | 88, regular | HT | 5 feet–3 inches |
| RR | 15, not labored | WT | 203 lbs |

***Patient Case Question 6.*** Which *two* clinical signs from Table 54.1 should arouse the most concern?

## Skin

- Dry and cool with tenting/poor skin turgor
- Significant xerosis on both feet with cracking
- Erythematous scaling rash in the axilla bilaterally
- (−) petechiae, ecchymoses, moles, or tumors upon careful inspection
- Normal capillary refill throughout

## Head, Eyes, Ears, Nose, and Throat

- PERRLA
- EOMI
- Pink conjunctiva
- R & L funduscopic exams showed mild arteriolar narrowing but without hemorrhages, exudates, or papilledema
- Non-icteric sclera
- TMs intact
- Nares and oropharynx clear without exudates, erythema, or lesions
- Mucous membranes dry

## Neck and Lymph Nodes

- Supple
- (−) thyromegaly, adenopathy, JVD, or nodules
- (+) bruit auscultated over right carotid artery

## Chest and Lungs

- No chest deformity; chest expansion symmetric
- Clear to auscultation and percussion throughout

## Heart

- Regular rate and rhythm with no murmurs, gallops, or rubs
- Apical impulse normal at 5th ICS at mid-clavicular line
- Normal $S_1$ and $S_2$
- No $S_3$, $S_4$

## Abdomen

- Soft, NT with prominent central obesity
- (+) BS in all four quadrants
- (−) organomegaly, distension, or masses
- Faint abdominal bruit auscultated

***Patient Case Question 7.*** What is the significance of the two bruits auscultated in the neck and abdomen?

## Breasts

No masses, discoloration, discharge, or dimpling of skin or nipples

## Genitalia/Rectum

- (−) vaginal discharge, erythema, and lesions
- (−) hemorrhoids
- Good anal sphincter tone
- Stool is guaiac-negative

## Musculoskeletal and Extremities

- Normal ROM in upper extremities
- Reduced ROM in knees
- (−) edema or clubbing
- Peripheral pulses diminished to 1+ in both feet
- Feet are cold to touch and dry with cracking, but no ulceration observed
- Strength 5/5 throughout except 2/5 in left foot

***Patient Case Question 8.*** What is the significance of this patient's cold feet and diminished peripheral pulses in the lower extremities?

## Neurologic

- Alert and oriented × 3
- Cranial nerves II–XII intact (including good visual acuity)
- Sensory response to light touch, proprioception, and vibration subnormal in both feet with abnormalities greater in the left foot
- DTRs 2+ throughout
- Gait normal except for left foot weakness

**Patient Case Question 9.** Clinical *signs* are objective manifestations of a disease that can be identified by someone other than the patient. List a minimum of *six* signs from the case study *above* that support a diagnosis of type 2 diabetes in this patient.

## Laboratory Blood Test Results (After Overnight Fast)

See Patient Case Table 54.2

| Patient Case Table 54.2 Laboratory Blood Test Results | | | | | |
|---|---|---|---|---|---|
| Na | 139 meq/L | Ca | 9.8 mg/dL | T. cholesterol | 246 mg/dL |
| K | 4.0 meq/L | PO$_4$ | 3.3 mg/dL | HDL | 28 mg/dL |
| Cl | 102 meq/L | Mg | 1.9 mg/dL | LDL | 168 mg/dL |
| HCO$_3$ | 22 meq/L | AST | 19 IU/L | Trig | 458 mg/dL |
| BUN | 14 mg/dL | ALT | 13 IU/L | HbA$_{1c}$ | 8.2% |
| Cr | 0.9 mg/dL | Alk phos | 43 IU/L | Ins | 290 μU/mL |
| Glu | 168 mg/dL | T. bilirubin | 1.0 mg/dL | | |

## Urinalysis

See Patient Case Table 54.3

| Patient Case Table 54.3 Urinalysis | | | | | |
|---|---|---|---|---|---|
| *Appearance* | Pale yellow and clear | *Bilirubin* | Negative | *Microalbuminuria* | Negative |
| *pH* | 5.8 | *Ketones* | Negative | *Glucose* | Positive |
| *SG* | 1.008 | *Protein* | Negative | *Microscopy* | Negative for microbes, red cells, and white cells |

## Electrocardiogram

Findings consistent with early left ventricular hypertrophy

**Patient Case Question 10.** List a minimum of *five* risk factors that predispose this patient to type 2 diabetes mellitus.

**Patient Case Question 11.** Clinical *symptoms* are subjective manifestations of a disease that can only be reported by the patient. List a minimum of *seven* symptoms that support a diagnosis of type 2 diabetes in this patient.

**Patient Case Question 12.** What has probably caused this patient's left ventricular hypertrophy?

**Patient Case Question 13.** Which *single* urinalysis test result is more suggestive of type 2 than type 1 diabetes?

**Patient Case Question 14.** Which *three* blood chemistry test results strongly support a diagnosis of diabetes?

*Patient Case Question 15.* Why do *stress* and *infection* promote hyperglycemia in patients with diabetes?

*Patient Case Question 16.* Why should medications other than glipizide or glyburide be considered for management of diabetes in this patient?

*Patient Case Question 17.* List *four* signs of *dehydration* in this patient.

*Patient Case Question 18.* What is the significance of xerosis and cracking of the feet in this patient?

# 55

## HYPERPARATHYROID DISEASE

 *For the Disease Summary for this case study, see the CD-ROM.*

## PATIENT CASE

### ▬▬ Chief Complaints

"I have been constipated for nearly a week and feel tired all the time."

### ▬▬ HPI

J.T. is a 48-year-old woman who presented to her PCP with a 3-day history of fatigue, hypersomnolence, and constipation. She states that she has "not felt herself for the past three days." Her last bowel movement was five days ago despite increased use of a laxative.

### ▬▬ PMH

- Migraine headaches, 1–2/month
- Calcium oxalate renal stone, 5 weeks ago, passed spontaneously
- HTN diagnosed 4 years ago
- Tonsillectomy at age 7 years

### ▬▬ FH

- Mother has DM type 2
- Remainder of FH unremarkable

*Patient Case Question 1.* Identify *four* manifestations of hyperparathyroid disease in the case study directly above.

### ▬▬ SH

J.T. is one of five children. She completed college and received a Bachelor of Science degree in chemistry. She has been teaching high school chemistry for 19 years. She denies using street drugs or OTC medications. She admits to drinking 1–2 glasses of wine when she is nervous. She smokes about 5 cigarettes per day and sometimes drinks up to 9 cups of coffee daily.

## ROS

The patient states that she is a little nauseated and feels very tired. Her husband confirms that his wife has been very tired, constipated, and nauseated lately. The patient states that she has unintentionally lost about 6 pounds during the past 1½ months. J.T. denies bone and joint pain and has no other complaints.

## Meds

- Ergotamine, 1 mg + caffeine, 100 mg, 2 tablets po at onset of migraine
- Metoclopramide, 10 mg po at onset of migraine
- Hydrochlorothiazide, 25 mg po Q AM
- Milk of Magnesia, 30 mL po QD PRN bowel movement; increased to BID 3 days ago

*Patient Case Question 2.* Why is this patient taking metoclopramide for migraine headaches?

*Patient Case Question 3.* For which condition is this patient taking hydrochlorothiazide?

## ALL

- NKDA
- Food allergies to hazelnuts and tofu (both cause wheezing and hives)

## PE and Lab Tests

### Gen

Patient does not appear to have any discomfort.

### VS

BP 115/70; P 80; RR 15; T 98.6°F; Wt 110 lbs; Ht 5′3″

*Patient Case Question 4.* Are any of the patient's vital signs abnormal?

### Skin

- Warm and dry
- No rashes or ulcers
- Normal turgor

## HEENT

- NC/AT
- Clear sclera
- PERRLA
- EOMI
- TMs intact
- No oral or nasal lesions
- Moist mucous membranes
- Oropharynx clear and without exudates or erythema

## Neck/LN

- No cervical, supraclavicular, or axillary adenopathy
- Normal thyroid
- No palpable neck masses
- No JVD or carotid bruits

## Heart

- RRR
- $S_1$, $S_2$ normal
- No m/r/g

## Lungs

- CTA bilaterally with clear, normal breath sounds
- No rales or rhonchi

## Abd

- Firm, distended, non-tender
- High-pitched BS
- No abdominal masses, bruits, or organomegaly

## Genit/Rect

Deferred

## Breasts

- Normal
- No lumps, discoloration, or dimpling

## Ext

- Pulses 2+ bilaterally
- No CCE

## Neuro

- Lethargic
- Oriented × 3 (self, location, year)
- Speech clear but slow
- Language normal

- Follows simple commands
- Answers questions appropriately
- Cranial nerves grossly intact
- Moves all extremities, but mild LLE and RLE weakness is present

**Patient Case Question 5.** How is "mild LLE and RLE weakness" related to the diagnosis?

## Laboratory Blood Test Results

See Patient Case Table 55.1

| Patient Case Table 55.1 Laboratory Blood Test Results | | | | | | | | | |
|---|---|---|---|---|---|---|---|---|---|
| Na | 137 meq/L | PO$_4$ | 1.9 mg/dL | RBC | $4.8 \times 10^6$/mm$^3$ | Bilirubin, total | 1.2 mg/dL |
| K | 4.3 meq/L | BUN | 20 mg/dL | WBC | 7300/mm$^3$ | Bilirubin, direct | 0.4 mg/dL |
| Cl | 109 meq/L | Cr | 1.1 mg/dL | Plt | 190,000/mm$^3$ | Alb | 3.4 g/dL |
| HCO$_3$ | 23 meq/L | Glu, fasting | 107 mg/dL | AST | 24 IU/L | Protein, total | 7.0 g/dL |
| Ca | 12.5 mg/dL | Hb | 13.7 g/dL | ALT | 37 IU/L | PTH | 115 pg/mL |
| Mg | 1.8 mg/dL | Hct | 44% | Alk phos | 99 IU/L | Vit D, 25OH | 32 ng/mL |

**Patient Case Question 6.** From the laboratory test data in Table 55.1, identify *three* abnormal findings that are consistent with a diagnosis of hyperparathyroid disease.

## Imaging Studies

Scintigraphy and ultrasound of the neck were both positive for a 1.3-cm mass in the left superior parathyroid gland. CT scans of the thorax and abdomen were negative. Standard x-rays were negative for bone lesions.

**Patient Case Question 7.** What is the most likely cause of hyperparathyroidism in this patient?

**Patient Case Question 8.** Would you expect that the patient has primary or secondary hyperparathyroid disease? Why?

**Patient Case Question 9.** What is the most appropriate therapy for this patient?

**Patient Case Question 10.** Why is it advisable in this patient to replace hydrochlorothiazide with another medication?

**Patient Case Question 11.** When polyuria and polydipsia are present in a patient with hyperparathyroid disease, the cause is usually:

a. diabetes mellitus type 1

b. diabetes mellitus type 2

c. nephrogenic diabetes insipidus

d. central (neurogenic) diabetes insipidus

**Patient Case Question 12.** What is the significance of this patient's serum 25OH-vitamin D determination?

# 56 HYPERPROLACTINEMIA

 *For the Disease Summary for this case study, see the CD-ROM.*

# PATIENT CASE

## ■ History of Present Illness

C.R. is a 24-year-old woman with a regular menstrual history (period every 28 days) since menarche at age 13. She presents to her gynecologist five days after missing her period. There has been a small amount of milky discharge from both breasts that she first noticed about two weeks ago. She and her husband have not been using birth control for the past six months so that they can start a family. However, she has not been able to get pregnant. "Do you think that I am finally pregnant?" she asks her physician. "All of the early pregnancy tests that I have taken so far have been negative."

## ■ Past Medical History

- One episode of bacterial pneumonia, 6 years ago, hospitalized
- 3-year Hx leg cramps
- Chickenpox as a child

## ■ Family History

- Father died at age 46 from liver cancer believed to be the result of alcoholism
- Mother with type 1 DM × 36 years
- Brother killed in Iraq in car bombing

## ■ Social History

- No tobacco, EtOH, or recreational drug use
- Married 3 years with no children and lives with husband
- Sexually active with husband only
- Employed as administrative assistant at local college

## ■ Review of Systems

- Bilateral galactorrhea
- No headaches, neck stiffness, or recent changes in vision
- Denies recent significant changes in appetite and thirst

## ■ Medications

- OTC multivitamin tablet QD
- St. John's Wort, 1 tablet, QD
- Ginseng tea occasionally HS to relieve stress

## ■ Allergies

NKDA

## ■ Vaccinations

Unknown

## ■ Physical Examination and Laboratory Tests

### General

The patient is a WDWN white female who appears to be slightly anxious and talkative, but otherwise in NAD.

### Vital Signs

BP 104/80, HR 70, RR 15, T 98.7°F, Wt 123 lbs, Ht 5′5½″

---

***Patient Case Question 1.*** At this point in the patient's profile, are there any *risk factors* that are consistent with a diagnosis of hyperprolactinemia?

***Patient Case Question 2.*** At this point in the patient's profile, are there any *clinical manifestations* that are consistent with a diagnosis of hyperprolactinemia?

***Patient Case Question 3.*** Are any of the patient's vital signs abnormal?

***Patient Case Question 4.*** Is this patient technically *underweight, overweight, obese,* or is this patient's weight considered *normal and healthy*?

---

### Skin

- Intact with no lesions
- Normal turgor and color
- Warm and dry
- No hirsutism noted

## Head, Eyes, Ears, Nose, and Throat

- NC/AT
- PERRLA
- Normal funduscopic exam
- Non-erythematous TMs
- Nose clear and non-erythematous
- Examination of the oral cavity reveals no lesions in the tonsils, palate, and floor of the mouth
- No ulcers in the oral cavity
- Teeth and gums appear healthy

**Patient Case Question 5.** What is the significance of the abbreviation NC/AT in this patient?

## Neck and Lymph Nodes

- Neck supple
- No lymphadenopathy
- Normal thyroid
- No bruits in carotid arteries
- No JVD

## Cardiac

RRR with no murmur

## Chest

Normal breath sounds

## Breasts

- Bilateral galactorrhea, mild
- No masses, tenderness, discoloration, or dimpling of the nipples

## Abdomen

- Soft with BS present
- No tenderness, masses, bruits, or organomegaly

## Genitourinary

- LMP 33 days ago
- Normal pelvic exam and Pap test

## Musculoskeletal and Extremities

- Muscle strength and tone 5/5
- No CCE
- Moves all extremities well
- Peripheral pulses 2+ bilaterally
- DTRs 2+

## Neurologic

- Alert and oriented
- CNs II–XII intact
- Gait normal
- No significant deficits noted

## Laboratory Blood Test Results

See Patient Case Table 56.1

### Patient Case Table 56.1 Laboratory Blood Test Results

| | | | | | | β-HCG undetectable | |
|---|---|---|---|---|---|---|---|
| Na | 141 meq/L | BUN | 10 mg/dL | Total bilirubin | 0.9 mg/dL | | |
| K | 4.3 meq/L | Cr | 1.1 mg/dL | TSH | 5.3 μU/mL | Hct | 44% |
| Ca | 8.5 mg/dL | Glu, fasting | 84 mg/dL | $T_3$ | 150 ng/dL | WBC | 5,600/mm$^3$ |
| Cl | 104 meq/L | AST | 26 IU/L | Total $T_4$ | 6.9 μg/dL | Plt | 380,000/mm$^3$ |
| HCO$_3$ | 24 meq/L | ALT | 41 IU/L | Free $T_4$ | 15.7 pmol/L | Alk phos | 67 IU/L |

## Other Tests

A series of three serum prolactin assays on three separate days revealed concentrations of 64 ng/mL, 65 ng/mL, and 68 ng/mL. An MRI of the pituitary gland and hypothalamus was negative for lesions. A chest x-ray was also negative.

*Patient Case Question 6.* What is the significance of the results from the BUN and Cr tests?

*Patient Case Question 7.* What is the significance of the results from the AST, ALT, and total bilirubin tests?

*Patient Case Question 8.* What is the significance of the results from the TSH, $T_3$, total $T_4$, and free $T_4$ tests?

*Patient Case Question 9.* Which of the four tests listed in *Question 8* would be expected to be abnormally high if the patient had developed primary hypothyroid disease?

*Patient Case Question 10.* What is the significance of the serum β-HCG test?

*Patient Case Question 11.* What is an appropriate diagnosis for this patient?

*Patient Case Question 12.* What is an appropriate initial approach to therapy for this patient?

## ■ Clinical Course

The patient returns one month later for a serum prolactin test. Concentration was 36 ng/mL. Galactorrhea has been absent for three weeks following initiation of therapy. There have been no bothersome side effects from the therapy.

*Patient Case Question 13.* Has response to therapy been positive?

*Patient Case Question 14.* Has the patient's prolactin level normalized?

# 57 HYPERTHYROID DISEASE

*For the Disease Summary for this case study,*
*see the CD-ROM.*

## PATIENT CASE

### ■ Patient's Chief Complaints

"I was jogging in the park like I do most mornings. Suddenly, I couldn't catch my breath and I felt very dizzy. When I sat down on a park bench for a minute, I noticed a weird feeling in my chest—like a strong fluttering sensation. I called 911 with my cellular phone and here I am."

### ■ History of Present Illness

B.G. is a 52 yo man who was brought to the emergency room by paramedics following symptoms of dyspnea, dizziness, and palpitations. When questioned about his recent medical history, he reports a sudden, unintentional loss in weight of approximately 10 pounds over the past two months and nearly 15 pounds over the last four months. "I've been eating like an elephant, but I've been losing weight," he reports. A few months ago, he began experiencing palpitations that came and went, but were not associated with chest pain. However, he notes that, sometimes, his "heart seems to beat too fast and too hard" and disproportionate to the activity in which he is engaged. Sometimes, it begins when he is sitting and watching TV or reading a magazine. He has also noticed that it has been "difficult getting some kinds of food down for the past week" and that he "had planned to see a doctor about that soon."

"My wife also tells me that I have been on edge and a bit short with her lately. I agree that I have not been myself mentally."

### ■ Past Medical History

- Migraine headaches × 9 years
- History of herpes simplex infections on lips and corners of mouth
- HTN × 3 years

### ■ Family History

- Paternal grandfather and father diagnosed with prostate cancer; father's cancer is currently in remission

- Half-sister had "thyroid problems with a goiter"
- Mother had arthritis and hyperthyroid disease
- One brother with type 2 DM who "takes pills"

## Social History

- Married and lives with wife of 30 years
- They had one daughter who was kidnapped and murdered in Aruba 6 months ago. The authorities have made no arrests to date and there are no suspects at this time.
- Works as an auto mechanic
- Previous smoker but quit 11 years ago
- Has an occasional beer with friends
- Denies use of illicit drugs, although he reports history of heroin and cocaine use as a young adult
- Admits to drinking "too much coffee" every day
- Physically very active and jogs 1–2 miles 3 or more days each week; also works out at the gym 1 day/week

## Review of Systems

- (+) occasional insomnia plus increased sensitivity to heat, fatigue, and decreased exercise tolerance for 1 week
- Reports that "hair seems to be falling out faster than usual" for past month
- (−) headache, cough, blurred or double vision, eye pain or sensitivity to light, excessive tearing or discomfort in the eyes, fever or chills, muscle weakness, diarrhea, chest pain, changes in libido or sexual performance, concentration problems, "shakiness," rashes or other skin lesions, painful swallowing, tenderness/pain in the neck, difficulty with urination, edema, recent fainting spells, and recent respiratory infection

## Medications

- Acetaminophen 500 mg + aspirin 500 mg + caffeine 130 mg po QD PRN
- Atenolol 25 mg po QD
- Multivitamin 1 tab po QD

## Vaccinations

Unknown

## Allergies

Morphine → intense pruritus

## Physical Examination and Laboratory Tests

### General

The patient is a thin, tanned, white male who appears slightly short of breath. He is cooperative and answers all questions appropriately.

## Vital Signs

See Patient Case Table 57.1

| Patient Case Table 57.1 Vital Signs | | | | | |
|---|---|---|---|---|---|
| BP | 98/70 supine | RR | 20 | HT | 5 ft–10 in |
| P | 130–170 irregular | T | 98.8°F | WT | 124 lbs |

## Integument

- Skin very warm, soft, intact, and moist
- Normal turgor and color
- Hyperpigmented lesions on upper back and lower extremities
- Hair is fine, velvety, and sparse on crown of head
- No evidence of rash, ecchymoses, petechiae, edema, or cyanosis

## Head, Eyes, Ears, and Throat

- PERRLA
- EOMI
- (+) eyelid lag bilaterally, R > L
- (+) mild proptosis bilaterally
- Fundi benign
- TMs intact
- Tongue and oral mucous membranes moist without erythema, exudates, or lesions
- Cold sore on right upper lip

## Neck and Lymph Nodes

- Neck supple
- (+) smooth, diffusely enlarged thyroid
- (−) JVD, carotid bruits, or cervical/axillary/inguinal adenopathy

## Lungs

- CTA bilaterally
- (−) wheezes or crackles

## Heart

- Irregular rhythm
- Tachycardic without murmurs
- No $S_3$ or $S_4$ heard
- No rubs heard

## Abdomen

- Soft, non-tender, and non-distended
- (+) BS in all four quadrants
- (−) HSM, masses, or bruits

## Genitalia/Rectum

- Normal male genitalia
- Prostate slightly enlarged, but no nodules noted
- Guaiac-negative stool

## Musculoskeletal and Extremities

- 2+ DP pulses bilaterally
- (−) joint tenderness, peripheral edema, cyanosis, or clubbing
- Full ROM
- No muscle weakness in proximal muscle groups
- No femoral bruits

## Neurologic

- A & O × 3
- DTRs 3+ at knees
- No tremor observed with fingers extended
- CNs II–XII intact
- Negative Babinski
- Sensory and motor levels appear intact

## Laboratory Blood Test Results

See Patient Case Table 57.2

| Patient Case Table 57.2 Laboratory Blood Test Results | | | | | |
|---|---|---|---|---|---|
| Na | 142 meq/L | Hb | 14.6 g/dL | Ca | 8.6 mg/dL |
| K | 4.0 meq/L | RBC | 4.9 million/mm³ | Mg | 1.8 mg/dL |
| Cl | 108 meq/L | MCV | 88 fL | ESR | 6 mm/hr |
| HCO$_3$ | 27 meq/L | WBC | 7.7 × 10³/mm³ | Total cholesterol | 68 mg/dL |
| BUN | 11 mg/dL | Plt | 378 × 10³/mm³ | Total T$_4$ | 26.5 µg/dL |
| Cr | 0.6 mg/dL | AST | 34 IU/L | Total T$_3$ | 508 ng/dL |
| Glu | NA | ALT | 31 IU/L | TSH | 0.016 µU/mL |
| Hct | 42% | Total bilirubin | 1.0 mg/dL | FT$_4$ | 57 pmol/L |

## Electrocardiogram

- Atrial fibrillation
- Sinus tachycardia
- (−) left ventricular hypertrophy

## Thyroid Ultrasound

Marked vascularity of the thyroid

## Radioactive Iodine Uptake Test

53% $^{123}$I absorbed after 5.9 hours

## Thyroid-Stimulating Hormone Receptor Antibody Test

Positive

## Chest X-Rays

Clear

## Exophthalmometry

- 20% greater than expected, R eye
- 11% greater than expected, L eye

***Patient Case Question 1.*** Identify the *single greatest risk factor* for hyperthyroid disease in this patient.

***Patient Case Question 2.*** Does this patient have *only hyperthyroid disease, only thyrotoxicosis,* or *both hyperthyroid disease and thyrotoxicosis*?

***Patient Case Question 3.*** Which is a more appropriate diagnosis and why: *primary* hyperthyroidism, *secondary* hyperthyroidism, or *tertiary* hyperthyroidism?

***Patient Case Question 4.*** What is the *cause* of hyperthyroid disease in this patient?

***Patient Case Question 5.*** Why is this cause atypical for this particular patient?

***Patient Case Question 6.*** List *four* clinical findings that are *specific to the cause* that you identified in Question 4.

***Patient Case Question 7.*** Which *two* clinical findings are *most specific* for the cause that you identified in Question 4?

***Patient Case Question 8.*** Why can a *pituitary tumor* be excluded as a potential cause of hyperthyroid disease in this patient?

***Patient Case Question 9.*** Why can a *thyroid adenoma* be excluded as a potential cause of hyperthyroid disease in this patient?

***Patient Case Question 10.*** Why can *subacute thyroiditis* be excluded as a potential cause of hyperthyroid disease in this patient?

***Patient Case Question 11.*** Clinical *symptoms* are subjective expressions of a disease that *can only be reported by the patient*. List a minimum of *eight* symptoms reported by the patient that are common to many patients with hyperthyroidism.

***Patient Case Question 12.*** Clinical *signs* are objective expressions of a disease that can be observed by someone other than the patient. Laboratory test results are also considered *signs* of a disease. List a minimum of *fifteen* signs observed in this patient that are common to many patients with hyperthyroidism.

***Patient Case Question 13.*** Why is this patient taking a combination drug regimen of acetaminophen, aspirin, and caffeine?

***Patient Case Question 14.*** Why is this patient taking atenolol?

***Patient Case Question 15.*** Why does Graves disease present with a diffuse or generalized and symmetric goiter, whereas Plummer disease presents as an asymmetric and nodular goiter?

# 58  HYPOPARATHYROID DISEASE

 *For the Disease Summary for this case study, see the CD-ROM.*

## PATIENT CASE

### ■ History of Present Illness

A.W. is a 52-year-old white female whose chief complaints to her primary care provider are recurrent and painful muscle spasms of the hands and feet and dry, scaly, puffy skin. She also states that "I have not been myself for the past 4–5 weeks." When asked to describe what she meant by that statement, she said that she has felt very irritable, aggressive, and even combative in recent weeks. She had been involved in several serious arguments with family members and close long-term friends.

### ■ Past Medical History

- Diagnosed with SLE 20 years ago
- Chronic history of alcohol abuse with one 2-week admission to alcohol detoxification and rehabilitation unit at the hospital
- Hospitalized for leaking cerebral aneurysm 4 years ago
- Multiple malignant melanomas surgically removed, primarily on arms and face
- Hospitalized in the psychiatric unit 2× for attempted suicide
- Tubal ligation following birth of son 29 years ago

### ■ Family History

- Father died at age 70 from pancreatic cancer with bone metastases
- Mother died 2 weeks after father from heart failure
- Younger sister with history of bipolar disorder and suicidal tendencies
- One older sister and one younger sister alive and well
- Brother died at age 38 from acute myocardial infarction
- Two brothers died from lung cancer
- One brother died soon after birth from hydrocephalus
- Family history of alcohol abuse, all children placed in foster homes
- Personal history of both sexual and physical abuse

## ■ Social History

The patient is a former certified nursing assistant and self-employed home health nurse's aide. She has not worked for six years, is technically disabled, and is receiving Social Security benefits for her disability. She has been divorced twice and is living with a female friend. She has two children, a son and daughter, both of whom are estranged and living in other states. She smokes 1½ packs of cigarettes (34-year smoking history) and drinks 5–6 cans of beer every day. She does not eat much because she is seldom hungry.

## ■ Medications

- OTC medications for occasional heartburn
- NSAIDs for flare-ups of arthralgia secondary to lupus

## ■ Allergies

- No known drug allergies
- Sunlight causes erythematous and macular rash on sun-exposed skin (related to SLE)

*Patient Case Question 1.* Which clinical manifestations in the patient's extensive histories above can be linked to hypoparathyroid disease?

## ■ Review of Systems

- Patient denies any thyroid or other types of neck surgery
- *Constitutional:* significant fatigue and weakness; poor appetite
- *Ear, nose, throat:* vision satisfactory; no eye pain, tinnitus, ear pain, or dysphagia
- *Cardiovascular:* no shortness of breath, chest pain, or dyspnea with exertion
- *Respiratory:* no cough or sputum production
- *Gastrointestinal:* no emesis, diarrhea, constipation, or nausea
- *Genitourinary:* no increase in urinary frequency, nocturia, painful urination, blood in the urine, painful menstruation, or vaginal bleeding
- *Musculoskeletal:* no joint pain or bone pain
- *Skin:* no rashes, nodules, or itching
- *Neurologic:* occasional headaches and dizziness; no fainting spells, unsteady gait, or seizures
- *Lymph nodes:* no swollen glands

## ■ Physical Examination and Laboratory Tests

### General Appearance

The patient is a very thin, weak- and frail-appearing white female in no apparent distress. She appears to be significantly undernourished but in good spirits. She is cooperative, alert, and attentive. The patient is wearing eyeglasses.

### Vital Signs

See Patient Case Table 58.1

| **Patient Case Table 58.1 Vital Signs** | | | | | |
|---|---|---|---|---|---|
| BP | 130/85 mm Hg | RR | 15/min, unlabored | Ht | 65 in |
| HR | 80/min | T | 98.5°F | Wt | 97 lbs |

*Patient Case Question 2.* What is the patient's body mass index (BMI) and what is the significance of this BMI?

## Head, Eyes, Ears, Nose, and Throat

- Right pupil normally reactive to light and accommodation, left pupil no light reflex (suspect Adie's pupil)
- Extra-ocular muscles intact
- Anicteric sclera
- Fundi normal
- Conjunctiva normal bilaterally
- Tympanic membranes intact and clear
- No exudates or erythema in oropharynx

## Skin

- Very pale, dry with flakiness
- No ecchymoses or purpura

## Neck

- Supple without masses or bruits
- Thyroid normal
- No lymphadenopathy

## Lungs

Clear to auscultation and percussion

## Heart

- Regular rate and rhythm
- $S_1$ and $S_2$ sounds clear with no additional heart sounds
- No murmurs or rubs

## Abdomen

- Soft, non-tender, and non-distended
- No guarding or rebound with palpation
- No masses, bruits, hepatomegaly, or splenomegaly
- Normal bowel sounds

## Rectal/Genitourinary

- Pap smear pending
- Stool is guaiac-negative

## Breasts

- No lumps or discoloration
- No dimpling or discharge

## Extremities

- Multiple scars from previous surgical excisions on lower and upper limbs bilaterally
- Negative for cyanosis or clubbing
- Mild edema of the hands and feet
- Normal range of motion throughout
- Joint exam reveals no active arthritis
- 2+ dorsalis pedis and posterior tibial pulses bilaterally

## Neurologic

- Alert and oriented ×3
- No sensory or motor abnormalities
- CNs II–XII intact
- DTRs 2+ throughout
- Muscle tone 4/5 throughout
- Positive Chvostek sign bilaterally

## Laboratory Test Results

See Patient Case Table 58.2

| Patient Case Table 58.2 Laboratory Test Results | | | | | | | |
|---|---|---|---|---|---|---|---|
| Na | 134 meq/L | Plt | 260,000/mm³ | Mg | 0.8 mg/dL |
| K | 3.5 meq/L | RBC | 4.2 million/mm³ | $PO_4$ | 5.3 mg/dL |
| Cl | 100 meq/L | WBC | 8,400/mm³ | PTH | 4 pg/mL |
| Ca | 6.8 mg/dL | AST | 36 IU/L | Uric acid | 3.9 mg/dL |
| $HCO_3$ | 25 meq/L | ALT | 56 IU/L | Glu, fasting | 94 mg/dL |
| BUN | 9 mg/dL | Alk phos | 83 IU/L | TSH | 2.9 µU/mL |
| Cr | 0.8 mg/dL | GGT | 114 IU/L | Folate | 120 ng/mL |
| Hb | 9.8 g/dL | T bilirubin | 1.1 mg/dL | B12 | 63 pg/mL |
| Hct | 31.7% | Alb | 3.4 g/dL | $PO_4$, urine | 0.2 g/day |
| MCV | 110 fL | T protein | 5.9 g/dL | ECG | Prolonged QT interval |

*Patient Case Question 3.* Identify the *twelve* abnormal laboratory test results in Table 58.2.

*Patient Case Question 4.* Identify *five* of the *twelve* abnormal test results in Table 58.2 that are consistent with hypoparathyroid disease.

*Patient Case Question 5.* Why might this patient's serum GGT level be abnormal?

*Patient Case Question 6.* What is the most likely cause of hypoparathyroid disease in this patient?

*Patient Case Question 7.* What is the likely cause of this patient's low hematocrit and hemoglobin concentration?

*Patient Case Question 8.* What would a peripheral blood smear show?

*Patient Case Question 9.* How might this patient be managed pharmacologically?

# 59

# HYPOTHYROID DISEASE

 *For the Disease Summary for this case study, see the CD-ROM.*

# PATIENT CASE

## ▬▬ Initial Presentation

Mrs. K.G. is a 29-year-old white female who was eight months pregnant at the onset of her illness. She is 5'2" tall and weighs 140 pounds. She has a son and daughter from a previous marriage. She has also suffered one miscarriage previously.

Upon calling her PCP's office and complaining of a severely sore throat, a temperature of 102° F, and the initiation of mild uterine contractions, she was instructed to go immediately to the emergency room. The ER physician chose to hospitalize her and treat her with antibiotics and IV magnesium sulfate to stop the contractions. Three days later, the fever resolved and there were no more contractions. K.G. felt much better and she was released from the hospital.

## ▬▬ Medical History

Up to this time, the patient had been in excellent health. The only medications that she was taking were prenatal vitamins. She had no known allergies, did not drink or smoke, and did not use illegal drugs.

## ▬▬ Clinical Course

Four weeks later after an uncomplicated delivery, K.G. gave birth to a healthy female child. Approximately six weeks later, K.G. saw her PCP with multiple clinical manifestations. She complained of being tired and weak. She also complained of lots of aches (both joint and muscle pain), that she was cold all the time, and that she had gained 30 pounds since her last delivery. When asked specific questions by her PCP, she also admitted (since her last delivery) to having recurrent headaches, mild constipation, and a lack of a menstrual period. "Could I be pregnant again?" she asked. A pregnancy test was conducted but determined to be negative. It was recommended that she take ibuprofen for her joint and muscle pain. A preliminary diagnosis of rheumatoid arthritis was considered, but a blood test for rheumatoid factor was negative.

K.G. returned to her PCP two weeks later. She noted that the ibuprofen had been somewhat effective for pain but not completely. The PCP ordered an ESR (which was 60 mm/hr). K.G. also mentioned that she was having difficulty hearing and comprehending and that she often felt "closed off in another world oblivious to what was going on around her." She also told her PCP that she "felt physically and mentally sluggish all the time." The PCP noted that her speech was very slow and deliberate, her voice was hoarse, her hands were swollen and her face puffy, and her skin was extremely dry and flaky. Heart rate was 46 beats/minute. There was no thyromegaly. K.G. told the PCP that she could not drive anymore because her "alertness was gone" and her reaction time was slow. Because of her poor mental state, she also could not care for her two young children anymore and her mother was providing care for them.

***Patient Case Question 1.*** Clinical *symptoms* are subjective manifestations of disease that may only be conveyed by the patient. List a minimum of 6 *symptoms* that this patient has conveyed that are consistent with a diagnosis of hypothyroid disease.

***Patient Case Question 2.*** Clinical *signs* are objective manifestations of disease that may be observed or measured by someone other than the patient, often a nurse or primary care provider. List a minimum of 5 *signs* that this patient demonstrates that are consistent with a diagnosis of hypothyroidism.

***Patient Case Question 3.*** Explain the pathophysiology underlying the patient's abnormal ESR.

***Patient Case Question 4.*** Explain the pathophysiology underlying the patient's swollen hands and puffy face.

***Patient Case Question 5.*** Explain the pathophysiology behind the patient's abnormal heart rate.

Three days following her last visit with her PCP, K.G. was thoroughly evaluated at a large medical facility. X-rays were taken of her hands and chest. CT scans were conducted of her neck, chest, and abdomen. She was given another ESR and pregnancy test, and a complete blood chemistry panel was run. During her clinical assessment, she received frequent hot compress applications to her hands, neck, and shoulders from a physical therapist and received daily hot whirlpool baths for her many aches and pains.

## Laboratory Blood Test Results

See Patient Case Table 59.1

### Patient Case Table 59.1 Laboratory Blood Test Results

| | | | | | |
|---|---|---|---|---|---|
| Na$^+$ | 128 meq/L | WBC | 11,500/mm$^3$ | ESR | 55 mm/hr |
| K$^+$ | 3.5 meq/L | Plt | 250,000/mm$^3$ | Thyroperoxidase antibodies | $(-)$ |
| Ca$^{+2}$ | 12.0 mg/dL | WBC differential: 45% neutrophils, 45% lymphocytes, 6% monocytes/macrophages, 3% eosinophils, 1% basophils | | Thyroglobulin antibodies | $(-)$ |
| Cl$^-$ | 101 meq/L | T$_4$, total | 3 µg/dL | Pregnancy test | $(-)$ |
| Glucose, fasting | 108 mg/dL | FT$_4$ | 6 pmol/L | Cholesterol | 260 mg/dL |
| RBC | 3.9 million/mm$^3$ | T$_3$ | 80 ng/dL | Calcitonin | 0 pg/mL |
| Hct | 33% | TSH | 25 µU/mL | | |

***Patient Case Question 6.*** List *six* blood laboratory test results that are *lower than normal* but consistent with a diagnosis of hypothyroid disease.

***Patient Case Question 7.*** Based on the laboratory blood test results in Table 59.1, does this patient have *primary* or *secondary* hypothyroid disease? Explain why.

*Patient Case Question 8.* Why might the patient's serum $Ca^{+2}$ concentration be abnormal?

*Patient Case Question 9.* Why was Hashimoto thyroiditis excluded as the cause of hypothyroidism in this patient?

*Patient Case Question 10.* A diagnosis of hypothyroid disease, possibly the result of suppurative (i.e., bacterial) thyroiditis, was established. Based upon which information was this diagnosis made?

# ■ Treatment

K.G. was prescribed oral 75 μg levothyroxine daily and she noticed a dramatic improvement in her personal health within 72 hours. There was a marked improvement in her alertness and thought processes and she felt considerably less tired and weak. Within four weeks of initiating therapy, all her aches, pains, and edema subsided and she felt normal again.

*Patient Case Question 11.* What is the significance of the patient's medical history with respect to levothyroxine use?

*Patient Case Question 12.* Why is this patient's abnormal serum cholesterol level consistent with hypothyroid disease?

# CHROMOSOME ABNORMALITY DISORDERS

# DOWN SYNDROME

 *For the Disease Summary for this case study, see the CD-ROM.*

## PATIENT CASE

### ■ History of Present Illness

Mrs. H.I. is a 42-year-old Caucasian $G_3P_{2-0-2}$ who was admitted to the delivery unit with labor pains. She was accompanied by her 44-year-old husband. Mrs. I. had been in relatively good health before her pregnancy. However, while pregnant she was diagnosed with gestational diabetes. Furthermore, her dose of thyroid hormone had to be adjusted several times during the last two trimesters. Mrs. I. also had several episodes of morning sickness during her first trimester. At time of admission, Mrs. I.'s blood pressure was 130/70 and her pulse was 75. Fetal heart rate was 145 beats/minute. Four hours after admission, Mrs. I. delivered a 37-week, 7-pound, 1-ounce baby girl. The Apgar score was **8** at 1 minute and **9** at 5 minutes after birth.

*Patient Case Question 1.* What information is provided by the designation $G_3P_{2-0-2}$?

*Patient Case Question 2.* Are Apgar scores within normal limits?

The delivery room physician and nurse immediately noticed that the baby had a rather small head with a flat occiput, a broad and flat nasal bridge, folds of skin in the corners of the eyes, an upward slant to the eyes, a protruding tongue, and short fingers. There also was an excess amount of skin on the back of her neck.

*Patient Case Question 3.* Which of the following explanations below is accurate and appropriate?

a. Episodes of morning sickness can create a disturbance in maternal metabolism that may interfere with embryonic development.

b. Drugs used to treat morning sickness can cause a variety of birth defects.

c. These physical characteristics are highly suggestive of some type of chromosome abnormality.

d. These phenotypic aberrations are pathognomonic (i.e., diagnostic) for Down syndrome.

When the baby is brought to the mother for feeding, Mrs. I. examines her new daughter carefully. She notices that her eyes, nose, and ears appear different from other babies. The baby's hands also have very short fingers, the "pinky" fingers are unusually curved, and both hands have a single crease extending the full width of the palms.

***Patient Case Question 4.*** Although many chromosome abnormalities occur due to abnormal cell division in the sperm or egg, they can also occasionally be inherited. The genetic basis for this baby's anomalies can *usually* be determined by:

a. analyzing the chromosomes in the baby's cells

b. analyzing the chromosomes in the mother's cells

c. analyzing the chromosomes in the father's cells

d. quantifying the number and severity of the baby's physical abnormalities

***Patient Case Question 5.*** The cause of this infant's physical characteristics is *most likely* the result of:

a. non-disjunction during meiosis I in the mother

b. non-disjunction during meiosis II in the mother

c. non-disjunction of the zygote sometime during embryogenesis

d. an inherited translocation involving chromosome 21 from the mother

***Patient Case Question 6.*** The parents struggle to understand what happened to their baby. "We don't smoke, drink, or take drugs, so why did this happen?" the mother asks. Which of the following represents the most accurate explanation?

a. Down syndrome is a genetically inherited disorder that is caused when both parents are carriers of a mutated gene.

b. Down syndrome is a genetically inherited disorder that may be caused when only one parent is a carrier of a mutated gene.

c. The risk for Down syndrome increases when the mother is older than age 35 and the egg is fertilized by multiple sperm.

d. The risk for Down syndrome increases when the mother is older than age 35 and chromosomes in her eggs fail to separate properly during cell division.

***Patient Case Question 7.*** During the first 36 hours after birth, nurses in the neonatal unit carefully watch the baby for irritability and abdominal distension. They note that she has passed no stool since birth. Which of the following has to be considered?

a. This is a common manifestation among most newborns and should not cause concern.

b. Down syndrome babies occasionally have a serious gastrointestinal blockage that requires surgery.

c. The baby may be showing signs of a gastrointestinal allergy to her mother's breast milk.

***Patient Case Question 8.*** Having just learned that their daughter has trisomy 21 and is not a mosaic, the parents are concerned about the possibility of severe mental retardation. Which of the following statements is most accurate?

a. Most children with Down syndrome are only minimally retarded and should be able to live a completely normal life.

b. Most children with Down syndrome are severely retarded and institutionalization is usually the best treatment option.

c. Every child with Down syndrome has some degree of mental retardation, but with early intervention affected individuals can live a long and relatively normal life.

***Patient Case Question 9.*** Upon examination of the new infant, the pediatrician detects a heart murmur. Which of the following is the most accurate and appropriate statement?

a. Heart murmurs are common to many infants and usually resolve within one month after birth.

b. Heart murmurs are benign and not a cause for concern.

c. A heart murmur in a child with Down syndrome may be a sign of a heart defect. However, further testing is necessary before a heart defect can be diagnosed.

d. A heart murmur in a child with Down syndrome is diagnostic for a heart defect and surgery should be performed as soon as possible to prevent the onset of heart failure and pneumonia.

***Patient Case Question 10.*** Conduct a literature search to determine the most common type of heart defect observed in children with Down syndrome.

# ■■■ Physical Examination and Laboratory Tests

## Laboratory Blood Test Results

See Patient Case Table 60.1

| Patient Case Table 60.1 Laboratory Blood Test Results | | | | | |
|---|---|---|---|---|---|
| Na | 140 meq/L | WBC | 6,500/mm³ | TSH | 5.3 µU/mL |
| K | 4.7 meq/L | Hct | 41% | $T_4$ total | 7 µg/dL |
| Cl | 107 meq/L | Hb | 14.1 g/dL | $HCO_3$ | 25 meq/L |
| Glu, fasting | 70 mg/dL | Plt | 297,000/mm³ | $PO_4$ | 3.0 mg/dL |

***Patient Case Question 11.*** Does the child have any abnormal laboratory blood test results and, if so, what condition might explain these findings?

## General

Full-term, Caucasian female infant of 37 weeks, weight 7 lb 1 oz, length 20 inches, delivered vaginally

## VS

- BP 70/35
- HR 155
- RR 35
- T 98.1°F

## Skin

Moist, pink, and well-perfused with good turgor

## Head, Eyes, Ears, Nose, and Throat

- Anterior fontanel flat and soft
- Sagittal sutures patent
- Microcephaly
- Epicanthal folds bilaterally
- Oblique palpebral fissures bilaterally
- Hypertelorism
- Broad, flat nasal bridge
- Oral pharynx normal
- Macroglossia with fissured tongue
- Protruding tongue

## Neck

- Supple with no masses
- Thyroid normal
- Clavicles intact

## Chest

- Chest wall rise symmetric
- Lungs clear bilaterally with auscultation

## Cardiac

- Regular sinus rhythm
- Systolic murmur prominent
- No rubs or gallops

## Abdomen

- Soft and non-distended
- (−) HSM
- (+) BS
- 3-vessel umbilical cord

## Genitalia/Rectum

- Normal female external genitalia
- Anus patent

## Spine

Straight and intact

## Extremities

- 20 digits
- Brachial pulses palpable
- Capillary refill WNL

- Significant hypotonia
- Brachydactyly
- Clinodactyly, fifth finger bilaterally
- Simian crease bilaterally
- Hyperextensible joints
- DTRs 3+ throughout

***Patient Case Question 12.*** Identify *fifteen* distinct clinical signs from the patient's physical examination that are consistent with a diagnosis of Down syndrome.

# CASE STUDY
# 61

## KLINEFELTER SYNDROME

 *For the Disease Summary for this case study,*
*see the CD-ROM.*

# PATIENT CASE

## ■ History of Present Illness

Mother's Communication: Mrs. C. presents to the pediatric clinic to discuss concerns about her 10-year-old son, M.C. "I am very concerned about my son, doctor. Teachers say that he daydreams a lot and that he is lazy and needs to focus more on his studies, but I think it is more than that. He has always been rather shy and quiet, but lately he seems to be slipping into some kind of depression. He doesn't seem to have any energy and has little enthusiasm for all those things that he has always enjoyed. He doesn't even want to go fishing anymore and he has always had a passion for fishing."

## ■ Past Medical History

Mother's Communication: "He was a very good baby, quiet and not at all demanding. He seemed very normal physically. As a toddler, he was somewhat shy and reserved. He began walking a little later than most children do, maybe 5–6 months later, but he did not talk until he was nearly 4½. The doctors always told us that he would talk when he was ready . . . and he did. He has always liked school. Teachers have commented that he has always been very well behaved, cooperative, and eager to please but also very shy and quiet. He has had a particularly difficult time learning to read and write. He also seems to have trouble sometimes finding the right word. His speech is definitely lagging behind other children his age. His teacher has told me that and I have noticed it with his friends in the neighborhood as well. My son can understand the conversations of other 10-year-olds, but his inability to use language the way other 10-year-olds use it makes him stand out. He only has a few close friends and those friends are getting into competitive athletics now. I think M. is becoming depressed because he feels left out. He's not very coordinated and not interested at all in playing competitive sports."

*Patient Case Question 1.* Identify four *significant* abnormalities above for which parents may have sought medical attention for their child much earlier.

*Patient Case Question 2.* What are *three* simple measures that parents and teachers might take with a KS boy to ensure his academic success?

## Medical Charts

- No major health problems
- Viral-like upper respiratory tract infection at age 8
- History of chronic left middle ear infections
- Immunizations current

## Family History

- Both parents alive and well
- Patient has two siblings who are alive and well

## Social History

- Attends the fifth grade and has not been set back any grades
- Enjoys fishing, checkers, helping father with yardwork and gardening, and playing with family pets
- Slightly above average student (C+)

## Medications

None

## Allergies

No known drug allergies

## Physical Examination and Laboratory Tests

### General Appearance

M.C. is an alert, appropriately anxious, quiet, cooperative white boy in no apparent distress

### Vital Signs

See Patient Case Table 61.1

| Patient Case Table 61.1 Vital Signs | | | | | |
|---|---|---|---|---|---|
| BP | 115/75 | RR | 14 | Height | *5′0″ |
| HR | 70 | T | 98.3°F | Weight | *119 lbs |

*Both height and weight are at the 95th percentile for a 10-year-old white boy.

### Skin

- Warm and dry with no lesions
- Normal turgor

### Head, Eyes, Ears, Nose, and Throat

- PERRLA
- EOMI
- TMs intact
- Mucous membranes moist and pink

## Neck

- Supple
- No thyromegaly or adenopathy

## Lungs

CTA bilaterally

## Heart

- RRR with no murmurs, gallops, or rubs
- $S_1$ and $S_2$ distinct and strong with no additional heart sounds

## Abdomen

- Soft, non-distended, with no palpable masses or bruits
- No HSM
- Positive bowel sounds
- No rebound or guarding

## Musculoskeletal/Extremities

- Peripheral pulses strong throughout
- No cyanosis, clubbing, or edema
- Strength 5/5 throughout
- Full range of motion

## Neurologic

- Alert and oriented $\times$ 3
- No signs of local deficit
- Negative Babinski reflex bilaterally
- Patellar deep tendon reflexes 2+
- Normal gait
- Sensory intact
- CNs II–XII intact

## Genitalia

Penis and testicles small for age

## Laboratory Test Results

See Patient Case Table 61.2

| Patient Case Table 61.2 Laboratory Test Results | | | | | |
|---|---|---|---|---|---|
| Na | 140 meq/L | Hb | 12.7 g/dL | Alb | 3.8 g/dL |
| K | 3.9 meq/L | Hct | 35% | Protein, total | 6.9 g/dL |
| Cl | 104 meq/L | Plt | 376,000/mm$^3$ | Alk phos | 79 IU/L |
| HCO$_3$ | 23 meq/L | WBC | 6,200/mm$^3$ | Testosterone | 24 ng/dL |
| BUN | 17 mg/dL | AST | 17 IU/L | FSH | 90 mU/mL |
| Cr | 0.8 mg/dL | ALT | 12 IU/L | LH | 135 mU/mL |
| Glu, fasting | 87 mg/dL | Bilirubin, total | 0.9 mg/dL | Karyotype | 47,XXY |

## ■ Clinical Course

The patient was referred to four different therapy specialists for management: a physical therapist, speech therapist, behavioral therapist, and mental health therapist.

*Patient Case Question 3.* Identify *seven* clinical manifestations from the physical examination and laboratory testing above that are consistent with Klinefelter syndrome.

*Patient Case Question 4.* Does this patient have the *most common form of Klinefelter syndrome,* a *mosaic form of the condition,* or an extremely *rare non-mosaic form*?

*Patient Case Question 5.* What is the probability that this patient will be able to have children?

*Patient Case Question 6.* What is the function of follicle-stimulating hormone in males?

*Patient Case Question 7.* What is the function of luteinizing hormone in males?

*Patient Case Question 8.* Which endocrine organ synthesizes and secretes follicle-stimulating hormone and luteinizing hormone into the circulation?

*Patient Case Question 9.* Would you suspect that this KS patient is a good candidate for immediate treatment with testosterone? Why or why not?

*For the Disease Summary for this case study,
see the CD-ROM.*

# PATIENT CASE

## ■ History of Present Illness

Mrs. A. presents at the clinic with her 13½-year-old daughter, P.A., for a thorough physical examination. P.A. has not had her first menstrual period and is showing no signs of breast development. P.A. is also very short for her age and has a peculiar webbing of the neck. She has a noticeably small lower jaw and skin folds in the corners of her eyes. She has never been tested for a chromosome disorder.

## ■ Past Medical History

With the exception of chronically recurring episodes of otitis media (i.e., middle ear infections) and a case of measles, P.A. has been a remarkably healthy child. She has had no surgeries. Her immunizations are current.

## ■ Family History

The patient's family history is unremarkable. P.A. is the last-born child of six children. Neither parent nor any of her siblings have been diagnosed with a genetic disease. At the time of her birth, P.A.'s mother was 34 years old and her father was 37 years old. Neither father nor mother has any chronic illnesses. The family lives on a farm 20 miles from town.

## ■ Social History

Despite dedication to her studies, the patient has always been a "C" student in school. She has passed all grades so far but has always had difficulty with mathematics, which has required the use of a math tutor for the past five years. She has learned to play the flute and wants to be an actress like her idol, Gwyneth Paltrow.

## ■ Current Medications

None

## ■ Allergies

She develops a rash as a reaction to several antibiotic medications (vancomycin, penicillin, and cephalexin).

*Patient Case Question 1.* Identify *seven* clinical manifestations that are consistent with Turner syndrome.

## ■ Physical Examination and Laboratory Tests

### General Appearance

The patient is an alert, friendly, relaxed, young white female in no apparent distress

### Vital Signs

See Patient Case Table 62.1

| Patient Case Table 62.1 Vital Signs | | | | | | | |
|---|---|---|---|---|---|---|---|
| Blood pressure | 145/95 | Respiratory rate | 15 | Height | | | 4'7" |
| Heart rate | 75 | Temperature | 98.2°F | Weight | | | 121 lbs |

*Patient Case Question 2.* Which of the patient's vital signs is abnormal and is this abnormality *consistent with* or *not related to* Turner syndrome?

*Patient Case Question 3.* Is the patient technically *underweight, overweight, obese,* or is her weight considered *healthy and normal*?

### Skin

The patient's skin is warm and dry with no rashes, tumors, or bruises. However, she has 15–20 small, dark brown moles on her chest and back. The turgor of the skin is normal.

*Patient Case Question 4.* How is skin turgor tested and what does a normal skin turgor suggest?

### Head, Eyes, Ears, Nose, and Throat

The patient's pupils are both 3 mm in diameter and react appropriately to light. Visual acuity is 20/50 in both eyes and she wears eyeglasses. No lesions were observed in the fundi and eye movements were normal. Tympanic membranes were intact, but the patient may have some hearing difficulties. A follow-up hearing test has been suggested. Mucous membranes are pink and moist. There was no exudate or erythema within the pharynx.

*Patient Case Question 5.* Are there any clinical manifestations seen in the skin or head that might be associated with Turner syndrome?

## Neck

The neck is supple with no pain during rotation or with up-and-down movement. The jugular veins are not distended, the thyroid gland is normal in size, no carotid bruits were heard with auscultation, and lymph nodes were not palpable.

## Lungs

Both lungs were clear with auscultation. Normal bronchial and vesicular sounds could be heard. No wheezes, rhonchi, or crackles could be heard.

## Heart

Heart rate and rhythm were regular. No murmurs, friction rubs, or gallops were heard. First and second heart sounds were strong. No additional heart sounds could be heard.

*Patient Case Question 6.* What is the significance of the cardiac exam?

## Abdomen

P.A.'s abdomen was soft, non-tender, and non-distended with no palpable masses, abdominal bruits, hepatomegaly, splenomegaly, rebound, or guarding. Bowel sounds were positive.

## Chest

There was complete absence of breast development. The chest was broad with widely spaced nipples.

## Musculoskeletal and Extremities

Peripheral pulses were strong bilaterally. There was no clubbing or cyanosis of the fingertips and no edema of the hands, feet, or ankles. Strength was optimal bilaterally and range of motion was excellent. Although the patient is short, extremities were proportional.

## Neurologic

The patient was alert and oriented to self, place, and time. There were no neurologic signs of a localized defect. There was no Babinski reflex bilaterally. Patellar deep tendon reflexes were active and equal bilaterally. Cranial nerves II–XII were intact. Sensation and gait appeared normal.

## Pelvic

External genitalia were female and appeared normal. Pubic hair development was normal. There was no vaginal discharge or lesions. A Pap test was done and the results were normal.

*Patient Case Question 7.* Identify *two* clinical manifestations in the breast, musculoskeletal extremity, and pelvic examinations that are consistent with Turner syndrome.

## Laboratory Blood Test Results

See Patient Case Table 62.2

## Patient Case Table 62.2 Laboratory Blood Test Results

| | | | | | |
|---|---|---|---|---|---|
| Sodium | 145 meq/L | Red blood cell count | 4.8 million/mm³ | Total cholesterol | 247 mg/dL |
| Potassium | 3.6 meq/L | Hematocrit | 40% | High-density lipoproteins | 41 mg/dL |
| Chloride | 111 meq/L | White blood cell count | 5,200/mm³ | Low-density lipoproteins | 171 mg/dL |
| Calcium | 8.9 mg/dL | Platelet count | 275,000/mm³ | Follicle-stimulating hormone | 130 mU/mL |
| Bicarbonate | 22 meq/L | Aspartate aminotransferase | 10 IU/L | Luteinizing hormone | 119 mU/mL |
| Blood urea nitrogen | 9 mg/dL | Alanine aminotransferase | 36 IU/L | Growth hormone | 4 ng/mL |
| Creatinine | 1.0 mg/dL | Total bilirubin | 1.2 mg/dL | Thyroid-stimulating hormone | 5.4 µU/mL |
| Glucose, fasting | 149 mg/dL | Albumin | 3.5 g/dL | Thyroxine | 10 µg/dL |

***Patient Case Question 8.*** Identify *five* abnormal laboratory blood test values and explain whether these are *consistent* or *inconsistent* with Turner syndrome.

***Patient Case Question 9.*** What is the significance of the two laboratory test findings in the last two rows of the third column in Table 62.2?

***Patient Case Question 10.*** How do you know that this patient's renal function is normal?

***Patient Case Question 11.*** How do you know that this patient's hepatic function is normal?

***Patient Case Question 12.*** What do you suspect a chromosome analysis will reveal?

# FEMALE REPRODUCTIVE SYSTEM DISORDERS

*For the Disease Summary for this case study, see the CD-ROM.*

# PATIENT CASE

## ▄▄ Patient's Chief Complaints

"My breasts have been naturally cystic, but I have a new lump in my right breast that has me concerned."

## ▄▄ History of Present Illness

G.S. is a 46 yo white, premenopausal woman who presents for her annual physical examination. Approximately six weeks ago, the patient noticed a small, painless lump in the upper outer quadrant of her right breast. At the time, she gave this observation little thought, assuming that the lump was like the many others that she tends to develop around her menses. She states that the lumps in her breasts become palpable and bothersome approximately 10 days before the start of menstruation. At present, she is approximately four days from this start date. There is no history of dysmenorrhea associated with her periods. However, the lump failed to resolve like the others and seemed to get larger with time. The patient denies tenderness, pain, nipple discharge, and skin changes in her breasts. She also denies any masses in the axillary region of the right arm.

The patient practices breast self-exams, but not routinely. She has never had a mammogram. Several years ago she had a breast biopsy that was consistent with fibrocystic changes. Her only Pap smear was done two years ago and the result was normal.

Mrs. S. is married and the mother of three children—ages 3, 8, and 10 years. She breastfed all three children. Her first full-term pregnancy occurred at age 35. She had been pregnant at age 15, but terminated the pregnancy with an elective abortion. She has also suffered a first-trimester miscarriage at age 20. She has had no pregnancies in which the delivery was conducted with caesarean section.

The patient's menarche occurred at age 11 years and 1 month. She has taken oral contraceptives for three years since the birth of her third child. Mrs. S. is the only child born to her parents late in life (father was 45, mother was 42).

## ▄▄ Past Medical History

- Asthma × 23 years
- Hypothyroidism × 8 years

# ■■■■ Family History

- Paternal grandmother was diagnosed with breast cancer before menopause at age 45
- Mother died from breast cancer 15 years ago at age 73; cancer was diagnosed before menopause at age 45; in long-term remission twice, but recurred again 16 years ago
- Father is alive at age 91 but suffers from HTN, CAD, DM type 2, and Alzheimer disease and is being cared for in a nursing home facility

# ■■■■ Social History

- Drinks 6–8 cups of coffee daily
- Denies tobacco, alcohol, or illegal drug use
- Exercises 3 times a week
- Graduated from a local university with a degree in journalism and has been a reporter for a local newspaper, but now works as a realtor
- Has been happily married for 21 years

# ■■■■ Review of Systems

- Unremarkable, except for complaints noted above
- Both asthma and hypothyroid disease have been well controlled with medication

# ■■■■ Medications

- Levothyroxine 100 μg po QD
- Albuterol inhaler PRN

# ■■■■ Allergies

Latex and adhesive tape produce rash

---

*Patient Case Question 1.* Identify this patient's major risk factors for breast cancer.

*Patient Case Question 2.* Which *single* risk factor has placed this patient at *extremely high risk* for developing breast cancer?

---

# ■■■■ Physical Examination and Laboratory Tests

## General

The patient appears well and is in no acute distress. She appears her stated age and is both alert and oriented.

## Vital Signs

See Patient Case Table 63.1

**Patient Case Table 63.1 Vital Signs**

| BP | 130/84 | RR | 13 | HT | 5 ft-4 in |
|----|--------|----|----|----|-----------|
| P | 74 | T | 98.2°F | WT | Stable at 125 lbs |

## HEENT

Head exam normal

## Neck/Lymph Nodes

- Neck supple with no JVD
- No palpable cervical, supraclavicular, or infraclavicular adenopathy
- One movable, firm, non-tender axillary lymph node of approximately 2 cm was palpated under the right arm
- Thyroid non-palpable

## Chest/Lungs

CTA and percussion

## Heart

- RRR
- No murmurs, rubs, or gallops

## Abdomen

- Soft, non-distended, and non-tender
- No HSM or masses
- BS normal

## Breast Examination

- Symmetric breasts
- No dimpling or erosion of the skin, nipple retraction or discharge, erythema or other discoloration, or swelling
- Multiple, diffuse, small (0.5–1.5 cm), mobile, apparently cystic lesions palpable throughout both breasts
- One 2- to 3-cm mass palpated in the upper outer quadrant of right breast; the mass felt firm, not fixed to the chest wall, and was not tender to the touch

## Spine

No tenderness to percussion

## Neurologic

No significant deficits noted

## Laboratory Blood Test Results

See Patient Case Table 63.2

| Patient Case Table 63.2 Laboratory Blood Test Results ||||||
|---|---|---|---|---|---|
| Na | 137 meq/L | Hb | 13.3 g/dL | • Monos | 6% |
| K | 4.2 meq/L | Hct | 38.5% | AST | 37 IU/L |
| Cl | 104 meq/L | Plt | 313 × 10³/mm³ | ALT | 30 IU/L |
| HCO₃ | 24 meq/L | WBC | 7.0 × 10³/mm³ | Alk phos | 97 IU/L |
| BUN | 8 mg/dL | • Neutros | 60% | T bilirubin | 0.3 mg/dL |
| Cr | 1.0 mg/dL | • Lymphs | 32% | T protein | 6.9 g/dL |
| Glu, fasting | 90 mg/dL | • Eos | 2% | Alb | 4.0 g/dL |

## Chest X-Rays

Lungs were clear

## Bilateral Mammogram

There were four 1.0–1.5 cm masses diffusely distributed throughout the left breast and three 0.5–1.0 cm masses in the right breast. There also was a 2.3 cm × 2.9 cm × 3.2 cm mass with irregular borders within the upper outer quadrant of the right breast. Associated with the suspicious lesion was diffuse skin thickening and an enlarged axillary lymph node of approximately 2.0 cm in greatest dimension. Six Y-shaped microcalcifications that extended toward the nipple were seen. There is some evidence of extension of the abnormal mass into pectoral muscle.

**Patient Case Question 3.** Identify *six* distinct clinical manifestations derived from the mammogram that strongly suggest that breast cancer is present.

## Ultrasound Right Breast and Right Axilla

* Three 0.5–1.0 cm cystic lesions diffusely distributed throughout the right breast
* Solid-appearing, non-cystic mass consistent with cancer in upper outer quadrant
* Ill-defined mass with abnormal vascularity
* The mass measures 2.3 cm × 2.9 cm × 3.2 cm
* There is some suggestion of skin thickening and mild tissue edema

## Core-Needle Biopsy of Large Right Breast Mass

* Pathology was consistent with that of infiltrating breast carcinoma
* Tubules were observed in 80–90% of the sample
* Approximately 3–5 cell divisions were seen per high-power field and there was only a mild degree of pleomorphism
* The tumor was positive for both estrogen and progesterone receptors

**Patient Case Question 4.** Based on the clinical information available to this point, to which *grade* has this patient's cancer progressed?

**Patient Case Question 5.** Based on the grade of the cancerous mass, what is this patient's expected 10-year survival rate?

## Ultrasound of Liver

- No masses suggesting metastasis were observed
- A 0.5 cm × 0.6 cm faintly visible region was observed to the left side and slightly cephalad of the ligamentum venosum. The appearance of this lesion is more consistent with that of a small hemangioma than with a metastatic nodule.

## Bone Scan

- No definitive evidence of bone metastasis was seen
- Positive for mild degenerative changes of the lower lumbar spine and multiple peripheral joints consistent with degenerative joint disease

# ▬▬ Clinical Course

The breast surgeon met with the patient and provided her with two treatment options:

(1) lumpectomy with sentinel node biopsy, followed by breast irradiation;
(2) modified radical mastectomy with sentinel node biopsy with or without reconstruction surgery.

The patient also met with a radiation oncologist who discussed with her the potential benefits and side effects of radiation therapy. The patient elected breast conservation therapy and sentinel lymph node biopsy with radiation therapy. The sentinel nodes were negative and all surgical margins were clear. The patient was treated with radiation and then placed on tamoxifen. The patient will be followed every 3–4 months for the first two years, then every six months for the next three years, and then annually.

*Patient Case Question 6.* Identify the *stage* to which this patient's breast cancer has advanced.

*Patient Case Question 7.* Based on the stage of this patient's breast cancer, what is this patient's expected 5-year survival rate?

*Patient Case Question 8.* Why was tamoxifen therapy initiated?

The patient did well with the therapeutic plan for the first 6½ years and all check-ups were negative for breast cancer. At 80 months after surgery and radiation, however, the patient returned to the clinic complaining of bone pain in her lower back and left hip and a severe headache that was not responding to OTC medications. The following tests were conducted: bone scan, chest x-ray, brain MRI scan, abdominal CT scan, and laboratory blood tests. The bone scan revealed lesions in the lumbar spine without impending fracture or spinal cord compression. The chest x-ray showed three small nodules in the upper lobe of the left lung. The right lung was clear. The MRI scan revealed a small mass in the right frontal lobe. The abdominal CT scan was negative. The patient's serum CEA level was elevated by 2-fold, the serum CA27-29 concentration by 2-fold, and the serum alkaline phosphatase level by 2.5-fold.

*Patient Case Question 9.* Identify the *stage* to which this patient's breast cancer has developed now.

*Patient Case Question 10.* Based on the stage of this patient's breast cancer, what is this patient's expected 5-year survival rate now?

*Patient Case Question 11.* Provide a minimum of *four* distinct types of therapy that may now benefit this patient.

# CASE STUDY
# 64 | CERVICITIS

 *For the Disease Summary for this case study, see the CD-ROM.*

# PATIENT CASE

## ■ History of Present Illness

M.F. is a 23-year-old woman who presents to the urgent care clinic complaining of three days of painful urination and increasing amounts of a yellow, creamy vaginal discharge. She is single, sexually active with two frequent partners and admits to unprotected sex at least twice in the past two weeks. She often insists that the guy wear a condom but "most times they don't use them because they don't like them." She rarely uses any type of barrier contraceptive and does not use spermicides. She denies intravenous drug use, oral or rectal intercourse, and has no active medical problems. She denies the presence of wart-like lesions or painful blisters in the genital region. She also denies each of the following:

- vaginal bleeding
- genital burning or itching
- malodorous discharge
- lower abdominal or pelvic pain
- use of douches, deodorant tampons, or perfumed products

Her last menstrual period occurred three days ago, approximately the same time as her symptoms developed.

*Patient Case Question 1.* What is the significance of the lack of wart-like lesions in the genital region?

*Patient Case Question 2.* What is the significance of the lack of painful blisters in the genital region?

*Patient Case Question 3.* What is the significance of the lack of use of spermicides, douches, or deodorant tampons?

*Patient Case Question 4.* What is the significance of the lack of use of any type of barrier contraceptive, like a diaphragm?

*Patient Case Question 5.* What is the significance of the lack of lower abdominal or pelvic pain?

## ■■ Past Medical History

- History of genital herpes, 2 years ago
- History of syphilis, 6 years ago
- Gravida 0
- No surgeries
- Immunizations current except for tetanus

***Patient Case Question 6.*** What is the significance of the patient's past medical history?

## ■■ Family History

- Father recently was treated with balloon angioplasty for peripheral vascular disease in femoral artery
- Mother has psoriasis, no other chronic conditions
- Two brothers are alive and healthy

## ■■ Social History

- Denies use of tobacco products
- Has several beers on weekends
- Works as a paralegal at local law firm
- Does not seek routine medical care because she "does not have very good health coverage at this time"

## ■■ Review of Systems

Patient denies headache, fever, rash, joint discomfort/redness/swelling, and muscle pain

***Patient Case Question 7.*** What is the significance of the information provided in the review of systems directly above?

## ■■ Medications

- Uses birth control pills
- Self-treats with acetaminophen for occasional menstrual cramps

## ■■ Allergies

- "Cedar fever" (allergy to mountain juniper)
- Demerol—"makes me goofy"

# ■■ Physical Examination and Laboratory Tests

## General Appearance

The patient is a healthy-looking, tall, slim, young white woman in no apparent distress; very talkative, quick to answer questions, and appears both slightly nervous and angry; wears glasses; alert and oriented

## Vital Signs

See Patient Case Table 64.1

| Patient Case Table 64.1 Vital Signs | | | | | | | |
|---|---|---|---|---|---|---|---|
| BP | 108/76 | RR | 12 | Ht | 5'11" |
| HR | 65 | T | 99.5°F | Wt | 117 lbs |

***Patient Case Question 8.*** Does the patient have any abnormal vital signs that could be related to her condition?

## Skin

- No rashes or other lesions
- Very warm and dry

## Head, Eyes, Ears, Nose, and Throat

- No signs of eye infection
- Funduscopic exam normal
- Tympanic membranes intact
- Mucous membranes moist and pink
- No erythema or edema of pharynx or oral ulcers
- Good dentition

***Patient Case Question 9.*** What is the significance of the finding that there are no signs of an eye infection?

## Neck and Lymph Nodes

- No cervical lymphadenopathy
- Neck supple
- No thyromegaly or carotid bruits

## Lungs

- Normal breath sounds
- Both lungs resonant
- Good air entry

## Cardiac

- Regular cardiac rate and rhythm
- Two clear heart sounds
- No murmurs

## Abdomen

- No tenderness, rebound, or guarding
- No hepatomegaly or splenomegaly

---

***Patient Case Question 10.*** What is the significance of the negative abdominal findings above?

---

## Genitalia

- No lesions visible on vulva
- Vagina with moderate amount of thick, yellow-white discharge and mild erythema
- Cervix shows erythema and moderate yellow-white discharge from cervical os
- No masses on bimanual exam
- Cervical motion tenderness present

## Musculoskeletal and Extremities

- No inguinal or axillary lymphadenopathy
- No rashes or other lesions, cyanosis, clubbing, or edema
- Muscle strength and tone normal
- Full range of motion throughout

## Neurologic

- Cranial nerves II–XII intact
- Patellar deep tendon reflexes grade 2+ bilaterally

## Laboratory Blood Test Results

See Patient Case Table 64.2

| Patient Case Table 64.2 Laboratory Blood Test Results | | | |
|---|---|---|---|
| Sodium | 137 meq/L | Glucose, fasting | 109 mg/dL |
| Potassium | 4.9 meq/L | Hemoglobin | 12.1 g/dL |
| Chloride | 107 meq/L | Hematocrit | 36% |
| Blood urea nitrogen | 19 mg/dL | Platelets | 410,000/mm$^3$ |
| Creatinine | 0.8 mg/dL | White blood cells | 12,750/mm$^3$ |

---

***Patient Case Question 11.*** Does the patient have any signs of renal failure?

***Patient Case Question 12.*** Which of the laboratory blood test results in Table 64.2 is abnormal and why is this abnormal finding consistent with the diagnosis?

# Examination of Cervical-Vaginal Discharge

- No yeast or hyphae seen
- Increased white blood cells
- Positive for intracellular gram-negative diplococci
- Ligase chain reaction positive for both *N. gonorrhoeae* and *C. trachomatis*

***Patient Case Question 13.*** Based on the information above, what is your assessment of this patient's condition?

***Patient Case Question 14.*** Is timing of possible exposure consistent with the incubation period for *N. gonorrhoeae*?

***Patient Case Question 15.*** How should this patient be treated pharmacologically?

***Patient Case Question 16.*** Is an HIV test appropriate in this patient?

# 65  ENDOMETRIOSIS

 *For the Disease Summary for this case study,
see the CD-ROM.*

## PATIENT CASE

### ■ Initial History

P.N. is a 29-year-old white female who presents to her gynecologist complaining of severe lower abdominal cramps that were poorly responsive to OTC ibuprofen or acetaminophen. She has been married for nine years and has two sons, ages 6 and 3 years. She and her husband would like to try to have a daughter as soon as possible. Menses began yesterday and the pain has lasted for about 72 hours. She reports that she had a similar episode of pain just before her last menses but that the pain subsided with the end of her period. She also complains of sharp, deep pain during sex, mild lower back pain, and pain with urination during the past two weeks. The patient denies blood in the stool, pain with defecation, heavy periods, intermenstrual bleeding, diarrhea, and constipation. P.N. began having her periods at 13 years of age.

### ■ Past Medical History

With the exception of typical childhood diseases like measles and chickenpox and one urinary tract infection four years ago, P.N. has been relatively healthy. She also had an episode of rheumatic fever at age 10, but there were no complications. Her mother has a history of hypertension and cancer. Her father has a history of hypertension, kidney stones, and genital herpes. Before her recent death, her maternal grandmother had a history of leukemia, breast cancer, and endometriosis.

### ■ Lifestyle History

P.N. eats a low-fat diet and tries to watch her weight. She exercises regularly (two 30-minute walks each day), plays softball, and participates in a women's bowling league. She does not smoke or drink alcohol. She is not taking any prescription medications, but occasionally uses naproxen for headaches. She has had some heartburn lately that is becoming more troublesome and will see her internal medicine physician about it next week.

# Physical Examination and Laboratory Tests

The patient is an alert female in mild acute distress. Her vital signs were: T = 37°C orally; P = 80 and regular; RR = 15 and unlabored; BP = 125/75 right arm, sitting; Wt = 115 lbs; Ht = 5′7″

---

***Patient Case Question 1.*** Are any of this patient's vital signs abnormal?

***Patient Case Question 2.*** Is the patient technically *underweight, overweight, obese,* or is this patient's weight considered *normal and healthy?*

---

## HEENT, Skin, Neck

- PERRLA and fundi are without hemorrhages or exudates
- Pharynx is clear
- Tympanic membranes intact
- Skin is dry and pink without rashes
- No cervical adenopathy

## Lungs, Cardiac

- Good chest excursion
- Lungs clear to auscultation and percussion
- RRR with distinct $S_1$ and $S_2$ sounds; no murmurs, rubs, or gallops

## Abdomen, Extremities

- Abdomen soft without organomegaly; tender in lower quadrant bilaterally
- Extremities with full pulses and without edema

## Breasts, Pelvic

- Breasts symmetric without masses, tenderness, discoloration, retraction of nipple, or nipple discharge; axillae without adenopathy
- Pelvic exam revealed tender cervical nodules; Pap pending

## Neurologic

- Oriented and alert; slightly anxious
- Strength 5/5 bilaterally
- Sensation normal and symmetric
- DTRs 2+ and symmetric
- Gait normal
- Cranial nerves II–XII intact

---

***Patient Case Question 3.*** Does this patient have any risk factors for endometriosis?

***Patient Case Question 4.*** Identify *two* clinical signs from the physical examination that are consistent with endometriosis?

## Laboratory Blood Test Results

See Patient Case Table 65.1

| Patient Case Table 65.1 Laboratory Blood Test Results | | | |
|---|---|---|---|
| Na$^+$ | 144 meq/L | RBC | 5.0 million/mm$^3$ |
| K$^+$ | 4.7 meq/L | WBC | 11,400/mm$^3$ |
| Ca$^{+2}$ | 9.1 mg/dL | WBC differential: Neutrophils 80%, Lymphocytes 14%, Monocytes/Macrophages 4%, Eosinophils 1%, Basophils 1% | |
| Glucose, fasting | 99 mg/dL | Plt | 300,000/mm$^3$ |
| Hct | 35% | ESR | 17 mm/hr |

*Patient Case Question 5.* Identify the *three* abnormal laboratory blood test results in Table 65.1.

*Patient Case Question 6.* Explain why the three abnormal laboratory test results identified above are consistent with a diagnosis of endometriosis.

*Patient Case Question 7.* Why might a magnetic resonance imaging scan be appropriate and beneficial to this patient?

*Patient Case Question 8.* Nafarelin is a nasal spray that is often prescribed for endometriosis to relieve pain. It acts by suppressing ovulation. What is the precise pharmacologic mechanism of action of this drug?

*Patient Case Question 9.* Explain the pathophysiology behind the lower back pain and pain with urination in this patient.

*Patient Case Question 10.* A magnetic resonance imaging scan clearly shows lesions in the ovaries, fallopian tubes, bladder, cervix, and uterine ligaments. The gynecologist suspects that the cause of P.N.'s pain is endometriosis. How might the gynecologist best confirm her diagnosis?

*Patient Case Question 11.* Explain the pharmacologic mechanism for why oral contraceptives may relieve the pain of endometriosis.

*Patient Case Question 12.* Why does danazol cause hirsutism, decreased breast size, and hot flashes as side effects of therapy for endometriosis?

*Patient Case Question 13.* Why is the patient's denial of diarrhea significant?

# CASE STUDY

# 66

## MENOPAUSE AND HORMONE REPLACEMENT THERAPY

 *For the Disease Summary for this case study, see the CD-ROM.*

# PATIENT CASE

## ■ Patient's Chief Complaints

"I've been having hot flashes for the last three or four months. They are becoming more frequent and definitely more annoying. Sometimes, they keep me up most of the night and then I am either dead tired or very irritable at work the next day. I can't have reached menopause already, can I? I'm only 45."

## ■ History of Present Condition

A.H. is a 45 yo white woman who reports experiencing hot flushes (sometimes associated with headache) that have been intensifying for the past 3–4 months. She has hot flushes several times each day and is frequently awakened at night with night sweats. Removing blankets from the bed and turning down the thermostat at night have not seemed to bring her any relief. She heard from several older friends that she can take medication for these symptoms, but she is most concerned about "getting her period back." Her LMP was 8–9 months ago after several months of erratic menstrual cycles.

*Patient Case Question 1.* Based on the information provided above, can a diagnosis of menopause be definitively established?

## ■ Past Medical History

- Menarche at age 12½ years
- Appendectomy at age 17 years
- 20-year history of alcohol abuse; has spent time in detoxification centers and sought help through personal counseling for alcohol use and Alcoholic Anonymous in the past
- Tubal ligation at age 24 years
- History of major depression with several suicide attempts (alcohol + pills); has been successfully treated in the past with fluoxetine

313

- 12-year history of systemic lupus erythematosus that has included multiple remissions and relapses; skin lesions (vasculitis), joint soreness, and sensitivity to sunlight have been especially problematic for her
- Normal mammogram and Pap smear 3 years ago
- Denies personal history of migraines, gallbladder disease, deep venous thrombosis, cerebrovascular disease, or heart disease
- Denies personal or family history of breast cancer

## ■■■ Family History

- Parents are deceased; father died from metastatic pancreatic cancer to bone and mother died from complications secondary to alcoholic cirrhosis
- Mother's menopause occurred at age 46 years
- Remaining family history is non-contributory

## ■■■ Social History

- Patient is seventh born of nine children
- Graduated from high school
- Parents were both alcoholics and, at one time, all children were removed from the home and placed in the custody of the state
- Patient was moved through several foster homes and one Catholic girls' home as an adolescent
- Claims that she had been beaten severely by one of her foster mothers and raped by an uncle
- Has been married and divorced twice with two children; son and daughter live with their father in another state
- Admits to realizing that she was gay at age 16; currently resides with lesbian girlfriend
- Drinks 4–5 beers and smokes 1 pack of cigarettes daily; has smoked since age 16
- Denies ever having used recreational drugs
- Works as a nursing assistant at a local nursing home
- Has no regular exercise program "(I get all the exercise I need running around at the nursing home everyday.")
- Does not take calcium or vitamin supplements

## ■■■ Review of Systems

- Denies vaginal itching, burning, or abnormal discharge
- Reports not having "much of an appetite most of the time"
- Denies shortness of breath, pain, urinary frequency, urinary urgency, bladder incontinence, recent genitourinary tract infections, chest pain, and transient ischemic attacks
- Has experienced intermittent episodes of transient migratory arthritis for years; her immunology specialist has told her that these attacks are related to lupus
- Admits to having "smoker's cough"

## ■■■ Medications

St. John's Wort, 300 mg po TID for the last 2 months (purchased at Walmart; someone told her that it would "make her feel happier")

*Patient Case Question 2.* Identify the *two* most likely risk factors for the patient's early menopause.

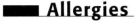

## Allergies

NKDA

## Physical Examination and Laboratory Tests

### General

The patient is a pale and thin white female who appears to be in NAD. She is alert and cooperative. There are multiple skin lesions on her arms.

### Vital Signs

See Patient Case Table 66.1

| Patient Case Table 66.1 Vital Signs | | | | | |
|---|---|---|---|---|---|
| BP | 132/86 | RR | 18 | HT | 5 ft–5½ in |
| HR | 76 | T | 97.5°F | WT | 113 lbs |

### Skin

- Pale, cool, and dry with multiple erythematous, scaling lesions on upper extremities
- Normal turgor

### Head, Eyes, Ears, Nose, and Throat

- Pupils equal, round, and responsive to light
- Fundi with sharp discs and without hemorrhages, exudates, or papilledema
- Extra-ocular muscles intact
- TMs intact
- Mucous membranes moist
- No pharyngeal edema or erythema
- No lateral deviation of tongue

### Neck, Lymph Nodes

- Neck supple
- No carotid bruits, cervical lymphadenopathy, or JVD
- No palpable thyroid masses or diffuse thyromegaly

### Chest, Lungs

- Good chest excursion
- Lungs clear to auscultation and percussion
- No wheezes, crackles, or rubs

### Heart

- RRR
- Normal $S_1$ and $S_2$

- No S$_3$ or S$_4$
- No m/r/g

## Abdomen

- Soft, NT/ND
- (+) BS
- (−) masses, organomegaly, or bruits
- Ovaries are not palpable

## Breasts

- Symmetric without masses, dimpling, discoloration, tenderness, or nipple discharge
- Axillae without adenopathy

## Genitalia, Rectum

- Normal female genitalia
- Pelvic exam normal except (+) for mild vaginal mucosal atrophy
- Stool guaiac (−)
- Normal sphincter tone
- Pap pending

## Musculoskeletal, Extremities

- (−) CCE
- Peripheral pulses full at 2+
- Joint examination reveals no active synovitis or arthritis
- Wrists, elbows, hips, shoulders, ankles, and knees have normal ROM

## Neurologic

- Oriented × 3
- Strength and sensation normal and symmetric
- DTRs (biceps, triceps, and patella) 2+ and symmetric
- Gait normal
- Memory intact
- CNs intact
- Negative Babinski

*Patient Case Question 3.* Clinical *symptoms* are subjective manifestations of a health condition that can only be reported by the patient (e.g., pain). Identify all of the clinical symptoms above that are consistent with a diagnosis of menopause.

*Patient Case Question 4.* Clinical *signs* are objective manifestations of a health condition that can be observed and reported by someone other than the patient, often a physician or nurse (e.g., rash). Identify all of the clinical signs above that are consistent with a diagnosis of menopause.

## Laboratory Blood Test Results

See Patient Case Table 66.2

## Patient Case Table 66.2 Laboratory Blood Test Results

| | | | | | |
|---|---|---|---|---|---|
| Na | 140 meq/L | WBC | $7.4 \times 10^3/mm^3$ | T bilirubin | 0.4 mg/dL |
| K | 4.1 meq/L | Plt | $361 \times 10^3/mm^3$ | Alb | 2.8 g/dL |
| Cl | 100 meq/L | Ca | 9.6 mg/dL | T protein | 5.7 g/dL |
| $HCO_3$ | 26 meq/L | Mg | 2.5 mg/dL | T cholesterol | 150 mg/dL |
| BUN | 55 mg/dL | $PO_4$ | 2.7 mg/dL | LDL | 128 mg/dL |
| Cr | 1.5 mg/dL | AST | 13 IU/L | HDL | 46 mg/dL |
| Glu, fasting | 86 mg/dL | ALT | 23 IU/L | Trig | 140 mg/dL |
| Hb | 12.0 g/dL | GGT | 60 IU/L | TSH | 2.2 μU/mL |
| Hct | 37.1% | Alk phos | 110 IU/L | FSH | 43.7 mU/mL |

## Urinalysis

See Patient Case Table 66.3

## Patient Case Table 66.3 Urinalysis

| | | | | | |
|---|---|---|---|---|---|
| *Color:* | Yellow-orange | *Bilirubin:* | (−) | *Protein:* | (+) |
| *Appearance:* | Mildly cloudy | *SG:* | 1.020 | *Blood:* | (+) |
| *Glucose:* | (−) | *pH:* | 5.5 | *Bacteria:* | (−) |
| *Ketones:* | (−) | *Nitrites:* | (−) | | |

## Mammogram

Consistent with perimenopause without masses or abnormal calcifications

## DEXA Scans

- Lumbar spine: L2–4, bone density = 671 mg/cm², T = −2.4
- Neck of right femur: bone density = 719 mg/cm², T = −2.2

*Assessment by radiologist*: DEXA scans are consistent with significant osteopenia bordering on osteoporosis

*Patient Case Question 5.* Does this patient have any laboratory evidence of hepatic disease?

*Patient Case Question 6.* Does this patient have any laboratory evidence of renal disease?

*Patient Case Question 7.* If the serum total protein concentration becomes too low, widespread swelling is often prominent. Briefly describe the pathophysiologic mechanism that underlies this phenomenon.

*Patient Case Question 8.* Does this patient have any laboratory evidence of thyroid disease?

*Patient Case Question 9.* Does the patient's CBC show any significant abnormalities?

*Patient Case Question 10.* Does this patient have any laboratory evidence of dyslipidemia?

*Patient Case Question 11.* What is the *single* most revealing laboratory evidence that menopause is imminent?

*Patient Case Question 12.* Identify *two* clinical indications for the justified use of hormone replacement therapy in this patient.

*Patient Case Question 13.* Identify *three* risk factors—other than menopause—that place this patient at increased risk over the general population for the development of osteoporosis.

*Patient Case Question 14.* Does this patient have any obvious contraindications for estrogen therapy?

# 67

# OVARIAN CANCER

 *For the Disease Summary for this case study, see the CD-ROM.*

## PATIENT CASE

### ■ HPI

W.D. is a 68-year-old woman who presented to the hospital emergency room three months ago with a 3-day history of acute abdominal pain. She also reported a weight gain of approximately 5 lbs during the previous three months despite a loss in appetite. Ultrasound and CT scans of the abdomen and pelvis revealed a relatively large, non-cystic, soft-tissue pelvic mass in the left lower quadrant. Multiple solid lesions were also seen in both kidneys and the liver. A chest x-ray was positive for several suspicious ½-inch masses in the lower lobe of the right lung. Laparoscopic surgery revealed a 3½-inch × 1¾-inch mass in the left ovary with positive involvement of the bilateral external iliac nodes. Tumor biopsies from the left ovary, kidneys, lymph nodes, and liver were positive for epithelial ovarian cancer. Serum CA-125 concentration was 190 units/mL. A hysterectomy, lymphadenectomy, and bilateral salpingo-oophorectomy were performed to debulk the tumor. Now she has been admitted to the Special Procedures Unit to undergo her first cycle of systemic chemotherapy.

*Patient Case Question 1.* Why is chemotherapy necessary if this patient has been recently treated with extensive surgery?

*Patient Case Question 2.* What combination of chemotherapeutic agents is appropriate for this patient?

### ■ PMH

- Menarche at age 11 years, menopause at age 54 years
- Asthma diagnosed at age 3 years, resolved at age 15 years
- Endometriosis diagnosed 15 years ago
- Hypertension diagnosed 6 years ago
- Seizure disorder beginning 4 years ago following a major motor vehicle accident in which patient sustained serious head trauma; she is currently well controlled with anti-seizure medication and has been seizure-free for 24 months
- Surgical history includes cholecystectomy for gallstones and cholecystitis

## FH

- Separated from husband of 27 years with no children
- Mother and maternal aunt passed away from ovarian cancer
- Father has hyperlipidemia, hypertension, and advanced coronary artery disease
- Maternal grandmother died from complications of cervical cancer at age 53

## SH

- Smokes 1 pack of cigarettes/day, has smoked for 9 years
- Lives alone
- Denies alcohol and drug abuse
- Has been a strict vegetarian for 6 years
- Currently not sexually active

## Meds

- Carbamazepine 200 mg po TID
- Amlodipine besylate 2.5 mg po QD

*Patient Case Question 3.* Identify *four* of this patient's risk factors for ovarian cancer.

*Patient Case Question 4.* Why is this patient taking carbamazepine?

*Patient Case Question 5.* Why is this patient taking amlodipine besylate?

## All

- Lupus-like syndrome with hydralazine
- Aspirin causes stomach cramps

## ROS

The patient denies fatigue, bloating, constipation, urinary urgency, vaginal bleeding, and sensation of pelvic pressure.

## PE and Lab Tests

### VS

See Patient Case Table 67.1

| Patient Case Table 67.1 Vital Signs | | | | | |
|---|---|---|---|---|---|
| BP | 128/84 | RR | 16 and unlabored | Wt | 130 lbs |
| P | 82 | T | 98.6°F | Ht | 5'3½" |

*Patient Case Question 6.* Are there any abnormal vital signs?

## Skin

Warm and dry without lesions, good turgor

## Neck/LN

Supple without adenopathy, masses, goiter, or bruits

## HEENT

- PERRLA
- EOMI
- Benign fundi
- TMs WNL bilaterally
- Moist and pink mucous membranes in oral pharynx
- Good dentition

---

***Patient Case Question 7.*** What is the significance of the *benign fundi* finding?

---

## Breasts

No masses, discharge, axillary adenopathy, nipple or skin abnormalities

## Lungs

Clear to auscultation bilaterally and resonant throughout all lung fields

## Cardiac

RRR with normal $S_1$ and $S_2$; no murmurs, friction rubs, or gallops

## Abd

- Soft with normal BS
- No bruits or organomegaly

## Genit/Rec

- Normal female genitalia
- Heme (−) dark brown stool
- No rectal wall tenderness or masses
- No vaginal discharge or lesions

## Ext

No CCE

## Neuro

- Speech, normal
- CNs II–XII intact

- Strength 5/5 throughout
- Reflexes 2+ and symmetric throughout
- Negative Babinski
- Cerebellar: finger-to-nose normal
- Rapid movements normal
- Fine motor coordination WNL
- Good sitting and standing balance
- Gait: normal speed and step length
- Cognition: A & O × 3
- Short- and long-term memories intact

*Patient Case Question 8.* Why is this comprehensive neurologic examination appropriate?

## Laboratory Blood Test Results

See Patient Case Table 67.2

| Patient Case Table 67.2 Laboratory Blood Test Results | | | | | |
|---|---|---|---|---|---|
| Na | 138 meq/L | Cr | 1.8 mg/dL | WBC | 7,800/mm³ |
| K | 4.7 meq/L | Glu, fasting | 105 mg/dL | AST | 32 IU/L |
| Cl | 100 meq/L | Hb | 12.7 g/dL | ALT | 30 IU/L |
| HCO₃ | 24 meq/L | Hct | 43% | T bilirubin | 0.9 mg/dL |
| BUN | 26 mg/dL | Plt | 160,000/mm³ | CA-125 | 93 units/mL |

*Patient Case Question 9.* With the exception of CA-125, identify *two* laboratory blood test results that are abnormal and suggest a reasonable explanation.

*Patient Case Question 10.* Which *three* test results suggest that liver function is normal?

*Patient Case Question 11.* Explain the altered CA-125 with respect to the patient's first CA-125 test.

# 68

# PELVIC INFLAMMATORY DISEASE

 *For the Disease Summary for this case study,*
*see the CD-ROM.*

## PATIENT CASE

### ■ Patient's Chief Complaints

"I've had increasing pain in my stomach for almost two days now and I think that I have a fever. I've also had occasional chills and I threw up once last night. I think that I have a virus of some kind."

### ■ HPI

Ms. P.C. is a 19-year-old white female who reports a 2-day history of lower abdominal pain, nausea, emesis × 1, and a heavy, malodorous vaginal discharge. She states that she is single, heterosexual, and that she has been sexually active with only one partner for the past eight months. She has no previous history of genitourinary infections or sexually transmitted diseases. She denies IV drug use. Her LMP ended three days ago. Her last intercourse (vaginal) was eight days ago and she states that they did not use a condom. She admits to unprotected sex "every once in a while." She noted an abnormal vaginal discharge yesterday and she describes it as "thick, greenish-yellow in color, and very smelly." She denies both oral and rectal intercourse. She does not know if her partner has had a recent genitourinary tract infection, "because he has been away on business for five days."

### ■ PMH

* Seizure disorder × 3 years
* Migraine headaches, 1–2 per month for 2½ years
* Denies any pregnancies, elective abortions, and miscarriages

### ■ FH

Both parents and older sister are "all healthy as far as I know"

## ■■■ SH

- Denies nicotine, caffeine, and recreational drug use
- Occasional glass of wine or wine cooler
- Uses birth control pills and occasional use of a condom for "double protection," but no diaphragms, IUDs, or spermicides
- No routine medical care because she "doesn't have a good health insurance plan yet"
- Denies that sexual partner sleeps with other women
- Admits to vaginal douching, but only "once in a while"

## ■■■ ROS

Occasional painful menses

## ■■■ Meds

- Phenytoin 100 mg po TID
- Sumatriptan 50 mg po PRN
- Acetaminophen ES PRN for headaches and menstrual cramps
- Ortho-Novum 1/35 28

***Patient Case Question 1.*** Why is this patient taking phenytoin?

***Patient Case Question 2.*** Why is this patient taking sumatriptan?

***Patient Case Question 3.*** Why is this patient taking Ortho-Novum 1/35 28?

***Patient Case Question 4.*** Identify *two* risk factors that predispose this patient to PID.

## ■■■ All

- PCN → allergy as a child
- NSAIDs → GI intolerance

## ■■■ PE and Lab Tests

### Gen

- Alert, WDWN white female with moderate-to-severe lower abdominal pain
- Appears to be her stated age
- Pain index at 7–8/10

### VS

See Patient Case Table 68.1

| Patient Case Table 68.1 Vital Signs | | | | | | | |
|---|---|---|---|---|---|---|---|
| BP | | 150/95 | RR | | 15 | HT | 5'4½" |
| P | | 125 | T | | 102.6°F | WT | 117 lbs |

***Patient Case Question 5.*** Briefly describe the pathophysiology for the *three* abnormal vital signs in Table 68.1.

## Skin

* Diffuse pallor
* Warm and slightly diaphoretic with no lesions or rashes

***Patient Case Question 6.*** Briefly describe the pathophysiology for the pale and slightly diaphoretic skin observed in this patient.

## HEENT

* Head is NC/AT
* PERRLA, pupils at 3 mm
* EOMI
* TMs intact
* Nares are clear bilaterally
* Throat shows no erythema, exudates, or lesions
* Mucous membranes in oropharynx are moist

## Neck/LN

* Neck supple and non-tender
* Shotty cervical and submandibular lymphadenopathy
* Thyroid not enlarged

***Patient Case Question 7.*** In view of this patient's illness, briefly describe the pathophysiology that underlies lymphadenopathy in this case.

## Chest

Good, clear breath sounds throughout

## Breasts

Mild fibrocystic changes, otherwise unremarkable

## Cardiac

* Sinus tachycardia
* Normal $S_1$ and $S_2$
* No $S_3$ or $S_4$ heard
* No murmurs

## Abd

- Guarding of both right and left lower quadrants with palpation
- (+) bilateral adnexal tenderness
- Bowel sounds present in all quadrants
- (−) HSM and bruits

## Genit/Rec

- Vulva: moderate erythema with no lesions visible
- Vagina: large amount of thick, malodorous, yellow-green discharge and moderate erythema with no lesions visible
- Cervix: moderate-to-severe erythema and significant yellow-green discharge around os with no lesions visible
- (+) cervical motion tenderness

## MS/Ext

- Pedal pulses 2+
- Shotty inguinal adenopathy
- No lesions or rashes
- Normal ROM
- Muscle strength 5/5 throughout

## Neuro

- A & O × 3
- CNs II–XII intact
- Sensory and motor levels intact
- (−) Babinski
- DTRs 2+
- Normal gait

***Patient Case Question 8.*** Can a diagnosis of PID be made based on the clinical manifestations of the illness at this point? Why or why not?

## Laboratory Test Results

See Patient Case Table 68.2

| Patient Case Table 68.2 Laboratory Test Results | | | | | |
|---|---|---|---|---|---|
| Na | 140 meq/L | Hb | 14.2 g/dL | • Neutros | 73% |
| K | 4.4 meq/L | Hct | 39% | • Bands | 10% |
| Cl | 104 meq/L | Plt | $270 \times 10^3/mm^3$ | • Lymphs | 13% |
| $HCO_3$ | 30 meq/L | ESR | 21 mm/hr | • Monos | 3% |
| BUN | 20 mg/dL | CRP | 2.3 mg/dL | • Eos | 1% |
| Cr | 1.1 mg/dL | Ca | 8.4 mg/dL | Complement fixation test for *C. trachomatis* | (−) |
| Glu, fasting | 125 mg/dL | WBC | $14.75 \times 10^3/mm^3$ | Urine pregnancy test | (−) |

*Patient Case Question 9.* Why is the patient's serum glucose concentration abnormal?

*Patient Case Question 10.* What does the abnormal white blood cell differential suggest?

*Patient Case Question 11.* Define "band cells" and describe the pathophysiology that underlies their abnormal number in the blood.

*Patient Case Question 12.* What is the significance of this patient's ESR and CRP?

## UA

See Patient Case Table 68.3

| Patient Case Table 68.3 Urinalysis | | | | | |
|---|---|---|---|---|---|
| pH | 6.4 | WBC/HPF | 2 | Gram stain | (−) |
| SG | 1.021 | RBC/HPF | 0 | | |

*Patient Case Question 13.* What is the significance of this patient's urinalysis?

## Microscopic Examination of Vaginal Discharge

- (−) yeast or hyphae
- (−) flagellated microbes
- (+) white blood cells
- (+) gram-negative intracellular diplococci

*Patient Case Question 14.* Which type of infection is suggested by microscopic examination of the vaginal discharge and other laboratory tests: chlamydial, gonococcal, or mixed chlamydial/gonococcal?

*Patient Case Question 15.* Should this patient be hospitalized and promptly given IV antibiotics? Why or why not?

## ▬ HPI: Patient's Sexual Partner

Upon return from his business trip, the patient's sexual partner, Mr. Y.V., presented to a health clinic with complaints of "several days of painful urination and an increasing amount of a thick, yellowish fluid from my penis." He admits to being sexually active with three frequent partners and to unprotected sex at least twice in the past two weeks. His PMH includes two episodes of urethritis secondary to an STD in the last two years. With the exception of a thick urethral discharge that was positive for WBC and showed gram-negative intracellular diplococci, the patient's limited physical examination was unremarkable.

*Patient Case Question 16.* Based on this sexual partner's history of present illness, identify one more very significant risk factor for PID.

PREMENSTRUAL SYNDROME

*For the Disease Summary for this case study,
see the CD-ROM.*

# PATIENT CASE

## ■ Patient's Chief Complaints

"I've really been feeling out of sorts lately. Just before my period, I feel irritable and my breasts are very sore. This has been going on now for three months."

## ■ History of Present Illness

P.E. is a 34 yo woman who was referred to the PMS clinic by her OB-GYN specialist. She states that she has a 3-month history of premenstrual symptoms that include irritability and breast tenderness. When questioned further, she also confirms that she has had cravings for salty snacks lately and, generally, she dislikes them. These symptoms have been recurrent and predictable for the last three menstrual periods, usually occur during the entire week prior to menses, and invariably resolve approximately two days after her menstrual flow has begun. She states that she has not been bothered by these symptoms during the remainder of her menstrual cycle. Her menstrual cycle has been remarkably predictable at 27–28 days for the last two years. She brought to the clinic the daily calendar that she has been asked to complete as documentation of her symptoms.

## ■ Patient's Documentation

For patient's 3-month documentation of clinical manifestations (August through October), see Patient Case Table 69.1.

## ■ Past Medical History

- Severe UTI, 14 years ago
- Tubal ligation after her second child, 10 years ago
- Ovarian cyst removed 8 years ago
- S/P ultrasonic renal lithotripsy secondary to nephrolithiasis, 5½ years ago
- Eczema × 5 years
- GERD × 2 years
- Acute sinusitis, 1 year ago

## Patient Case Table 69.1 Patient's 3-Month Documentation of Clinical Manifestations (August through October)

(Adapted with permission from Freeman EW, DeRubeis RJ, Rickels K. Reliability and validity of a daily diary for premenstrual syndrome. Psychiatry Res 1996;65:97–106.)

### August

| DAY | A | B | C | D | E | F | G | H | I | J | K | L | M | N | O | P | Q | R | S | T | U | V | W | X |
|---|---|---|---|---|---|---|---|---|---|---|---|---|---|---|---|---|---|---|---|---|---|---|---|---|
| 1 | | | | | | | | | | | | | | | | | | | | | | | | |
| 2 | | | | | | | | | | | | | | | | | | | | | | | | |
| 3 | | | | | | | | | | | | | | | | | | | | | | | | |
| 4 | | | | | | | | | | | | | | | | | | | | | | | | |
| 5 | | | | | | | | | | | | | | | | | | | | | | | | |
| 6 | | | | | | | | | | | 1 | | | | | | | | | 1 | | | | 2 |
| 7 | | | | | | | | | | | 1 | | 1 | | | | | | | 1 | | | | 3 |
| 8 | | | | | | | | | | | 2 | | 1 | | | | | | | 1 | | | | 4 |
| 9 | | | | | | | | | | | 2 | | 2 | | | | | | | 2 | | | | 6 |
| 10 | | | | | | | | | | | 2 | | 2 | | | | | | | 3 | | | | 7 |
| 11 | | | | | | | | | | | 3 | | 3 | | | | | | | 4 | | | 3 | 13 |
| 12* | | | | | | | | | | | 4 | | 2 | | | | | | | 4 | | | | 10 |
| 13 | | | | | | | | | | | 2 | | | | | | | | | 2 | | | | 4 |
| 14 | | | | | | | | | | | | | | | | | | | | | | | | |
| 15 | | | | | | | | | | | | | | | | | | | | | | | | |
| 16 | | | | | | | | | | | | | | | | | | | | | | | | |
| 17 | | | | | | | | | | | | | | | | | | | | | | | | |
| 18 | | | | | | | | | | | | | | | | | | | | | | | | |
| 19 | | | | | | | | | | | | | | | | | | | | | | | | |
| 20 | | | | | | | | | | | | | | | | | | | | | | | | |
| 21 | | | | | | | | | | | | | | | | | | | | | | | | |
| 22 | | | | | | | | | | | | | | | | | | | | | | | | |
| 23 | | | | | | | | | | | | | | | | | | | | | | | | |
| 24 | | | | | | | | | | | | | | | | | | | | | | | | |
| 25 | | | | | | | | | | | | | | | | | | | | | | | | |
| 26 | | | | | | | 2 | | | | | | | | | | | | | | | | | 2 |
| 27 | | | | | | | | | | | | | | | | | | | | | | | | |
| 28 | | | | | | | | | | | | | | | | | | | | | | | | |
| 29 | | | | | | | | | | | | | | | | | | | | | | | | |
| 30 | | | | | | | | | | | | | | | | | | | | | | | | |
| 31 | | | | | | | | | | | | | | | | | | | | | | | | |

### September

| DAY | A | B | C | D | E | F | G | H | I | J | K | L | M | N | O | P | Q | R | S | T | U | V | W | X |
|---|---|---|---|---|---|---|---|---|---|---|---|---|---|---|---|---|---|---|---|---|---|---|---|---|
| 1 | | | | | | | | | | | | | | | | | | | | | | | | |
| 2 | | | | | | | | | | | | | | | | | | | | | | | | |
| 3 | | | | | | | | | | | 1 | | | | | | | | | | | | | 1 |
| 4 | | | | | | | | | | | 1 | | 1 | | | | | | | 1 | | | | 3 |
| 5 | | | | | | | | | | | 1 | | 1 | | | | | | | 2 | | | | 4 |
| 6 | | | | | | | | | | | 2 | | 1 | | | | | | | 2 | | | | 5 |
| 7 | | | | | | | | | | | 3 | | 2 | | | | | | | 3 | | | | 8 |
| 8 | | | | | | | | | | | 3 | | 3 | | | | | | | 4 | | | | 10 |
| 9* | | | | | | | | | | | 4 | | 2 | | | | | | | 3 | | | | 9 |
| 10 | | | | | | | | | | | 1 | | | | | | | | | 1 | | | | 2 |
| 11 | | | | | | | | | | | | | | | | | | | | | | | | |

*(Continued)*

## Patient Case Table 69.1 (*Continued*)

| DAY | A | B | C | D | E | F | G | H | I | J | K | L | M | N | O | P | Q | R | S | T | U | V | W | X |
|-----|---|---|---|---|---|---|---|---|---|---|---|---|---|---|---|---|---|---|---|---|---|---|---|---|
| 12 |  |  |  |  |  |  |  |  |  |  |  |  |  |  |  |  |  |  |  |  |  |  |  |  |
| 13 |  |  |  |  |  |  |  |  |  |  |  |  |  |  |  |  |  |  |  |  |  |  |  |  |
| 14 |  |  |  |  |  |  |  |  | 3 |  |  |  |  |  |  |  |  |  |  | 2 |  |  |  | 5 |
| 15 |  |  |  |  |  |  |  |  | 3 |  |  |  |  |  |  |  |  |  |  | 2 |  |  |  | 5 |
| 16 |  |  |  |  |  |  |  |  |  |  |  |  |  |  |  |  |  |  |  |  |  |  |  |  |
| 17 |  |  |  |  |  |  |  |  |  |  |  |  |  |  |  |  |  |  |  |  |  |  |  |  |
| 18 |  |  |  |  |  |  |  |  |  |  |  |  |  |  |  |  |  |  |  |  |  |  |  |  |
| 19 |  |  |  |  |  |  |  |  |  |  |  |  |  |  |  |  |  |  |  |  |  |  |  |  |
| 20 |  |  |  |  |  |  |  |  |  |  |  |  |  |  |  |  |  |  |  |  |  |  |  |  |
| 21 |  |  |  |  |  |  |  |  |  |  |  |  |  |  |  |  |  |  |  |  |  |  |  |  |
| 22 |  |  |  |  |  |  |  |  |  |  |  |  |  |  |  |  |  |  |  |  |  |  |  |  |
| 23 |  |  |  |  |  |  |  |  |  |  |  |  |  |  |  |  |  |  |  |  |  |  |  |  |
| 24 |  |  |  |  |  |  |  |  |  |  |  |  |  |  |  |  |  |  |  |  |  |  |  |  |
| 25 |  |  |  |  |  |  |  |  |  |  |  |  |  |  |  |  |  |  |  |  |  |  |  |  |
| 26 |  |  |  |  |  |  |  |  |  |  |  |  |  |  |  |  |  |  |  |  |  |  |  |  |
| 27 |  |  |  |  |  |  |  |  |  |  |  |  |  |  |  |  |  |  |  |  |  |  |  |  |
| 28 |  |  |  |  |  |  |  |  |  |  |  |  |  |  |  |  |  |  |  |  |  |  |  |  |
| 29 |  |  |  |  |  |  |  |  |  |  |  |  |  |  |  |  |  |  |  |  |  |  |  |  |
| 30 |  |  |  |  |  |  |  |  |  |  |  |  |  |  |  |  |  |  |  |  |  |  |  |  |

### October

| DAY | A | B | C | D | E | F | G | H | I | J | K | L | M | N | O | P | Q | R | S | T | U | V | W | X |
|-----|---|---|---|---|---|---|---|---|---|---|---|---|---|---|---|---|---|---|---|---|---|---|---|---|
| 1 |  |  |  |  |  |  |  |  |  |  | 1 |  |  | 1 |  |  |  |  | 2 |  |  |  |  | 4 |
| 2 |  |  |  |  |  |  |  |  |  |  | 2 |  |  | 1 |  |  |  |  | 2 |  |  |  |  | 5 |
| 3 |  |  |  |  |  |  |  |  |  |  | 2 |  |  | 1 |  |  |  |  | 2 |  |  |  |  | 5 |
| 4 |  |  |  |  |  |  |  |  |  |  | 3 |  |  | 2 |  |  |  |  | 2 |  |  |  |  | 7 |
| 5 |  |  |  |  |  |  |  |  |  |  | 3 |  |  | 3 |  |  |  |  | 3 |  |  |  |  | 9 |
| 6 |  |  |  |  |  |  |  |  |  |  | 4 |  |  | 3 |  |  |  |  | 4 |  |  |  |  | 11 |
| 7* |  |  |  |  |  |  |  |  |  |  | 4 |  |  | 2 |  |  |  |  | 4 |  |  |  |  | 10 |
| 8 |  |  |  |  |  |  |  |  |  |  | 2 |  |  |  |  |  |  |  | 1 |  |  |  |  | 3 |
| 9 |  |  |  |  |  |  |  |  |  |  |  |  |  |  |  |  |  |  |  |  |  |  |  |  |
| 10 |  |  |  |  |  |  |  |  |  |  |  |  |  |  |  |  |  |  |  |  |  |  |  |  |
| 11 |  |  |  |  |  |  |  |  |  |  |  |  |  |  |  |  |  |  |  |  |  |  |  |  |
| 12 |  |  |  |  |  |  |  |  |  |  |  |  |  |  |  |  |  |  |  |  |  |  |  |  |
| 13 |  |  |  |  |  |  |  |  |  |  |  |  |  |  |  |  |  |  |  |  |  |  |  |  |
| 14 |  |  |  |  |  |  |  |  |  |  |  |  |  |  |  |  |  |  |  |  |  |  |  |  |
| 15 |  |  |  |  |  |  |  |  |  |  |  |  |  |  |  |  |  |  |  |  |  |  |  |  |
| 16 |  |  |  |  |  |  |  |  |  |  |  |  |  |  |  |  |  |  |  |  |  |  |  |  |
| 17 |  |  |  |  |  |  |  |  |  |  |  |  |  |  |  |  |  |  |  |  |  |  |  |  |
| 18 |  |  |  |  |  |  |  |  |  |  |  |  |  |  |  |  |  |  |  |  |  |  |  |  |
| 19 |  |  |  |  |  |  |  |  |  |  |  |  |  |  |  |  |  |  |  |  |  |  |  |  |
| 20 |  |  |  |  |  |  |  |  |  |  |  |  |  |  |  |  |  |  |  |  |  |  |  |  |
| 21 |  |  |  |  |  |  | 3 |  |  |  |  |  |  |  |  |  |  |  |  |  |  |  |  | 3 |
| 22 |  |  |  |  |  |  |  |  |  |  |  |  |  |  |  |  |  |  |  |  |  |  |  |  |
| 23 |  |  |  |  |  |  |  |  |  |  |  |  |  |  |  |  |  |  |  |  |  |  |  |  |
| 24 |  |  |  |  |  |  |  |  |  |  |  |  |  |  |  |  |  |  |  |  |  |  |  |  |
| 25 |  |  |  |  |  |  |  |  |  |  |  |  |  |  |  |  |  |  |  |  |  |  |  |  |
| 26 |  |  |  |  |  |  |  |  |  |  |  |  |  |  |  |  |  |  |  |  |  |  |  |  |

*(Continued)*

| DAY | A | B | C | D | E | F | G | H | I | J | K | L | M | N | O | P | Q | R | S | T | U | V | W | X |
|-----|---|---|---|---|---|---|---|---|---|---|---|---|---|---|---|---|---|---|---|---|---|---|---|---|
| 27 | | | | | | | | | | | | | | | | | | | | | | | | |
| 28 | | | | | | | | | | | | | | | | | | | | | | | | |
| 29 | | | | | | | | | | | | | | | | | | | | | | | | |
| 30 | | | | | | | | | | | | | | | | | | | | | | | | |
| 31 | | | | | | | | | | | | | | | | | | | | | | | | |

**Patient Case Table 69.1 (Continued)**

A Overeating
B Lack of energy
C Poor coordination
D Feeling overwhelmed
E Feeling out of control
F Crying spells
G Headache
H Swelling of ankles
I Anxiety
J Body aches

K Irritability
L Mood swings
M Bloating
N Food cravings
O Nervous tension
P Decreased interest in activities
Q Cramps
R Sadness, hopelessness, worthlessness
S Breast tenderness
T Sleep problems

U Difficulty concentrating
V Anger
W Interpersonal conflict
X Total daily score
1 Mild
2 Moderate
3 Severe
4 Very severe
*First day of menses

## Family History

- Father, 61, has hypercholesterolemia, HTN, CAD, glaucoma, and colonic polyps
- Mother, 55, had PMDD; became menopausal at age 44
- One brother, 31, is alive and well
- One sister, 30, has PMS

## Social History

- Married, mother of two healthy sons, ages 10 and 12
- Completed nursing school at a local hospital and is a registered nurse
- She walks on her treadmill three times each week and eats healthy
- She does not smoke and drinks alcohol only around holidays
- One cup decaffeinated coffee every morning and does not drink caffeinated soft drinks
- Socially active and volunteers extensively in the community
- Has had a strained relationship with her mother and a colleague at work for the past three months

## Physical Examination and Laboratory Tests

### General

- WDWN attractive, healthy-looking white female
- Appearance is well kept
- In conversation she seems alert, friendly, and courteous

### Vital Signs

See Patient Case Table 69.2

**Patient Case Table 69.2 Vital Signs**

| BP | 122/86 | RR | 15 | HT | 5′6½″ |
|----|--------|----|----|----|-------|
| P | 78 | T | 98.5°F | WT | 123 lbs |

## Skin

- Warm and dry with no rashes or lesions
- Fair complexion
- Color and turgor good

## HEENT

- NC/AT
- PERRLA
- EOMI
- Funduscopic exam shows no arteriolar narrowing, hemorrhages, or exudates
- TMs WNL bilaterally
- Nose and throat clear w/o exudates or lesions
- Mucous membranes moist

## Neck/Lymph Nodes

- Neck supple
- No palpable nodes
- Thyroid in mid-line and not enlarged
- No bruits or JVD

## Chest/Lungs

Clear to A & P bilaterally

## Heart

- RRR
- $S_1$ and $S_2$ normal
- No $S_3$ or $S_4$ heard
- No murmurs or rubs

## Abdomen

- Soft, NT/ND
- (+) BS
- No masses or organomegaly
- No guarding

## Breasts

Mild fibrocystic changes

## Genitalia/Rectum

Patient declined exam as she just had normal pelvic exam three weeks ago

## Musculoskeletal/Extremities

- Full ROM in all extremities
- Pedal pulses strong at 2+
- (−) CCE
- Muscle strength 5/5 throughout

## Neurologic

- WNL
- A & O × 3
- CNs II–XII intact
- DTRs 2+ and equal bilaterally
- Normal sensory and motor function
- Negative Babinski

## Laboratory Blood Test Results

See Patient Case Table 69.3

### Patient Case Table 69.3 Laboratory Blood Test Results

| Hb | 13.2 g/dL | MCHC | 33.7 g/dL | • Monos | 6% |
|---|---|---|---|---|---|
| Hct | 38.1% | Plt | $155 \times 10^3/mm^3$ | • Eos | 2% |
| RBC | $4.7 \times 10^6/mm^3$ | WBC | $5.2 \times 10^3/mm^3$ | • Basos | 1% |
| MCV | 97.7 fL | • Neutros | 62% | TSH | 1.7 µU/mL |
| MCH | 33.0 pg | • Lymphs | 29% | Glu, fasting | 98 mg/dL |

## Pap Smear

WNL

## Mammogram

WNL

***Patient Case Question 1.*** Identify this patient's most significant risk factor for premenstrual syndrome.

***Patient Case Question 2.*** Is hypothyroid disease possibly contributing to this patient's symptoms?

***Patient Case Question 3.*** Is anemia possibly contributing to this patient's symptoms?

***Patient Case Question 4.*** Provide either positive *or* negative evidence for a diagnosis of premenstrual syndrome.

***Patient Case Question 5.*** Provide either positive *or* negative evidence for a diagnosis of premenstrual dysphoric disorder.

***Patient Case Question 6.*** Which of the following treatment regimens would be most appropriate for this patient during the premenstrual week of each month?

a. fluoxetine + frequent, small meals + medroxyprogesterone acetate

b. fluoxetine + ginger + chasteberry

c. fluoxetine + black cohosh + evening primrose oil

# PART 10

# MALE REPRODUCTIVE SYSTEM DISORDERS

# 70

# BENIGN PROSTATIC HYPERPLASIA

 *For the Disease Summary for this case study, see the CD-ROM.*

## PATIENT CASE

### ■■ Patient's Chief Complaints

"I've not been getting much sleep at night and it's making me irritable during the day. It's also starting to affect my performance at work. I'm up five or six times every night to urinate and then when I get to the bathroom all that comes out is a little bit. Sometimes I get a sudden urge to urinate and I don't make it to the bathroom on time. Somebody told me that I might have something called 'neurogenic bladder' or the 'gotta-go-all-the-time syndrome.'"

### ■■ HPI

W.M. is a 76 yo man with a recent history of recurrent UTIs. He has been hospitalized three times in the last two years with acute pyelonephritis. Today, he presents with complaints of recent-onset urinary frequency, urgency, occasional incontinence, and nocturia.

### ■■ PMH

- Hypothyroidism, × 24 years
- Adenomatous colonic polyps, removed 21 years ago
- Varicocele above left testicle, surgically treated 18 years ago
- Lipoma, left anterior chest, surgically removed 10 years ago
- COPD, × 5 years
- Iron deficiency anemia, × 1 year
- DJD, hip fracture, 1 year ago
- Obesity

### ■■ FH

- Father had alcoholic cirrhosis and died in MVA at age 49
- Mother had DM type 2 and died at age 53 secondary to chronic renal failure

- Two sisters in good health, one son in good health, one grandson with cystic fibrosis, one grandson in good health

# SH

- Did not complete high school
- Lives by himself, divorced twice
- Worked for 35 years as a maintenance man at a local community college
- Currently employed part-time as a Walmart greeter
- He states that his "family cares about me, but they all live so far away now"
- Occasional social alcohol use; heavy alcohol abuse for 8 years
- 4 cups coffee/day
- 1 ppd smoker for 40 years, continues to smoke 5 cigarettes/day ("too expensive to smoke these days")
- No illicit drug or smokeless tobacco use

# ROS

- Often needs to strain to initiate urination
- Sometimes urinary flow stops and then starts again
- Complains of post-void dribbling "for about a year"

# Meds

- Ipratropium bromide MDI 2 puffs QID
- Ibuprofen 800 mg po BID for hip pain
- Levothyroxine 0.075 mg po QD
- Ferrous sulfate 325 mg po QD

**Patient Case Question 1.** For what condition is the patient probably taking ipratropium bromide?

**Patient Case Question 2.** For what condition is the patient probably taking levothyroxine?

# All

- Penicillin ("I break out with a terrible rash")
- Sulfa drugs (hives)
- Morphine (intense itching)

# Patient's Prostate Symptom Questionnaire

See Patient Case Table 70.1

**Patient Case Question 3.** Based on the patient's IPSS, is his condition of prostatic enlargement considered *mild, moderate,* or *severe*?

## Patient Case Table 70.1 Patient's Prostate Symptom Questionnaire

(Adapted with permission from Barry MJ et al. The American Urological Association symptoms index for benign prostatic hyperplasia. J Urol 1992;148:1549.)

| QUESTION Over the past month ... | NOT AT ALL (0) | LESS THAN 1 TIME IN 5 (1) | LESS THAN HALF THE TIME (2) | ABOUT HALF THE TIME (3) | MORE THAN HALF THE TIME (4) | ALMOST ALWAYS (5) |
|---|---|---|---|---|---|---|
| 1. How often have you had a sensation of not emptying your bladder completely after you finish urinating? | | | X | | | |
| 2. How often have you had to urinate again less than 2 hours after you finished urinating? | | | | X | | |
| 3. How often have you found you stopped and started again several times when you urinated? | | | | X | | |
| 4. How often have you found it difficult to postpone urination? | | | | X | | |
| 5. How often have you had a weak urinary stream? | | | | | | X |
| 6. How often have you had to push or strain to begin urination? | | | X | | | |
| 7. How many times do you most typically get up to urinate from the time you go to bed at night until you get up in the morning? | None | 1 time | 2 times | 3 times | 4 times | 5 times X |

| | | | | | | |
|---|---|---|---|---|---|---|
| 8. If you were to spend the rest of your life with your urinary condition just the way it is now, how would you feel about it? | Delighted | Pleased | Mostly satisfied | Mixed | Mostly dissatisfied | Unhappy | Terrible X |

## ■■■ PE and Lab Tests

### Gen

- Elderly, overweight, white male in NAD
- Well groomed and well dressed
- Alert, friendly, courteous, and conversant

### VS

See Patient Case Table 70.2

| **Patient Case Table 70.2 Vital Signs** | | | | | |
|---|---|---|---|---|---|
| BP | 135/85 (R arm, seated) 130/85 (L arm, seated) | RR | 16 and unlabored | HT | 6'0" |
| P | 80 and regular | T | 98.6°F | WT | 249 lbs |

*Patient Case Question 4.* Based on the patient's body mass index, is he technically *overweight* or *obese*?

# Skin

- Warm and dry with normal distribution of body hair
- No significant lesions or discoloration
- Well-healed, 2-inch surgical incision is visible on the left anterior chest wall from lipoma resection

# HEENT

- NC/AT
- PERRLA
- EOMI
- Eyes anicteric
- TMs intact
- No mouth lesions
- Oral mucosa is moist
- Throat without lesions or erythema
- Tongue normal size

# Neck/LN

- Neck supple
- No cervical, supraclavicular, or axillary adenopathy
- No thyromegaly or JVD

# Chest

- CTA & P bilaterally
- No wheezes or crackles

# Heart

- RRR
- $S_1$ and $S_2$ normal
- No murmurs, gallops, or rubs

# Abd

- Obese with multiple striae
- NT/ND without rebound or guarding
- HSM (–)
- BS (+)

- No palpable masses or bruits
- Slightly distended bladder

## Genit/Rect

- Normal male genitalia, circumcised penis without discharge, erythema, or lesions
- No inguinal adenopathy
- No inguinal hernia
- DRE: large prostate with smooth surface, no distinct nodules or induration, approximately 70 grams
- Heme (–)
- Hemorrhoids (–)
- Normal anal sphincter tone

## MS/Ext

- No clubbing, cyanosis, or edema
- Lower extremity varicose veins prominent bilaterally
- Limited ROM in both knees with patient discomfort bilaterally
- 2+ dorsalis pedis and posterior tibial pulses bilaterally

## Neuro

- A & O × 3
- CNs II–XII intact
- Romberg and Babinski signs (–)
- Motor 5/5 upper and lower extremity bilaterally
- Sensation intact
- DTRs active at 2+ and equal

## Urinary Function Tests

- Uroflowmetry: $Q_{max}$ = 7 mL/sec
- Transabdominal ultrasound: Residual urine volume = 110 mL
- Pressure flow study: Bladder voiding pressure = 74 cm $H_2O$

---

*Patient Case Question 5.* Which urinary function test(s) is/are consistent with an enlarged prostate?

## UA

See Patient Case Table 70.3

| Patient Case Table 70.3 Urinalysis | | | | | | |
|---|---|---|---|---|---|---|
| *Color* | Straw-colored | *Bilirubin* | (–) | *WBC* | | 2/HPF |
| *Appearance* | Clear | *Ketones* | (–) | *RBC* | | 2/HPF |
| *SG* | 1.017 | *Blood* | (–) | *Bacteria* | | Trace |
| *pH* | 6.4 | *Urobilinogen* | (–) | *Crystals* | | (–) |
| *Glucose* | (–) | *Nitrites* | (–) | *Culture* | | Not indicated |

*Patient Case Question 6.* Identify all abnormal results of this patient's urinalysis.

## Laboratory Blood Test Results

See Patient Case Table 70.4

### Patient Case Table 70.4 Laboratory Blood Test Results

| | | | | | |
|---|---|---|---|---|---|
| Na | 141 meq/L | MCHC | 31.8 g/dL | LDH | 219 IU/L |
| K | 3.9 meq/L | Plt | 282,000/mm$^3$ | Bilirubin, total | 1.2 mg/dL |
| Cl | 109 meq/L | WBC | 8,700/mm$^3$ | Protein, total | 5.9 g/dL |
| HCO$_3$ | 32 meq/L | • Neutros | 65% | Cholesterol | 255 mg/dL |
| BUN | 15 mg/dL | • Lymphs | 27% | Ca | 8.7 mg/dL |
| Cr | 0.8 mg/dL | • Monos | 5% | Mg | 2.2 mg/dL |
| Glu, fasting | 119 mg/dL | • Eos | 2% | PO$_4$ | 2.8 mg/dL |
| Hb | 13.9 g/dL | • Basos | 1% | Uric acid | 6.3 mg/dL |
| Hct | 41% | AST | 31 IU/L | T$_4$, total | 3.5 µg/dL |
| MCV | 97 fL | ALT | 41 IU/L | TSH | 10.79 µU/mL |
| MCH | 28.7 pg | Alk phos | 52 IU/L | PSA* | 5.2 ng/mL |

\* PSA 13 months ago was 5.0 ng/mL

*Patient Case Question 7.* Is this patient experiencing an electrolyte imbalance?

*Patient Case Question 8.* Is renal function *normal* or *abnormal*?

*Patient Case Question 9.* Is hepatic function *normal* or *abnormal*?

*Patient Case Question 10.* What is the significance of the test results for Hb, Hct, MCV, MCH, and MCHC?

*Patient Case Question 11.* What is the significance of the test results for T$_4$ and TSH?

*Patient Case Question 12.* What is the *single* most significant laboratory blood test result in Table 70.4?

*Patient Case Question 13.* Provide *three* strong lines of evidence that this patient does not have prostate cancer.

*Patient Case Question 14.* Provide a short commentary whether pharmacotherapy or surgery would be more appropriate treatment for this patient.

*Patient Case Question 15.* When a patient with mild-to-moderate BPH does not respond to pharmacotherapy with $\alpha_1$-blockers or $5\alpha$-reductase inhibitors, what can be inferred?

# CASE STUDY

# 71

# ERECTILE DYSFUNCTION

 *For the Disease Summary for this case study, see the CD-ROM.*

## PATIENT CASE

### ▬▬ Patient's Chief Complaints

"I've been having some problems in matters of the bedroom."

### ▬▬ HPI

T.R. is a 61-year-old man who presents to his PCP with the complaint noted above. Upon questioning, he states that for the last 5½ months he has only been able to achieve temporary, partial erections that are insufficient for intercourse. This has been distressing both to him and his wife and has resulted in significant marital discord. The patient's IIEF-5 score was 5, consistent with a diagnosis of severe ED. He notices occasional nocturnal, morning, and spontaneous penile tumescence, but these erections are also incomplete in nature. The patient denies any feelings of diminished sexual desire, but performance anxiety is becoming a problem. He has not had a problem with premature ejaculation since he was a young adult. He also denies discomfort or pain with ejaculation and feelings of depression. He and his wife agree that they would like to have sex at least twice a week and foreplay has been adequate, but results continue to be negative. The patient has tried several alternative treatments recommended by friends (including arginine, flaxseed meal, and Ginkgo biloba) with little improvement in erectile function. He does not want to have surgery or injections, but he would like to try "some of those little blue pills that everyone is talking about." On a scale of 0–5, he rates the importance of determining the cause of his problem as "5."

**Patient Case Question 1.** What evidence so far suggests that this patient has *primarily* organic or psychogenic erectile dysfunction?

### ▬▬ PMH

- DM type 2 × 18 years
- HTN × 9 years
- Post-traumatic stress disorder s/p Vietnam War veteran (no current symptoms)
- No other history of psychiatric illness

- GSW to upper left arm during the war
- Fractured left arm due to bicycle accident at age 12
- Had tetanus booster 6 years ago
- H/O kidney infections

## FH

- Father died recently at age 83 from COPD and cardiac arrest
- Mother still alive and well at age 79
- Maternal history (+) for stroke and vascular disease
- No siblings
- 3 children are alive and well

## SH

- Patient has been married for 37 years and lives at home with his spouse
- Has a 50 pack-year smoking history but quit smoking 8 years ago
- Only drinks alcohol socially and has no long-term history of alcohol or recreational drug abuse
- He recently retired from construction work and plays golf 1–2 times per week; he also walks 1 mile on days that he does not golf
- He watches what he eats because of his DM
- He denies non-compliance with his medications

## ROS

- Denies significant life stressors other than mild performance anxiety
- Denies recent weight loss
- Denies blurry vision, chest pain, episodes of dizziness or blackouts, unsteady gait, polyphagia, polydipsia, nocturia, dysuria, hematuria, urinary urgency, or increased urinary frequency
- Complains of "constantly cold feet" and seasonal allergies (not active at present)

## Meds

- Metformin 850 mg po TID
- Amlodipine 2.5 mg po QD
- Docusate sodium 100 mg po HS
- Enalapril 10 mg po QD
- Glyburide 1.25 mg po Q AM
- Furosemide 40 mg po BID

## All

- PCN (maculopapular rash above the waist)
- Molds (watery eyes, sneezing)

***Patient Case Question 2.*** Does the patient have *primary* or *secondary* erectile dysfunction?

***Patient Case Question 3.*** Which medications is the patient taking for diabetes?

***Patient Case Question 4.*** Which medications is the patient taking for hypertension?

***Patient Case Question 5.*** In addition to diabetes and hypertension, does this patient have any other risk factors for erectile dysfunction?

***Patient Case Question 6.*** Does erectile dysfunction in this patient appear to be primarily *neurogenic, vascular, hormonal,* or *drug-induced?*

## ■■■ PE and Lab Tests

### Gen

- WDWN, alert and oriented, but slightly anxious male in NAD
- Pleasant and cooperative
- Appears healthy and looks his stated age
- Weight appears to be within healthy range

### VS

See Patient Case Table 71.1

| Patient Case Table 71.1 Vital Signs | | | | | |
|---|---|---|---|---|---|
| BP | 124/80 | RR | 18 | HT | 5′11″ |
| P | 90 regular | T | 97.7°F | WT | 168 lbs |

***Patient Case Question 7.*** Was the primary care provider's observation correct that the patient's weight was within a healthy range?

### Skin

- Marked "crow's feet" wrinkling around the eyes consistent with long-term smoking
- Some dry, yellow scales on forehead, in nasal folds, and on upper lip
- Warm and dry without obvious tumors, moles, or other lesions
- Normal turgor and skin tone normal in color
- Normal nail beds
- (–) for diaphoresis
- Distribution of hair WNL

### HEENT

- NC/AT
- EOMI
- PERRLA
- Wears bifocals
- Funduscopic exam shows no arteriolar narrowing, hemorrhages, or exudates
- TMs WNL bilaterally
- Nose clear
- Significant dental work but has most of his permanent teeth
- Throat without erythema
- Moist mucous membranes

# Neck/LN

- Supple without cervical, axillary, or femoral lymphadenopathy or masses
- Faint left carotid artery bruit
- Thyroid normal size without nodules
- (–) JVD

# Lungs/Chest

- Clear to A & P bilaterally
- No additional sounds

# Cardiac

- RRR
- Normal $S_1$ and $S_2$
- No m/r/g
- (–) $S_3$ or $S_4$

# Abd

- Soft and ND
- Normal bowel sounds
- No masses or organomegaly
- Faint bruit

# Genit/Rect

- Normal scrotum
- Normal size testes
- Non-tender testes without nodules
- Penis, circumcised and without discharge, scarring, or other abnormalities
- Digital rectal exam showed mildly enlarged prostate but without nodules
- (–) occult blood in stool

# Spine

No tenderness to percussion

# MS/Ext

- Muscle strength 5/5 throughout
- Full ROM in all extremities
- Peripheral pulses 2+ in upper extremities, 1+ in lower extremities
- Ingrown toenail on right great toe
- No clubbing or edema
- Feet are cold to touch but not cyanotic
- No bone pain elicited with palpation

# Neuro

- A & O × 3
- CNs II–XII intact
- DTRs 2+ and equal bilaterally
- No sensory/motor deficits

- Fixes and follows well with conjugate eye movements
- Hearing appears intact
- Gait is essentially normal
- Babinski downgoing bilaterally

*Patient Case Question 8.* Did the physical examination reveal any clinical manifestations consistent with a diagnosis of erectile dysfunction?

## Laboratory Blood Test Results (Fasting)

See Patient Case Table 71.2

| Patient Case Table 71.2 Laboratory Blood Test Results (Fasting) | | | | | |
|---|---|---|---|---|---|
| Na | 141 meq/L | Hb | 13.9 g/dL | Cholesterol | 265 mg/dL |
| K | 4.1 meq/L | Hct | 39.5% | HDL | 38 mg/dL |
| Cl | 102 meq/L | WBC | $8.9 \times 10^3/mm^3$ | LDL | 120 mg/dL |
| $HCO_3$ | 24 meq/L | Plt | $271 \times 10^3/mm^3$ | Trig | 270 mg/dL |
| BUN | 14 mg/dL | Ca | 8.8 mg/dL | $HbA_{1c}$ | 11.8% |
| Cr | 1.1 mg/dL | Mg | 2.0 mg/dL | Testosterone | 700 ng/dL |
| Glu | 195 mg/dL | Phos | 2.9 mg/dL | PSA | 4.0 ng/mL |

## UA

- Clear, dark amber color
- SG 1.028
- pH 6.0
- (–) leukocyte esterase, nitrites, ketones, bilirubin
- Protein, trace
- Urobilinogen WNL
- RBC 2/HPF
- WBC 0/HPF

*Patient Case Question 9.* Are there any laboratory blood test or urinalysis results that support a diagnosis of erectile dysfunction?

## Duplex Ultrasound, Penis

- Peak systolic velocity = 0.28 m/sec
- End diastolic velocity = 0.13 m/sec

*Patient Case Question 10.* The results of the ultrasound study of the penis support a diagnosis of . . .

a. neurogenic erectile dysfunction

b. vascular erectile dysfunction

c. both neurogenic and vascular dysfunction

d. none of the above

*Patient Case Question 11.* Is there any reason why the patient should not be prescribed a phosphodiesterase 5 inhibitor?

# 72

# PROSTATE CANCER

*For the Disease Summary for this case study, see the CD-ROM.*

# PATIENT CASE

## ■ Initial History

J.A. is a 53-year-old, married, African American male who has come into the clinic for his annual physical examination. He has no specific complaints and denies any difficulties with urination, pain, or swelling. He has no known drug or other allergies and is not currently taking any medications other than naproxen for an occasional headache. There is a significant positive family history for cancer as both the patient's father and maternal grandfather had a history of prostate cancer. He has a 75 pack-year smoking history and continues to smoke. (Pack-years can be calculated from the product of number of packs of cigarettes smoked daily and number of years as a smoker. For example, 75 pack-years can be the result of 3 packs smoked daily for 25 years.) He uses alcohol occasionally. His diet is healthy and includes few saturated fats and many fresh fruits, vegetables and whole grain products.

## ■ Physical Examination and Laboratory Tests

### Vital Signs

T = 98.0°F; BP = 118/75 sitting, left arm, 120/78 sitting, right arm; P = 90 beats/minute, normal rhythm; RR = 17 breaths/minute, unlabored; Ht = 6′2″; Wt = 193 lbs

### HEENT, Neck, Lungs, Cardiac

- HEENT unremarkable, fundi without lesions
- Neck supple with no adenopathy, thyromegaly, or bruits
- Bilateral, symmetric, and normal chest expansion with vesicular and bronchial breath sounds
- $S_1$ and $S_2$ clear with no rubs, gallops, or murmurs

### Abdomen, Neurologic

- Positive bowel sounds throughout; abdomen neither tender nor distended
- Alert and oriented; cranial nerves II–XII intact; strength 5/5 throughout; DTRs 2+ and symmetric; sensation intact

## Skin, Extremities

- Skin intact and warm
- All peripheral pulses palpable
- No bruits or edema

## Digital Rectal Examination

- Prostate mildly enlarged overall with one distinct, 2-cm indurated nodule on surface

## PSA History

- 4 years ago: 1.7 ng/mL
- 3 years ago: 1.8 ng/mL
- 2 years ago: 1.7 ng/mL
- Last year: 2.0 ng/mL
- Last week: 4.7 ng/mL

## Laboratory Blood Test Results

See Patient Case Table 72.1

| Patient Case Table 72.1 Laboratory Blood Test Results | | | |
|---|---|---|---|
| Na$^+$ | 146 meq/L | WBC count | 6,000/mm$^3$ |
| K$^+$ | 4.0 meq/L | Hct | 48% |
| Cl$^-$ | 103 meq/L | RBC count | 6.0 million/mm$^3$ |
| Ca$^{+2}$ | 9.9 mg/dL | Plt | 440,000/mm$^3$ |
| Glucose, fasting | 70 mg/dL | Albumin | 3.5 g/dL |

***Patient Case Question 1.*** Identify this patient's *two* major risk factors for prostate cancer.

***Patient Case Question 2.*** Is J.A. *underweight, overweight, obese,* or is his weight considered *healthy* and *normal*?

***Patient Case Question 3.*** Which *two* clinical manifestations shown in the physical examination above should concern the primary care provider?

***Patient Case Question 4.*** Which type of test is the PCP likely to order to establish a definitive diagnosis?

***Patient Case Question 5.*** A thorough clinical workup with biopsy shows that J.A. has a well-differentiated *prostatic adenocarcinoma.* What do the following lab data suggest?

- Alkaline phosphatase: 70 IU/L
- BUN: 18 mg/dL
- Creatinine: 0.7 mg/dL
- AST: 8 IU/L
- ALT: 15 IU/L
- Total bilirubin: 0.9 mg/dL
- Negative radionuclide bone scan

***Patient Case Question 6.*** Transrectal ultrasonography revealed that the primary tumor was located in less than one-half of one lobe of the prostate gland. MRI scans showed that prostate cancer had not spread to any lymph nodes or other organs but had remained confined exclusively to the prostate. Furthermore, there was no sign that the tumor had penetrated the capsule of the prostate. To which stage has this prostate cancer progressed?

***Patient Case Question 7.*** List *three* appropriate treatment procedures for J.A.

***Patient Case Question 8.*** Why wouldn't treatment with the drug ketoconazole be an appropriate treatment for this patient?

***Patient Case Question 9.*** What is this patient's expected 5-year survival rate?

*For the Disease Summary for this case study,*
*see the CD-ROM.*

## PATIENT CASE

### ■■ Patient's Chief Complaints

"It hurts to urinate and it seems that I am going to the bathroom every hour, if not more. I was up again last night at least a half-dozen times to use the bathroom and this has been going on now for several days."

### ■■ History of Present Illness

Mr. E.D. is a 63-year-old retired pharmacist who visits the family practice clinic for a routine follow-up for hypertension. He complains of a three-day history of dysuria, increased urinary frequency, and nocturia. He denies fever, chills, and recent sexual activity. On examination, his temperature is 99.5°F, pulse 75 and regular, respiratory rate 16 and unlabored, and blood pressure 135/85. He does not appear acutely ill and is in no apparent distress. Examination of the abdomen was normal. A digital rectal exam revealed a moderately enlarged, firm, non-tender prostate gland.

### ■■ Past Medical History

- History of "heart attack" per patient report approximately 15 years ago (no records available)
- Sciatica on right side × 10 years following lifting injury; several steroid floods and laminectomy with no long-term pain relief
- Hepatitis B carrier detected at age 53
- HTN diagnosed at age 56
- BPH × 5 years
- UTI and/or prostatitis, 3 episodes in last 5 years, last attack 20 months ago
- Prostatic calculi detected with ultrasonography 4 years ago

### ■■ Family History

- Father died from prostate cancer at age 77
- Mother currently undergoing treatment for ovarian cancer at age 84

# ■■■ Social History

* Divorced and lives alone
* Previous smoker of ½ to 1 ppd for 35 years, quit 8 years ago
* Has 2–4 beers on weekends
* May be unreliable in keeping follow-up appointments, because he states "I don't like doctors"

# ■■■ Medications

* Atenolol 25 mg po QD
* HCTZ (25 mg) + triamterene (37.5 mg) po QD
* Oxycodone (4.88 mg) + aspirin (325 mg) 2 tablets po PRN

# ■■■ Allergies

NKDA

# ■■■ Clinical Workup

Symptoms suggest that cystitis, urethritis, and/or prostatitis are the most likely diagnoses. The patient was immediately referred to a urologist at the clinic who conducted a 3-cup bacterial localization test, CBC, blood culture for bacteremia, and renal function studies.

## 3-Cup Bacterial Localization Results

See Patient Case Table 73.1

| Patient Case Table 73.1 3-Cup Bacterial Localization Results | | |
|---|---|---|
| SAMPLE | WBC TYPES | CULTURE RESULTS |
| First-void (V1) | 1 WBC/HPF | (–) for bacteria |
| Second-void (V2) | 1 WBC/HPF | (–) for bacteria |
| Prostatic fluid only | TNTC/HPF Macrophages + lymphocytes predominant | (+) for E. coli; strain sensitive to TMP-SMX and fluoroquinolones |
| Post-prostatic massage void (V3) | TNTC/HPF Macrophages + lymphocytes predominant | (+) for E. coli; strain sensitive to TMP-SMX and fluoroquinolones |

## Other Laboratory Test Results

See Patient Case Table 73.2

| Patient Case Table 73.2 Other Laboratory Test Results | | | | | |
|---|---|---|---|---|---|
| Hct | 40.6% | • PMNs | 48% | • Basos | 1% |
| Hb | 15.4 g/dL | • Lymphs | 40% | BUN | 25 mg/dL |
| WBC | 10,700/mm³ | • Monos | 10% | Cr | 1.4 mg/dL |
| Plt | 189,000/mm³ | • Eos | 1% | Blood culture: | Negative |

***Patient Case Question 1.*** Why did the primary care provider ask the patient if he was sexually active?

***Patient Case Question 2.*** Based on the results of the 3-cup bacterial localization test, is urethritis and/or cystitis associated with prostatitis in this patient?

*Patient Case Question 3.* Cite *three* major risk factors that may play key roles in the development of prostatitis in this patient.

*Patient Case Question 4.* Which subtype of prostatitis does this patient have or is prostatodynia a more appropriate assessment of the condition?

*Patient Case Question 5.* Provide a brief rationale for your answer to *Question 4* above.

*Patient Case Question 6.* Which antibiotic regimen do you think the urologist prescribed for this patient?

*Patient Case Question 7.* Why was hospitalization considered unnecessary at this point in the clinical course of the illness?

## ■ Clinical Course

The patient returns 48 hours later with continued dysuria. He has also noted severe urgency and greater difficulty with passage of urine. "I hardly peed at all since I saw you last and I feel worse." On examination, temperature was 100.8°F and the suprapubic area was tender. A repeat BUN was 35 mg/dL and serum creatinine concentration was 2.1 mg/dL.

*Patient Case Question 8.* What is causing the progressive nature of this condition?

*Patient Case Question 9.* Provide at least *four* management approaches that are appropriate at this time.

*Patient Case Question 10.* Provide several reasons why chronic inflammation is a logical progression from acute inflammation.

# CASE STUDY

# 74

# TESTICULAR CANCER

 *For the Disease Summary for this case study, see the CD-ROM.*

## PATIENT CASE

### ■ HPI

L.A. is a 29-year-old white male who presented to his PCP because he recently felt a "heavy sensation" in his scrotum and subsequently discovered a small, but distinct, lump on the surface of his right testicle. He is accompanied by his wife, who appears to be very supportive.

### ■ PMH

- Appendicitis, 18 years ago
- Asthma, since age 5 years
- Vasectomy, 5 years ago
- Last PE was 5 years ago

### ■ FH

Adopted, none available

### ■ SH

- Works full-time as a janitor in a home for the mentally disabled
- Before that served 3 years in the U.S. Army
- Has been married for 7 years and has twin daughters, age 8
- Smoked ½ pack cigarettes/day for 8 years but quit 5 months ago
- Denies alcohol consumption and IV drug use
- Has used cocaine several times in the past year

### ■ Meds

Albuterol inhaler PRN

***Patient Case Question 1.*** Briefly describe the mechanism of action for the drug albuterol.

## All

- Aspirin causes swelling in the face and tongue
- Latex causes a rash
- Sulfa drugs cause a rash

## ROS

The patient denies any swelling or abnormal lumps in locations other than his right testicle. He also denies fatigue, headaches, changes in vision, dizziness, cough, coughing up of blood, abdominal or chest pain, difficulty breathing, seizures, difficulty swallowing, and back pain.

***Patient Case Question 2.*** Why has the primary care provider questioned the patient about these specific clinical manifestations?

## Immunizations

- Patient unsure about immunization status
- Remembers tetanus vaccine last year when he stepped on a rusty nail

***Patient Case Question 3.*** Based on the information provided above, does this patient have any risk factors for testicular cancer?

## PE and Lab Tests

### Gen

Thin, alert but anxious, healthy-looking, young, white male in NAD

### VS

BP 115/75; P 80, regular; RR 16 and unlabored; T 98.6°F; Wt 141 lbs; Ht 5'10"

### Skin

- Soft, intact, warm, and dry
- No evidence of rash, ecchymosis, petechiae, cyanosis, or other lesions

***Patient Case Question 4.*** What is the layman's commonly used term for *ecchymosis*?

***Patient Case Question 5.*** What are *petechiae*?

## HEENT

- PERRLA
- Funduscopic exam normal
- Ears and nose clear
- Normal-looking TMs
- Throat normal

## Neck

- Supple
- No swelling, bruits, or nodal enlargement
- Thyroid normal

## Chest

- Normal breath sounds
- Chest CTA
- (–) for gynecomastia

## Cardiac

- $S_1$, $S_2$ normal with regular rate and rhythm
- No $S_3$, $S_4$, or murmurs

---

*Patient Case Question 6.* Fill in the blank in the following sentence. A heart that beats with an abnormal rhythm is known as a **d**_____ heart.

## Abd

- Soft, NT/ND
- Normoactive BS
- No HSM, masses, or bruits

## Genit/Rect

- External genitalia normal with no enlarged inguinal lymph nodes
- Uncircumcised male
- No rectal/prostate exam conducted

## Ext

- Pulses 2+ throughout
- Full ROM in all extremities
- No CCE
- Poor nail care with some overgrown toenails
- No muscle weakness perceived

## Neuro

- Oriented to self, place, current president
- CNs II–XII intact

- Motor and sensory systems intact throughout
- Deep tendon reflexes normal

## Laboratory Blood Test Results

See Patient Case Table 74.1

| Patient Case Table 74.1 Laboratory Blood Test Results | | | | | |
|---|---|---|---|---|---|
| RBC | 4.8 million/mm³ | LDH | 100 IU/L | Chloride | 106 meq/L |
| WBC | 8,100/mm³ | Albumin | 4.6 g/dL | Glucose, fasting | 99 mg/dL |
| Plt | 41,000/mm³ | Sodium | 138 meq/L | Bicarbonate | 25 meq/L |
| AFP | 71 ng/mL | Potassium | 3.9 meq/L | BUN | 19 mg/dL |
| β-HCG | 3 mU/mL | Calcium | 10.1 mg/dL | Cr | 0.7 mg/dL |

***Patient Case Question 7.*** Identify *one* abnormal laboratory blood test result that is consistent with a diagnosis of testicular cancer.

***Patient Case Question 8.*** Identify *one* abnormal laboratory blood test result that is not consistent with a diagnosis of testicular cancer but suggests another health problem for the patient.

***Patient Case Question 9.*** Which laboratory blood test results indicate that the patient's renal function is normal?

## ▬ Clinical Course

Ultrasound of the right testicle revealed a 2-cm solid, non-cystic mass. A chest x-ray and CT scans of the chest and abdomen were negative. An orchiectomy was performed of the right testicle. Microscopic analysis of the tumor revealed a mixed population of malignant cells that had not invaded the tunica albuginea, epididymis, or spermatic cord, but was confined exclusively to the testicle. Diagnosis was consistent with *mixed cell tumor*.

***Patient Case Question 10.*** Based on the information provided, why is a diagnosis of *non-seminoma* more likely than *seminoma*?

***Patient Case Question 11.*** Do you suspect that this cancer is in an *early, intermediate,* or *advanced stage*? Explain your answer.

***Patient Case Question 12.*** What is the probability that orchiectomy alone will be curative in this patient?

***Patient Case Question 13.*** What is the probability that, following treatment, this patient will be disease-free for 5 years?

***Patient Case Question 14.*** Would chemotherapy be an appropriate follow-up treatment to surgery in this patient? Explain your answer.

# IMMUNOLOGIC DISORDERS

# CASE STUDY

# 75

# ACQUIRED IMMUNODEFICIENCY SYNDROME

 *For the Disease Summary for this case study, see the CD-ROM.*

## PATIENT CASE

### ■■■ Patient's Chief Complaints

"I've been out of breath, I've had a cough, and I feel run down. I think that I may also have a fever. This came on fast and it has been going on now for almost a full week."

### ■■■ History of Present Illness

M.C. is a 29-year-old white male who tested positive for HIV 2½ years ago. He visits the HIV clinic at regular 2- to 3-month intervals for routine follow-up, most recently six weeks ago. He has been stable on antiretroviral treatment consisting of tenofovir, emtricitabine, and lopinavir-ritonavir for the last 11 months. Prior to that, the patient had developed drug resistance to his initial combination regimen of zidovudine, lamivudine, and efavirenz. He presents today complaining of moderate dyspnea, a persistent and non-productive cough, and fatigue.

### ■■■ Past Medical History

* Respiratory syncytial virus infection at 7 months old
* Forehead laceration that required stitches from falling vase at age 4 years
* Seroconversion to PPD 11 years ago; treated for 12 months with isoniazid
* Perianal ulceration that cultured positive for herpes simplex, topically treated with acyclovir and zinc oxide, 3 years ago
* Oral candidiasis, resolved with fluconazole, 2½ years ago
* Tested positive for HIV with both ELISA and Western blot, 2½ years ago
* Oral candidiasis, resolved with fluconazole, 20 months ago
* Two episodes of anemia, treated with erythropoietin, 10 months and 14 months ago
* Cytomegalovirus retinitis in right eye, tested positive for IgG to CMV, received induction therapy with IV ganciclovir twice daily for 21 days, followed by IV ganciclovir maintenance therapy for 10 weeks until discontinued due to recurrent central line infections, subsequent placement of intra-ocular ganciclovir implant in right eye, 6 months ago

- Catheter line infections, 2 episodes in 10 weeks
- Hospitalized for *Pneumocystis* pneumonia, developed allergic reaction to trimethoprim-sulfamethoxazole, effectively treated with IV pentamidine for 14 days and discharged, 6 weeks ago

## ■■ Family History

Non-contributory

## ■■ Social History

- Homosexual, admitted to engaging in both unprotected anal and oral intercourse with multiple partners since age 22, one partner died 8 months ago from AIDS-related complications
- He has since lived with his 51 yo mother who has DM type 2 and rheumatoid arthritis
- Currently, the patient is unemployed and receiving Social Security disability checks, but sells T-shirts and sweat shirts on the street near the HIV clinic to pay for his medication and healthcare
- Previously worked for 5 years as forest ranger
- Smoked 3 ppd for 10 years before quitting 2 years ago
- Past history of alcohol abuse, cocaine sniffing, and IVDU

## ■■ Immunizations

- Patient had tetanus shot about 10 years ago but otherwise is unsure of his immunization status
- "Had some vaccinations as a child"

## ■■ Review of Systems

- (−) nausea, vomiting, diarrhea, chills, night sweats, headache, urinary frequency, nocturia, or pain with urination
- (+) loss of appetite with weight loss of "about 4 or 5 pounds in the last week"

## ■■ Medications

- Tenofovir 300 mg po QD
- Emtricitabine 300 mg po QD
- Lopinavir-ritonavir, 400 mg/100 mg po BID
- Ganciclovir implant, right eye
- Ganciclovir, 1 g po TID
- Vitamins
- Dapsone, 50 mg po QD (ran out 2 weeks ago and did not have enough money to refill his prescription)

## ■■ Allergies

Trimethoprim-sulfamethoxazole → bright red rash that covered his torso and face; also, fever of 102°F

*Patient Case Question 1.* Identify this patient's *two most significant risk factors* for developing HIV disease.

*Patient Case Question 2.* Why do you think that this patient had been taking dapsone?

# ■ Physical Examination and Laboratory Tests

## General

Thin, slightly anxious, acutely ill-appearing, young white male with tachypnea

## Vital Signs

See Patient Case Table 75.1

| Patient Case Table 75.1 Vital Signs | | | | | |
|---|---|---|---|---|---|
| BP | 130/87 | RR | 30 | HT | 6 ft–2 in |
| P | 90 | T | 101.9°F | WT | 155 lbs |

## Skin

- Soft, intact, warm, and dry
- No visible lesions, rash, ecchymoses, petechiae, or cyanosis

## Head, Eyes, Ears, Nose, and Throat

- PERRLA
- Funduscopic exam of left eye reveals new fluffy, white retinal patches with focal hemorrhages consistent with CMV retinitis; right eye reveals no new lesions
- Ears and nose clear
- Sinuses non-tender
- Oral cavity negative for thrush, erythema, exudates, or lesions

## Neck and Lymph Nodes

- Neck supple with no masses or bruits
- Slight cervical lymphadenopathy
- Thyroid normal

## Chest and Lungs

- Mild axillary lymphadenopathy
- Bibasilar crackles with auscultation

## Heart

- Normal sinus rhythm
- Normal $S_1$ and $S_2$
- (−) rubs, murmurs, or gallops

# Abdomen

- Soft and non-distended
- (−) pain or tenderness
- (−) hepatosplenomegaly
- (+) BS
- Mild-to-moderate inguinal lymphadenopathy

# Genitalia/Rectum

- Guaiac-negative stool
- Anal sphincter function normal
- (−) visible genital or anal lesions
- Prostate exam deferred

# Musculoskeletal and Extremities

- Neuromuscular intact
- Pedal pulses 2+
- (−) edema or wasting
- Nails normal
- Full ROM

# Neurologic

- A & O × 3
- (−) Babinski reflex
- (−) cranial nerve abnormalities
- Normal DTRs
- (−) focal neurologic signs

***Patient Case Question 3.*** Identify the *two most specific clinical signs* in the physical examination that support a diagnosis of pneumonia.

# Serial Laboratory Values

For the serial laboratory values beginning nine months prior to the present visit, see Patient Case Table 75.2

***Patient Case Question 4.*** Relative to his previous two visits to the HIV clinic, what do the patient's HIV markers indicate at this time?

# Chest X-Rays

- Bilateral diffuse interstitial disease without hilar adenopathy
- Mild cystic changes noted
- No consolidation or nodules

| Patient Case Table 75.2 Serial Laboratory Values Beginning Nine Months Prior to Present Visit | | | | |
|---|---|---|---|---|
| | **9 Months Ago** | **6 Months Ago** | **3 Months Ago** | **This Visit** |
| *GENERAL* | | | | |
| Weight (lbs) | 167 | 167 | 162 | 155 |
| Blood pressure (mm Hg) | 125/72 | 120/65 | 120/72 | 130/87 |
| *HEMATOLOGY* | | | | |
| Hb (g/dL) | 13.6 | 13.5 | 11.5 | 10.9 |
| Hct (%) | 38.9 | 38.0 | 33.4 | 32.0 |
| Plt ($\times10^3$/mm$^3$) | 376 | 390 | 287 | 260 |
| WBC ($\times10^3$/mm$^3$) | 3.8 | 4.1 | 3.3 | 3.8 |
| Lymphs (%) | 24.7 | 32.0 | 36.4 | 18.2 |
| Monos (%) | 14.5 | 14.1 | 10.2 | 11.4 |
| Eos (%) | 2.5 | 2.4 | 3.7 | 1.5 |
| Basos (%) | 1.0 | 0.6 | 1.0 | 1.1 |
| Neutros (%) | 57.3 | 50.9 | 48.7 | 67.8 |
| *HIV MARKERS* | | | | |
| CD4 cells (%) | 18 | 27 | 26 | 15 |
| CD4 cells/mm$^3$ | 163 | 353 | 359 | 119 |
| CD8 cells (%) | 33 | 37 | 35 | 29 |
| CD8 cells/mm$^3$ | 307 | 470 | 350 | 214 |
| HIV RNA (copies/mL)* | >750,000 | <500 | <500 | 67,600 |
| *CHEMISTRY* | | | | |
| Na (meq/L) | 141 | 140 | 135 | 136 |
| K (meq/L) | 4.2 | 4.0 | 3.5 | 4.3 |
| Cl (meq/L) | 107 | 107 | 103 | 108 |
| BUN (mg/dL) | 7 | 8 | 7 | 10 |
| Cr (mg/dL) | 0.9 | 0.9 | 0.7 | 0.9 |
| Glu, fasting (mg/dL) | 95 | 90 | 104 | 115 |
| T Bili (mg/dL) | 0.5 | 0.6 | 1.2 | 0.5 |
| T Prot (g/dL) | 6.3 | 6.5 | 6.0 | 6.1 |
| Alb (g/dL) | 3.2 | 2.9 | 3.0 | 2.7 |
| AST (IU/L) | 25 | 30 | 28 | 34 |
| ALT (IU/L) | 50 | 55 | 54 | 51 |
| Ca (mg/dL) | 8.8 | 8.6 | 8.9 | 7.8 |
| Phos (mg/dL) | 3.5 | 3.1 | 3.9 | 3.8 |
| Mg (mg/dL) | 1.9 | 1.9 | 1.8 | 2.0 |

*Determined with reverse transcriptase-polymerase chain reaction assay

## Other Tests

- Sputum specimen obtained with inhalation of 3% saline by ultrasonic nebulizer
- Methenamine silver stain positive (consistent with *Pneumocystis* infection)
- Monoclonal antibody with immunofluorescence: + for *Pneumocystis*

## Arterial Blood Gas Analysis

- pH: 7.45
- $PaO_2$ = 69 mm Hg

- $PaCO_2$ = 30 mm Hg
- $SaO_2$ = 91.9%

***Patient Case Question 5.*** The correct assessment of this patient's arterial blood gas analysis is:

a. hypoxemia and hypercapnia

b. hypoxemia and hypocapnia

c. normal $PaO_2$ and hypercapnia

d. normal $PaO_2$ and hypocapnia

e. normal $PaO_2$ and normal $PaCO_2$

***Patient Case Question 6.*** Following seroconversion of this patient to HIV disease, which AIDS-defining clinical manifestations or complications has this patient developed?

***Patient Case Question 7.*** Direct HIV infection of renal cells may result in clinical manifestations of kidney disease. Do laboratory tests indicate that HIV has affected kidney function?

***Patient Case Question 8.*** Based on the CDC HIV Classification System, what is the current clinical category (or stage of HIV infection) for this patient?

# 76

# SYSTEMIC LUPUS ERYTHEMATOSUS

 *For the Disease Summary for this case study, see the CD-ROM.*

## PATIENT CASE

### ■ Current Status

A.B. is a married, 47-year-old white female homemaker with two children and an 18-year medical history of systemic lupus erythematosus. She has no known allergies. The patient takes an occasional naproxen for joint pain and antacid for heartburn but no other prescription or OTC medications. She neither smokes nor drinks alcohol. Except for lupus, the patient's medical history is unremarkable.

*Patient Case Question 1.* What is the relevance of this information to her disease?

She is 5 feet, 5 inches in height and weighs 102 pounds, a decrease in weight of 23 pounds since her last physical examination nearly 1 year ago. She has four brothers and three sisters. An older sister has rheumatoid arthritis, an aunt has pernicious anemia, and her deceased mother suffered from Graves disease.

*Patient Case Question 2.* What is the significance of the patient's family history?

*Patient Case Question 3.* Is this patient *underweight, overweight, obese,* or is this patient's weight considered *healthy and normal*?

The patient's **BP** is 110/70, **HR** 70, **RR** 15/unlabored, and oral temperature 99.8°F.

### ■ Medical History

Eighteen years ago, A.B. complained to her PCP of multiple rashes that developed on her arms and legs whenever she went out into the sun. She also complained of several small patches of hair loss on her head that she attributed to stress and an airplane trip that she took three months previously. Flying terrifies her. Furthermore, she mentioned at that time that she lacked energy, became tired very easily, and always needed to take at least one nap each day. She was also suffering from mild arthritic pain in her fingers and elbows but attributed the joint discomfort to "growing old." Her **ESR** was 25 mm/hr.

---

**Patient Case Question 4.** Explain the pathophysiology that underlies hair loss in this patient and the relevance of the abnormal ESR.

**Patient Case Question 5.** What might have caused the lack of energy in this patient, and what type of tests might be ordered to support this conclusion?

---

She had been aware of these problems for approximately four months. A physical examination was conducted during which the PCP noted multiple rash-like lesions on sun-exposed areas of the body, primarily on the arms and legs. A tissue biopsy of one of the lesions was taken and microscopic examination of the tissue revealed vasculitis (white blood cells within the walls of blood vessels). An ANA test was positive. The lungs were clear to auscultation, heart sounds were normal with a prominent $S_1$ and $S_2$, and there was no evidence of enlarged lymph nodes. Blood tests revealed an **Hct** of 23% and an **RBC** count of 3.5 million/mm³. She was also slightly jaundiced with some yellowing within the sclera. Microscopic examination of a peripheral blood smear revealed that red blood cells were normal in shape, size, and color, ruling out iron, folate, and vitamin B12 deficiencies. The total **WBC** count was 5,500/mm³ and her **Plt** count was 350,000/mm³. Urinalysis was normal. She was placed on prednisone for two months, during which time all signs and symptoms of disease resolved.

---

**Patient Case Question 6.** Vasculitis in lupus results from the trapping of antigen-antibody complexes in blood vessel walls followed by an intense inflammatory response to the immune complexes. Why is prednisone effective in relieving vasculitis?

**Patient Case Question 7.** What can be said about the patient's **Hct, RBC** count, **WBC** count, and **Plt** count?

**Patient Case Question 8.** What is the most likely cause of jaundice in this patient?

---

Five years ago, A.B. presented again to her PCP, this time complaining of a productive cough and stiffness and pain in her hands and feet that seemed to come and go and to affect different joints (*migratory polyarthritis*). She is afraid that she is developing rheumatoid arthritis like her older sister.

---

**Patient Case Question 9.** It is appropriate for her PCP to inform her that . . .

a. she clearly is showing signs of rheumatoid arthritis and probably has it.

b. the arthritis of lupus, which is a likely possibility, is relatively benign, unlike rheumatoid arthritis, which destroys cartilage in the joints and causes deformities.

c. the pain she is feeling in the joints is probably due to getting older and wear and tear (a condition known as *degenerative joint disease*) and is not likely related to her condition.

d. the pain that she is feeling in her joints is most likely the result of gout, and a serum uric acid test is appropriate.

---

Her **BP** at this time was 140/90, **HR** 105, and she had a temperature of 100°F. Auscultation of the lungs revealed abnormal lung sounds, suggesting that she had bronchitis. A chest x-ray revealed mild pulmonary edema but no white blood cell infiltrates in the terminal airways. The PCP was concerned about susceptibility for developing pneumonia. Axillary and inguinal lymph nodes were slightly enlarged.

*Patient Case Question 10.* Why might the PCP be concerned about the possibility for pneumonia?

*Patient Case Question 11.* What is the pathophysiology that underlies lymph node enlargement in this patient?

Blood tests revealed an **Hct** of 43%, a **Plt** count of 330,000/mm$^3$, and a total **WBC** count of 1,200/mm$^3$. A urinalysis was essentially normal.

*Patient Case Question 12.* Which of the three blood test results directly above would be of most concern? Give a likely cause for the abnormality.

*Patient Case Question 13.* The patient's **WBC differential** was: 75% neutrophils, 15% lymphocytes, 5% monocytes/macrophages, 4% eosinophils, and 1% basophils. Which one of these 5 white blood cell types has been specifically targeted by the patient's immune system?

*Patient Case Question 14.* What is the association between the abnormal blood test results, abnormal lung sounds, and productive cough?

*Patient Case Question 15.* Give a reasonable explanation for the cause of tachycardia and elevated blood pressure in this patient.

The patient was given a 10-day course of antibiotic therapy to prevent pneumonia and placed on prednisone again. All signs and symptoms resolved within three months. Now she returns to her PCP complaining of fatigue, anorexia, weight loss, and significant swelling within the abdomen, face, and ankles. The PCP notes that a "butterfly-shaped" rash is present across the bridge of her nose and cheeks. Blood tests reveal an **Hct** of 24%. The **WBC** count is 2,400/mm$^3$. A dipstick examination of the urine revealed an abnormal protein concentration and microscopy showed the presence of significant numbers of red and white blood cells. A 24-hour urine protein collection revealed excretion of 2.5 g protein/24 hr.

*Patient Case Question 16.* What is a likely cause of the abnormal blood test results now?

*Patient Case Question 17.* Explain the pathophysiology of swelling throughout the body.

*Patient Case Question 18.* Suggest *one* reasonable explanation for an association between systemic swelling and anorexia/weight loss in this patient.

*Patient Case Question 19.* Patients with SLE should receive an influenza vaccination every year and a pneumococcal vaccination every 5 years. Why?

*Patient Case Question 20.* Why is *hypocomplementemia* consistent with a diagnosis of SLE?

# MUSCULOSKELETAL DISORDERS

*For the Disease Summary for this case study, see the CD-ROM.*

# PATIENT CASE

## ■ Patient's Chief Complaints

"I woke up in the middle of the night last evening and my right big toe felt as if it was on fire. It's hot, swollen, and so tender that even the weight of a blanket on it is nearly intolerable. And there's no way that I can put a shoe on."

## ■ History of Present Illness

Mr. J.H. is a 47 yo male seen in the clinic by his new general internist for severe pain in his right great toe. The pain began last evening after his 47th birthday celebration and kept him awake much of the night. He has been taking extra-strength acetaminophen to keep the pain under control. He states that he is unable to bear any weight on his right foot. He came into the clinic wearing open-toed sandals. He denies any history of injury to his right foot.

## ■ Past Medical History

- Hypercholesterolemia × 9 years
- HTN × 9 years
- TIA 3 months ago, appears to have no residual neurologic deficits
- Chronic sinus drainage/rhinitis (S/P laryngoscopy)

## ■ Medications

- HCTZ 25 mg po QD with supper
- ASA 325 mg po Q AM
- Atorvastatin 10 mg po QD
- Flunisolide 2 sprays each nostril QD
- Pseudoephedrine 60 mg po Q6h PRN

**Patient Case Question 1.** Why should the use of pseudoephedrine by this patient be carefully monitored by the primary care provider?

## ■■ Family History

- Educated through high school
- Mother alive with type 2 DM
- Father died at age 68 from osteosarcoma
- No siblings
- Four adult children are all healthy

## ■■ Social History

- Non-smoker
- Uses alcohol weekly (5–6 drinks per week on average)
- Married twice with 4 adult children (1 from first marriage)
- Employed 17 years as a truck driver and is frequently away on the road
- Lives with wife of 22 years, happily married
- Diet is heavy on red meat and other high-purine foods

## ■■ Review of Systems

- Denies HA, dizziness, chest pain, SOB, and generalized swelling or tenderness of the joints
- Weight has increased approximately 15 lbs in the last year
- No previous episodes of joint pain

## ■■ Allergies

NKDA

## ■■ Physical Examination and Laboratory Tests

### General

White male in mild acute distress

### Vital Signs

See Patient Case Table 77.1

| Patient Case Table 77.1 Vital Signs | | | | | |
|---|---|---|---|---|---|
| BP | 145/85 | RR | 17 | HT | 6'1" |
| HR | 92 | T | 100.2°F | WT | 225 lbs |

**Patient Case Question 2.** Has an optimal target for blood pressure management been reached in this patient?

> *Patient Case Question 3.* Is this patient *underweight, overweight, obese,* or is this patient's weight considered *normal and healthy* for his height?
>
> *Patient Case Question 4.* Are any of this patient's vital signs consistent with a diagnosis of gout?
>
> *Patient Case Question 5.* Identify *eight* risk factors from the information provided above in this case study that predispose the patient to gout.

## Neck/Lymph Nodes

Normal with no swelling, thyromegaly, masses, or jugular venous distension

## Eyes

- Pupils equal at 3 mm, round, and reactive to light and accommodation
- Normal funduscopic examination

## Lungs

CTA

## Cardiac

- RRR
- $S_1$ and $S_2$ with no extra cardiac sounds
- No gallops, rubs, or murmurs

## Abdomen

- Non-tender and non-distended
- No HSM
- Normal bowel sounds

## Musculoskeletal/Extremities

- Pulses full throughout
- Muscle strength 5/5 throughout
- Right first metatarsophalangeal joint hot, tender, erythematous, swollen

## Neuro

- A & O to person, place, time
- CNs II–XII intact
- DTRs 2+
- Babinski (−)

## Laboratory Blood Test Results

See Patient Case Table 77.2

> *Patient Case Question 6.* Identify *five* laboratory blood test values that are consistent with a diagnosis of gout.

## Patient Case Table 77.2 Laboratory Blood Test Results

| Na | 140 meq/L | Uric acid | 13.1 mg/dL | • Bands | 3% |
|---|---|---|---|---|---|
| K | 4.2 meq/L | Glu, fasting | 120 mg/dL | • Monocytes | 3% |
| Cl | 106 meq/L | Hb | 15.6 g/dL | • Lymphocytes | 20% |
| HCO₃ | 27 meq/L | Hct | 47% | • Eosinophils | 1% |
| BUN | 14 mg/dL | WBC | $13.3 \times 10^3/mm^3$ | ESR | 15 mm/hr |
| Cr | 0.9 mg/dL | • Neutrophils | 73% | T chol | 189 mg/dL |

***Patient Case Question 7.*** What is the significance of this patient's fasting blood glucose concentration?

***Patient Case Question 8.*** Is there a need to adjust the patient's dose of atorvastatin upward at this time?

# 24-hour Urinary Uric Acid

985 mg/day

# X-Ray, Right Great Toe

Moderate soft tissue edema; normal joint space; no erosions or sclerosis

# Synovial Fluid Examination

- Significant PMN infiltration
- MSU crystals confirmed microscopically with polarized light

***Patient Case Question 9.*** Would probenecid, sulfinpyrazone, or allopurinol be a more appropriate medication for this patient? Why?

*For the Disease Summary for this case study,*
*see the CD-ROM.*

# PATIENT CASE

## ■■ Patient's Chief Complaints

"I'm really having trouble getting around. My joints have been killing me. Knees and lower back are the worst. Other doctors won't give me what I need to feel better."

## ■■ History of Present Illness

G.J. is a 71 yo overweight woman who presents to the Family Practice Clinic for the first time complaining of a long history of bilateral knee discomfort that becomes worse when it rains and usually feels better when the weather is warm and dry. "My arthritis hasn't improved a bit this summer though," she states. Discomfort in the left knee is greater than in the right knee. She has also suffered from low back pain for many years, but recently it has become worse. She is having difficulty using the stairs in her home.

The patient had recently visited a rheumatologist who tried a variety of NSAIDs to help her with pain control. The medications gave her mild relief but also caused significant and intolerable stomach discomfort. Her pain was alleviated with oxycodone. However, when she showed increasing tolerance and began insisting on higher doses of the medication, the physician told her that she may need surgery and that he could not prescribe more oxycodone for her. She is now seeking medical care at the Family Practice Clinic.

Her knees started to get significantly more painful after she gained 20 pounds during the past nine months. Her joints are most stiff when she has been sitting or lying for some time and they tend to "loosen up" with activity. The patient has always been worried about osteoporosis because several family members have been diagnosed with the disease. However, no clinical manifestations of osteoporosis have developed.

## ■■ Past Medical History

At age 23, the patient suffered a left knee injury in an MVA that did not require surgery. She also suffered a broken left hip 11 years ago when she fell on an icy sidewalk while visiting her sister in Michigan. Her hip seemed to have healed well as she has no significant symptoms that suggest hip joint involvement.

The patient has a 14-year history of OA, a 10-year history of HTN, a 4-year history of hypercholesterolemia, and a 4-year history of DM type 2. She also was hospitalized for an episode of diverticulitis two years ago. Her only surgery was a hysterectomy without oophorectomy 21 years ago. Menopause occurred at age 49, but she has never taken hormones.

## ■■■ Family History

- Father died from AMI at age 53
- Mother died from breast CA at age 80
- Patient has one brother, age 68, with HTN; one sister, age 74, who has severe allergies and has had two mitral valve replacements for rheumatic heart disease; and one sister, age 72, who also has OA
- Positive history of osteoporosis in mother and maternal grandmother

## ■■■ Social History

- Lives with her 72 yo sister in a 3-story townhouse near the beach
- Exercises regularly in the pool and, sometimes, in the ocean, but can no longer walk long distances daily as she has done in the past
- Has a well-balanced diet with plenty of fresh fruits and vegetables, whole grains, and dairy products, but admits to eating "too many sweets"
- Has Medicare but no other health insurance
- Does not smoke and drinks 1–2 cocktails or glasses of white wine every evening with her meal
- Hobbies include quilting, baking, and teaching piano to children

## ■■■ Review of Systems

- Mild pain in right shoulder with lifting, carrying
- Low back pain with occasional "shooting pains" radiating to back of thigh
- Deep, aching pain in the pretibial area bilaterally and extending distally to the ankles and toes
- Patient denies any swollen, red, or hot joints, but notes "hard lumps" at the margins of the interphalangeal joints
- Patient denies numbness or weakness in her legs
- Patient denies pain or discomfort in her wrists and elbows
- Negative for headaches, neck stiffness, SOB, chest pains, urinary frequency or dysuria, constipation, diarrhea, nausea, loss of appetite, or significant changes in the appearance of her urine or stools
- Finger-stick blood glucose levels are usually around 180 mg/dL
- Occasional polyuria but no changes in vision

***Patient Case Question 1.*** Why is the phrase "occasional polyuria but no changes in vision" relevant to this patient's overall health status?

## ■■■ Medications

- Zolpidem 10 mg po Q HS PRN
- Atorvastatin 20 mg po Q HS
- Atenolol 25 mg po QD
- Lisinopril 40 mg po QD
- Metformin 250 mg po QD

- Glipizide 2.5 mg po QD
- Acetaminophen 1000 mg po TID
- High-potency multivitamin supplement with calcium, iron, and zinc po QD
- Calcium 600 mg with Vitamin D 125 IU supplement po BID with meals

---

*Patient Case Question 2.* Why is this patient taking zolpidem?

*Patient Case Question 3.* Why is the patient taking both metformin and glipizide for diabetes mellitus type 2?

*Patient Case Question 4.* Why is the patient taking both atenolol and lisinopril for hypertension?

---

# ■■■ Allergies

No known drug allergies

# ■■■ Physical Examination and Laboratory Tests

## General

Alert, WDWN, overweight Caucasian female who appears slightly anxious but otherwise in NAD

## Vital Signs

See Patient Case Table 78.1

| Patient Case Table 78.1 Vital Signs | | | | | |
|---|---|---|---|---|---|
| BP sitting, left arm | 155/88 | RR | 15 and unlabored | HT | 5 ft–3 in |
| P | 72 and regular | T | 98.8°F | WT | 164 lbs |

---

*Patient Case Question 5.* Has an optimal target for blood pressure management been reached in this patient?

*Patient Case Question 6.* Rounded to the nearest 5 pounds, how many pounds should this patient minimally lose to achieve a healthy weight?

---

## Skin

- Warm and dry with normal turgor
- No petechiae, ecchymoses, or rash

## Head, Eyes, Ears, Nose, and Throat

- NC/AT
- PERRLA

- Funduscopic exam reveals sharp discs with no vascular abnormalities or papilledema
- (−) scleral icterus
- TMs intact
- Mucous membranes moist
- (−) lateral deviation of tongue, pharyngeal edema, or erythema

---

*Patient Case Question 7.* Why is the above statement "funduscopic exam reveals sharp discs with no vascular abnormalities or papilledema" relevant to this patient's overall health status?

---

## Neck/Lymph Nodes

- Neck supple
- (−) evidence of thyromegaly, adenopathy, masses, JVD, or carotid bruits

## Chest/Lungs

- Good chest excursion
- Lungs CTA & P

## Heart

- Normal $S_1$ and $S_2$
- PMI normal at 5th ICS
- RRR
- No m/r/g

## Abdomen

- Soft and non-tender without guarding
- (+) BS
- (−) organomegaly, bruits, and masses

## Breasts

- Symmetric
- No apparent masses, discharge, discoloration, or dimpling

## Genitalia/Rectum

- Normal female genitalia
- (+) mild vaginal atrophy
- Normal anal sphincter tone
- Stool heme-negative

## Musculoskeletal/Extremities

- Back with decreased flexion and extension
- Back pain radiating to right buttock with straight right leg raising >60°
- Full ROM at left shoulder, elbows, and ankles
- Mild left hip discomfort with flexion >90° and with internal and external rotation >45°

- Hips not tender to palpation
- Bilateral knee crepitus and enlargement but more pronounced in left knee
- Slight decrease in ROM and both Bouchard and Heberden nodes observed bilaterally during hand examination; no tenderness in finger joints
- No redness, heat, or swelling in joints
- Feet without breakdown, ulcers, erythema, or edema

***Patient Case Question 8.*** Why is the statement directly above "feet without breakdown, ulcers, erythema, or edema" relevant to this patient's overall health status?

## Neurologic

- Oriented × 3
- Cranial nerves intact
- Sensory exam normal and symmetric to pinprick and vibration
- DTRs 2+ and equal bilaterally except for 1+ Achilles reflexes bilaterally
- Strength 5/5 in both upper extremities; 4/5 in lower extremities
- Gait slow but without specific deficits
- Coordination WNL
- No focal deficits
- (−) Babinski bilaterally

## Laboratory Blood Test Results

See Patient Case Table 78.2

### Patient Case Table 78.2 Laboratory Blood Test Results

| | | | | | |
|---|---|---|---|---|---|
| Na | 137 meq/L | MCV | 87 fL | Protein, total | 7.9 g/dL |
| K | 4.4 meq/L | MCH | 27.7 pg | Alb | 4.2 g/dL |
| Cl | 108 meq/L | MCHC | 31.8 g/dL | Cholesterol | 248 mg/dL |
| $HCO_3$ | 23 meq/L | WBC | $5.2 \times 10^3/mm^3$ | $HbA_{1c}$ | 7.5% |
| BUN | 7 mg/dL | Plt | $239 \times 10^3/mm^3$ | Ca | 8.7 mg/dL |
| Cr | 0.6 mg/dL | AST | 31 IU/L | $PO_4$ | 2.9 mg/dL |
| Glu, fasting | 241 mg/dL | ALT | 19 IU/L | Mg | 1.9 mg/dL |
| Hb | 13.5 g/dL | Bilirubin, total | 0.6 mg/dL | ESR | 14 mm/hr |
| Hct | 39.1% | Alk phos | 97 IU/L | TSH | 1.9 μU/mL |

## Urinalysis

See Patient Case Table 78.3

### Patient Case Table 78.3 Urinalysis

| | | | |
|---|---|---|---|
| *Appearance* | Pale yellow, clear | *Leukocyte esterase* | Negative |
| *Specific gravity* | 1.017 | *Nitrites* | Negative |
| *pH* | 6.3 | *Bacteria* | Negative |
| *WBC* | 0/HPF | *Protein* | Negative |
| *RBC* | 0/HPF | *Ketones* | Negative |

# X-Rays

Lumbosacral spine

- Advanced degenerative changes with disk space narrowing and osteophyte formation at L3–4 and L4–5
- No evidence of compression fracture

Left hip

- Mild-to-moderate degenerative changes with mild osteophytosis of femoral head
- Slight narrowing in joint space

Right and left knees

- Moderate degenerative changes with joint space narrowing, subchondral sclerosis, and bone cysts
- No radiographic evidence of osteoporosis or joint effusions

Right shoulder

- Mild degenerative changes with bone spurs at head of humerus
- Slight narrowing in joint space

***Patient Case Question 9.*** In the context of osteoarthritis, define *crepitus.*

***Patient Case Question 10.*** Identify *four* risk factors that have predisposed this patient to osteoarthritis.

***Patient Case Question 11.*** Identify *three* abnormal laboratory blood test results in this case study.

***Patient Case Question 12.*** What types of therapeutic approach may be taken to bring the three abnormal laboratory blood test results that you identified in Question 11 above into a normal reference range?

***Patient Case Question 13.*** The primary cause of limited range of motion in a joint afflicted with osteoarthritis is/are:

a. bone spurs

b. loss of proprioceptive reflexes

c. formation of new bone

d. degeneration of articular cartilage

e. cysts that form in subchondral bone

***Patient Case Question 14.*** Identify a *single* blood chemistry test that is helpful in distinguishing if a patient has osteoarthritis or gouty arthritis.

***Patient Case Question 15.*** Are there any forms of complementary and alternative medicine available for treating osteoarthritis?

***Patient Case Question 16.*** What are the brand names of two topical pain creams that contain the pain reliever trolamine salicylate and have been widely promoted to temporarily relieve arthritis pain?

***Patient Case Question 17.*** Cockscomb is a garden plant commonly grown for its flowers. Name a medication derived from cockscomb that is used to treat osteoarthritis.

# CASE STUDY

# 79

# OSTEOPOROSIS

 *For the Disease Summary for this case study, see the CD-ROM.*

## PATIENT CASE

### ■ Patient's Chief Complaints

"I've had back pain now for more than 5 weeks and I can't stand it anymore. I've tried extra-strength ibuprofen, naproxen, and acetaminophen, and I've visited a chiropractor, but I don't get any long-term relief."

### ■ History of Present Illness

Mrs. I.A. is a very pleasant 63-year-old white woman of slight stature who has been referred to an orthopedic specialist by her PCP. She has been experiencing insidious back pain for 5–6 weeks. OTC analgesics provide temporary relief, but the pain is otherwise constant and aggravated by activity. She denies any obvious acute injury to her back, although she reports that she had a case of the flu with a prolonged and severe cough approximately one month ago. She also reports a vertebral fracture approximately five years ago.

The patient has been an avid gardener for many years. Following the death of her husband 18 months ago, she has continued to live in her house and do all the household chores. Since her back pain began, she has been limited in her ability to do her household chores and gardening.

### ■ Past Medical History

The patient entered natural menopause at 52 years and has never used hormone replacement therapy. Currently, she has mild hot flashes and vaginal dryness. At age 58, she suffered a vertebral fracture at T10 by simply carrying a shopping bag. DEXA scans conducted at that time revealed the onset of osteoporosis. Her bone mass density T-scores at that time were: $-3.33$ lumbar spine, $-2.24$ right femoral neck, and $-2.44$ right radius. These scans represented a 6.1%, 6.9%, and 6.2% decrease in bone mass density in the previous 19 months in the lumbar spine, right femoral neck, and right radius, respectively. Her serum calcium concentration was low-normal at 8.5 mg/dL and serum alkaline phosphatase level was moderately increased at 290 IU/L. She was prescribed alendronate and a calcium supplement daily.

The patient was diagnosed with a seizure disorder at age 22 years and is currently well controlled with phenytoin. She has had asthma since childhood. Her current asthma medications include a bronchodilator that she uses when needed, a daily steroid inhaler, and an oral corticosteroid that she uses about four times per year for 3–6 weeks when symptoms worsen. She also takes a daily multivitamin tablet and has 1–2 dairy servings every day. She has noticed a slight reduction in height in recent years, but denies any significant changes in weight. She had an appendectomy at 11 years of age.

*Patient Case Question 1.* Following her vertebral fracture at T10, the patient was prescribed alendronate and calcium. Which additional pharmacotherapeutic agent should have been prescribed?

*Patient Case Question 2.* At the time of her previous DEXA scans 19 months ago, was osteoporosis present in the spine, femur, and radius?

*Patient Case Question 3.* Based on the information provided so far, which type or types of osteoporosis does this patient have?

## ■ Family History

The patient has a positive family history of osteoporosis. Her older sister has experienced a hip fracture and her paternal aunt was diagnosed with an osteoporosis-related wrist fracture following a fall.

Her mother was diagnosed with breast cancer at age 56, but died from lung cancer at age 69. She also suffered from high blood pressure and "high blood sugar." Her father died at age 54 from AMI. Her brother (age 65) has HTN and high cholesterol, and her younger sister (age 57) has no known medical problems.

## ■ Social History

The patient smokes four cigarettes a day (down from 1½ ppd eight years ago) and drinks one glass of wine daily. Her main sources of dietary calcium are milk with her breakfast cereal and "some" cheese about three times a week. The patient is widowed and was married for 39 years until the death of her husband 1½ years ago. She has one son who is healthy. She had a miscarriage at age 19. She does most of her cooking and "watches what she eats." She denies non-compliance with her medications. She gets very little weight-bearing exercise. She uses SPF 30 sunscreen to protect herself from sunburn and skin cancer every time that she spends more than 15 minutes in the sun.

## ■ Review of Systems

The patient denies any unusual bleeding, weakness, back spasms, shortness of breath, chest pain, fever, chills, heat or cold intolerance, and changes in her hair, skin, and nails. She reports vaginal dryness, occasional hot flashes and night sweats "maybe once every 6 months."

## ■ Medications

- Alendronate 10 mg po QD
- Calcium carbonate 1.25 g (500 mg calcium) po BID
- Multivitamin tablet po QD
- Phenytoin 100 mg po TID
- Albuterol MDI 2 puffs BID PRN
- Triamcinolone MDI 2 puffs QID
- Prednisolone 5 mg po BID PRN

# ■ Allergies

- Codeine intolerance (nausea, vomiting)
- Sulfa drugs (rash)
- Aspirin (hives, wheezing)
- Cats (wheezing)

***Patient Case Question 4.*** Which risk factors does this patient have that have made her susceptible to bone loss?

# ■ Physical Examination and Laboratory Tests

## General

The patient is an alert and oriented, cooperative 63-year-old white female of slight stature who walks with a normal gait and is in no apparent distress. She appears somewhat anxious.

## VS

See Patient Case Table 79.1

| Patient Case Table 79.1 Vital Signs | | | | | |
|---|---|---|---|---|---|
| BP | 129/83 sitting, left arm | RR | 20 and unlabored | HT | 5'3½" |
| P | 88 and regular | T | 98.6°F oral | WT | 106 lbs |

## Skin

- Fair complexion
- Color and turgor good
- No lesions

## Head

- Normocephalic
- No areas of tenderness
- Slight hair thinning

## Eyes

- Conjunctiva clear
- PERRLA
- EOMI
- Funduscopic exam unremarkable

## Ears

TMs pearly without bulging or retraction

## Throat

- Mucous membranes moist
- Clear without drainage or erythema

## Neck and Lymph Nodes

- No obvious nodes
- Thyroid non-tender without thyromegaly and no masses palpable
- (−) JVD
- No bony tenderness
- Full ROM without pain elicited

## Chest

- Normal chest excursion
- Clear to A & P

## Breasts

- WNL
- Mammography normal (3 months ago)

## Cardiac

- RRR
- (−) murmurs
- Normal $S_1$ and $S_2$
- No $S_3$ or $S_4$

## Abdomen

- Soft, NT/ND
- (+) BS
- (−) organomegaly or masses

## Genitalia/Rectum:

Deferred

## Musculoskeletal/Extremities

- Good peripheral pulses bilaterally
- Point tenderness with palpation of bony prominence at L2
- Limited flexion and extension of the back
- Significant lumbar lordosis
- Lateral bending unlimited and non-painful
- (−) kyphosis
- (−) deformity or swelling of joints

## Neurologic

- A & O × 3
- Recent and remote memory intact

- Cranial nerves intact
- No focal motor deficits
- No gross sensory deficits
- DTRs 1+ and symmetric throughout
- Toes downgoing

*Patient Case Question 5.* Which findings in the physical examination above are consistent with a diagnosis of osteoporosis?

## Laboratory Blood Test Results

See Patient Case Table 79.2

| Patient Case Table 79.2 Laboratory Blood Test Results | | | | | |
|------|------|------|------|------|------|
| Na | 139 meq/L | Glu, fasting | 91 mg/dL | 25,OH vitamin D | 3 ng/mL |
| K | 4.4 meq/L | TSH | 1.42 μU/mL | Hb | 12.6 g/dL |
| Cl | 103 meq/L | Ca | 8.6 mg/dL | Hct | 39.5% |
| $HCO_3$ | 23 meq/L | $PO_4$ | 4.6 mg/dL | WBC | $8.8 \times 10^3/mm^3$ |
| BUN | 15 mg/dL | Mg | 1.8 mg/dL | Plt | $339 \times 10^3/mm^3$ |
| Cr | 1.0 mg/dL | Alk phos | 283 IU/L | PTH | 33 pg/mL |

## DEXA Scan Results

See Patient Case Table 79.3

| Patient Case Table 79.3 DEXA Scan Results | |
|------|------|
| **Site** | **T Score** |
| Lumbar spine L2–4 | −3.79 |
| Right femoral neck | −3.19 |
| Right radius | −2.97 |

*Patient Case Question 6.* Is *osteopenia* or *osteoporosis* the appropriate diagnosis in the . . .

a. lumbar spine

b. right femoral neck

c. right radius

## Spinal Radiographs

- Significant radiographic lucency suggestive of poor bone density
- Recent compression fracture at L2
- Healed compression fracture at T10
- Thoracic vertebrae are wedge shaped, consistent with progressive osteoporosis
- Lumbar vertebrae are biconcave, consistent with progressive osteoporosis

***Patient Case Question 7.*** Which single laboratory test in Table 79.2 was significantly high?

***Patient Case Question 8.*** Provide *three* reasons for this patient's abnormal serum 25, OH-vitamin D concentration.

***Patient Case Question 9.*** Provide *one* good reason for why this patient is not taking hormone replacement therapy for vaginal dryness and hot flashes and as prophylactic therapy for post-menopausal osteoporosis.

***Patient Case Question 10.*** Distinguish between *lordosis* and *kyphosis*.

***Patient Case Question 11.*** Is this patient's thyroid function *normal* or *abnormal*?

***Patient Case Question 12.*** Is this patient's parathyroid function *normal* or *abnormal*?

***Patient Case Question 13.*** Are there any indications that this patient also has type 2 osteoporosis?

# CASE STUDY

# 80

# RHEUMATOID ARTHRITIS

 *For the Disease Summary for this case study, see the CD-ROM.*

## PATIENT CASE

### Patient's Chief Complaints and History of Present Illness

M.L. is a 50-year-old white female who has been working in the front office of a medical clinic for the past five years. She has made an appointment to see her primary care provider because she has been feeling very tired for the past month and has also been suffering from stiffness, pain, and swelling in multiple joints.

"I ache all over," she told her PCP, "and I have pain in different places all the time. One day it is in my right shoulder, the next day in my right wrist, and the following day in my left wrist. I'm stiff everywhere when I get up in the morning or if I sit for any length of time. And I feel so tired, like I have a case of the flu that won't go away."

The patient is allergic to IV iron dextran from which she has developed shortness of breath. She rarely uses alcohol and does not smoke. She is taking an over-the-counter calcium supplement, levothyroxine sodium, and venlafaxine. There is no family history of rheumatoid arthritis.

### Physical Examination and Laboratory Tests

The patient is pleasant and alert, but appears very tired. She is in moderate acute distress from joint pain.

#### Vital Signs

BP = 125/80 left arm, sitting; P = 80; RR = 15; T = 100.0°F; Ht = 5′4″; Wt = 140 lbs.

*Patient Case Question 1.* Which of the vital signs above is consistent with a diagnosis of rheumatoid arthritis and why?

*Patient Case Question 2.* List *two* conditions for which the drug venlafaxine is often prescribed.

382

## HEENT

- Head atraumatic
- PERRLA
- Normal funduscopic examination
- EOMI
- TMs intact

## Skin

- Intact, warm, pink, and dry
- No rashes
- Normal turgor

## Neck

- Supple with no jugular vein distension or thyromegaly
- No bruits
- Mild lymphadenopathy bilaterally

## Lungs

- Clear to auscultation and percussion

## Heart

- RRR
- Normal $S_1$, $S_2$; no $S_3$ or $S_4$
- No murmurs, rubs, or gallops

## Abdomen

- Soft, non-tender, and non-distended
- Positive bowel sounds throughout
- No superficial veins or organomegaly

## Breasts

No lumps, dimpling, discharge, or discoloration

## Genitourinary

- Last menstrual period 16 months ago
- Normal pelvic exam and Pap smear

## Neurologic

- Alert and oriented × 3
- Cranial nerves II–XII intact
- Muscle strength: 5/5 upper extremities, 4/5 lower extremities
- DTRs 2+ in biceps, triceps, and patella

## Rectal

Heme-negative stool

> **Patient Case Question 3.** Identify *two* abnormal findings from the physical exam above that are consistent with rheumatoid arthritis.

## Musculoskeletal, Extremities

- No clubbing or ankle edema
- Hands: Swelling of the 3rd, 4th, and 5th PIP joints bilaterally; pain in the 4th and 5th MCP joints bilaterally; poor grip strength bilaterally
- Wrists: Good range of motion, fixed nodule at pressure point on left side
- Elbows: Good range of motion, fixed nodule at pressure point on right side
- Shoulders: Pain and decreased range of motion bilaterally
- Hips: Good range of motion
- Knees: Pain, significant edema, and decreased range of motion bilaterally
- Feet: No edema, full plantar flexion and dorsiflexion and full pedal pulse bilaterally

> **Patient Case Question 4.** What is the association between the "fixed nodule(s) at pressure point(s)" on the left wrist/right elbow and a diagnosis of rheumatoid arthritis?
>
> **Patient Case Question 5.** Why is it reasonable that this patient has no stiffness, pain, or swelling in the DIP joints of the fingers?

## Laboratory Blood Test Results

See Patient Case Table 80.1

### Patient Case Table 80.1 Laboratory Blood Test Results

| | | | | | | | | |
|---|---|---|---|---|---|---|---|---|
| Na$^+$ | 140 meq/L | ANA | *Negative* | Hct | 43% | Uric acid | 2.9 mg/dL |
| K$^+$ | 3.7 meq/L | ESR | 38 mm/hr | WBC | 15,100/mm$^3$ | Cholesterol | 189 mg/dL |
| Cl$^-$ | 104 meq/L | Cr | 1.0 mg/dL | Plt | 270,000/mm$^3$ | Albumin | 4.0 g/dL |
| HCO$_3^-$ | 23 meq/L | Glucose, fasting | 94 mg/dL | RBC | 4.7 million/mm$^3$ | TSH | 1.7 µU/mL |
| BUN | 18 mg/dL | Hb | 14.9 g/dL | Ca$^{+2}$ | 8.8 mg/dL | RF | *Positive* |

> **Patient Case Question 6.** Identify *three* abnormal laboratory tests in Table 80.1 that are consistent with a diagnosis of rheumatoid arthritis.
>
> **Patient Case Question 7.** Why is it entirely appropriate that the PCP has ordered a TSH test for this patient?
>
> **Patient Case Question 8.** Provide a reasonable explanation for the serum uric acid test result shown in Table 80.1.
>
> **Patient Case Question 9.** What is probably the first class of drugs that the PCP will prescribe for this patient?

## Urinalysis

Normal with no RBC, WBC, or protein

## Chest X-Ray

No fluid, masses, infection, or cardiomegaly

## Hand X-Ray

Soft tissue swelling and bone demineralization; no erosions

## Synovial Fluid Analysis (Left Knee)

- 7.4 mL volume
- Cloudy and yellow in appearance
- 14,000 WBC/mm³, primarily neutrophils
- Glucose: 60 mg/dL

*Patient Case Question 10.* In terms of the progression of the disease, what do the results of the hand x-ray suggest?

*Patient Case Question 11.* Which findings in the examination of the synovial fluid are consistent with a diagnosis of rheumatoid arthritis?

*Patient Case Question 12.* What causes limitation of joint motion that occurs early in the clinical course of rheumatoid arthritis?

*Patient Case Question 13.* What causes limitation of joint motion that occurs late in the clinical course of rheumatoid arthritis?

# DISEASES OF THE SKIN

# 81

## ACNE VULGARIS

 *For the Disease Summary for this case study, see the CD-ROM.*

## PATIENT CASE

### ◼ HPI

M.E. is a 21 yo woman with a Hx of facial acne since age 18. Thirty days ago she completed a 2½-month course of 500-mg erythromycin BID in combination with topical adapalene gel 0.1%. Her acne has flared up and she has presented to her primary care provider again for treatment. She also complains of irregular menses and increased facial hair.

### ◼ PMH

The patient is up-to-date with immunizations. There are no other chronic medical conditions and no other acute or recent illnesses. The patient first developed a mild case of acne three years ago. At that time she responded well to topical daily 0.5% salicylic acid and twice-daily 2.5% benzoyl peroxide. Despite the use of topical antibiotics during the past two years, the number of facial lesions has increased and lesions have progressed from comedones to pustules and cystic nodules with some scarring. Initially, oral tetracycline (500 mg BID) was beneficial and it controlled her condition for nearly 10 months, but then the acne worsened. Induction of a resistant strain of *P. acnes* was suspected. Doxycycline (100 mg BID) and clindamycin (150 mg BID) were also tried but were not successful in achieving a remission.

### ◼ FH

No family history of cystic acne. Both parents and an older brother are alive and well.

### ◼ SH

The patient is a non-smoker. No alcohol or IVDA. She has been under significant stress as she is working 20 hours/week, is enrolled in 15 credit hours of molecular biology, is involved in various extracurricular activities on campus including cheerleading, and is currently studying for the Pharmacy College Admissions Test. She is sexually active. Her boyfriend does not use condoms and she is not taking oral contraceptives or using a diaphragm. She has been involved in a monogamous relationship for three years. She enjoys movies, jogging, racquetball, canoeing, and reading.

## ■■■ Meds

None

## ■■■ All

Avoids cold medications (especially decongestants) and naproxen because they make her "feel irritable."

## ■■■ PE and Lab Tests

### Gen

Alert, moderately anxious, slim, young white female in NAD

### VS

BP 115/75, P 80, RR 14, T 98.6°F, Wt 114 lbs, Ht 5′4″

---

*Patient Case Question 1.* Are any of the patient's vital signs abnormal?

*Patient Case Question 2.* Is this patient considered *underweight, overweight, obese,* or does this patient have a *healthy weight* with respect to her height?

---

### Skin

- Warm and dry with no rashes, tumors, moles, or bruises
- Closed and open comedones on forehead, chin, and malar area
- Pustules and cystic nodules on nose and chin
- Facial hair prominent
- Normal turgor

### HEENT

- Pupils 3 mm bilaterally and properly reactive to light
- Visual acuity 20/20 bilaterally
- Funduscopic exam normal
- EOMI
- TMs intact
- Mucous membranes moist and pink

### Neck

- Supple
- No JVD, thyromegaly, carotid bruits or adenopathy

### Lungs

CTA bilaterally

## Heart

- RRR with no m/r/g
- $S_1$ and $S_2$ with no extra heart sounds

## Abd

- Soft with no palpable masses
- NT/ND
- No HSM
- (+) BS

## MS/Ext

- No joint or muscle aches or pains
- Peripheral pulses strong at 2+ throughout
- (−) CCE
- Strength 5/5 bilaterally
- Full ROM

## Neuro

- A & O × 3
- No signs of local deficit
- (−) Babinski reflex bilaterally
- Patellar DTRs active and equal bilaterally
- CNs II–XII intact
- Sensory intact
- Normal gait

## Pelvic

- No vaginal discharge or lesions
- LMP 5 days ago, abnormally light flow

## Laboratory Test Results

See Patient Case Table 81.1

| Patient Case Table 81.1 Laboratory Test Results | | | | | |
|---|---|---|---|---|---|
| Na | 139 meq/L | Plt | 290,000/mm³ | HDL | 41 mg/dL |
| K | 3.0 meq/L | WBC | 6,000/mm³ | Trig | 100 mg/dL |
| Cl | 101 meq/L | AST | 20 IU/L | DHEAS | 31 μmol/L |
| HCO₃ | 24 meq/L | ALT | 38 IU/L | Testosterone | 150 ng/dL |
| BUN | 11 mg/dL | Alk phos | 79 IU/L | Prolactin | 16 ng/mL |
| Cr | 0.9 mg/dL | T. bilirubin | 0.9 mg/dL | FSH follicular | 10 mU/mL |
| Glu, fasting | 90 mg/dL | Alb | 3.8 g/dL | LH follicular | 10 mU/mL |
| Hb | 17.5 g/dL | T. cholesterol | 175 mg/dL | MRI abdomen: (+) for 2.0-cm mass, superior pole, right adrenal |
| Hct | 49% | LDL | 120 mg/dL | |

***Patient Case Question 3.*** What might be a major concern with prescribing monocycline or isotretinoin for this patient?

***Patient Case Question 4.*** Would you suspect that this patient has *inflammatory* or *non-inflammatory* acne?

***Patient Case Question 5.*** In addition to acne, identify *eight* findings from the physical examination and laboratory tests that are abnormal.

***Patient Case Question 6.*** What condition is suggested by the vast majority of clinical manifestations that you identified in Question 5 above?

***Patient Case Question 7.*** Briefly discuss how stress may be a contributory factor to the patient's acne.

***Patient Case Question 8.*** What is the significance of this patient's current medication profile?

***Patient Case Question 9.*** What is a likely cause of this patient's progressive acne?

***Patient Case Question 10.*** How might this patient's acne be cured?

***Patient Case Question 11.*** Two of the patient's hematology tests were abnormal. Why are these values consistent with the diagnosis?

***Patient Case Question 12.*** Identify the *single* abnormal clinical manifestation that cannot be explained based on the available information.

***Patient Case Question 13.*** Is this patient's lipid profile considered *healthy* or *unhealthy*?

# BASAL CELL CARCINOMA

 *For the Disease Summary for this case study, see the CD-ROM.*

## PATIENT CASE

### ▄▄▄ Patient's Chief Complaints

"This lump on my face is getting bigger . . . and sometimes it bleeds."

### ▄▄▄ History of Present Illness

Mr. N.S. is a 49 yo white male, who was referred to the dermatology clinic by his PCP after complaining of a slowly growing lesion overlying his right cheekbone. He first noticed the abnormal growth approximately five months ago, but just recently became aware that it was increasing in size. He states that the growth bleeds occasionally after he has showered and dried his face with a towel.

### ▄▄▄ Past Medical History

* Tonsillectomy, age 6 years
* Appendectomy complicated with infection, age 10
* Duodenal ulcer, age 44, resolved with pharmacotherapy, no recurrence
* Hernia repair, age 45
* HTN diagnosed 2 years ago

### ▄▄▄ Family History

* Mother alive and healthy at age 71
* Father died from cardiac arrest at age 56
* Brother alive and well at age 46
* Maternal grandparents may have had CAD
* Two daughters, ages 23 and 26, are in good health
* No known history of cancer or chronic skin conditions

## ■■■ Social History

- Has worked full-time as a roofer for 19 years
- Hobbies include gardening, fishing, and working out with weights at the gym
- History of several blistering sunburns as a child and chronic exposure to the sun with daily sunbathing as a young man
- Lives with wife of 29 years
- Smoked ½–¾ pack of cigarettes/day for 25 years but quit 8 years ago
- Drinks several beers on Friday-Saturday evenings
- Denies current IV drug use although he has snorted heroin in the past

## ■■■ Review of Systems

- No changes in vision or hearing
- No headaches, cough, fevers, chills, night sweats, nausea, or vomiting
- No changes in bowel or bladder habits
- Denies weakness, tiredness, shortness of breath, bruising tendencies, and chest pain

## ■■■ Allergies

- Aspirin (diarrhea)
- Penicillin (skin rash as a child)

## ■■■ Medications

Nifedipine XL 60 mg po QD

*Patient Case Question 1.* Why is this patient taking nifedipine?

*Patient Case Question 2.* Explain why nifedipine is effective for the condition that you cited for Question 1?

## ■■■ Physical Examination and Laboratory Tests

### General

The patient is a well-developed, well-nourished, muscular, middle-aged white male with blue eyes and blond hair. He is of Scandinavian heritage. He is both alert and interactive.

### Vital Signs

See Patient Case Table 82.1

| Patient Case Table 82.1 Vital Signs | | | | | |
|---|---|---|---|---|---|
| BP | 125/80 | RR | 15 and unlabored | HT | 5′10″ |
| P | 65 and regular | T | 98.8°F | WT | 180 lbs |

***Patient Case Question 3.*** Including body mass index, should any of this patient's vital signs be a cause for concern?

***Patient Case Question 4.*** Identify a minimum of *four* significant risk factors for basal cell carcinoma that this patient has.

## Skin

* Warm and dry, but aged and poorly resilient from years of sun exposure
* Dark summer tan
* No signs of nevi, rash, ecchymoses, or petechiae
* 1.5-cm waxy, flesh-colored papule on the right cheek with some erosion centrally; telangiectases obvious upon close inspection; no pigmentation, erythema, or scar-like properties

***Patient Case Question 5.*** Based on the gross appearance of the neoplasm, which type of basal cell carcinoma does this patient probably have?

## Head, Eyes, Ears, Nose, and Throat

* Male pattern baldness
* Pupils equal at 3 mm, round, reactive to light/accommodation
* EOMI
* Sclera anicteric
* TMs clear
* No sinus drainage or tenderness
* Throat without lesions or erythema
* Oral mucosa moist and intact

## Neck and Lymph Nodes

* Supple and non-tender
* No lymphadenopathy
* Thyroid without masses
* No carotid bruits auscultated

## Lungs

CTA bilaterally without wheezes or crackles

## Cardiovascular

* RRR
* Normal $S_1$ and $S_2$
* No m/r/g
* No JVD

## Abdomen

* Soft and non-tender
* (+) BS
* No rebound, guarding, or distension
* No HSM

## Rectum

- Normal sphincter tone
- (−) heme
- Prostate normal size without nodules

## Musculoskeletal and Extremities

- No CCE
- Femoral pulses 2+ bilaterally
- No joint deformities
- ROM and muscle strength symmetric throughout
- No pain elicited with palpation

## Neurologic

- A & O × 3
- CNs II–XII intact
- Fixes and follows well with conjugate eye movements
- Hearing appears normal
- DTRs 2+ and symmetric throughout
- Cerebellar function intact (gait steady)
- Sensory levels grossly intact
- 5/5 motor strength throughout
- Facial strength appears symmetric and normal
- Babinski downgoing bilaterally

*Patient Case Question 6.* Other than the solitary neoplasm on the face, are there any other clinical findings in the physical examination that should raise concern?

## Biopsy Results

Cells have large, uniform, oval, hyperchromatic, relatively non-anaplastic nuclei with little cytoplasm. Nuclear-to-cytoplasmic ratio appears greater than that of normal basal cells. Tumor appears well differentiated. Mitotic figures are rare. Tumor cells are aligned in a palisade pattern at the periphery of cell aggregates. Consistent with basal cell carcinoma—nodular subtype.

*Patient Case Question 7.* Which type of treatment is preferred for this type of basal cell carcinoma?

*Patient Case Question 8.* Would it be appropriate for the primary care provider to order a chest x-ray or a CT scan for this patient?

*Patient Case Question 9.* Would it be appropriate for the primary care provider to order a complete blood count, chemistry panel, and urinalysis?

*Patient Case Question 10.* What is the probability that this patient will develop a basal cell carcinoma at another site within 5 years?

*Patient Case Question 11.* What is the single best piece of advice that can be provided by the patient's primary caregiver?

# MALIGNANT MELANOMA

 *For the Disease Summary for this case study, see the CD-ROM.*

## PATIENT CASE

### ■ HPI

R.S. is a 38-year-old white male who presents to his PCP after his wife noticed a suspicious-looking, dark brown mole in his scalp while giving him a haircut. He was referred to the dermatology clinic.

### ■ PMH

- Lipoma over left ribcage, surgically removed 10 years ago, no recurrence
- Episode of major depression with suicidal tendency 8 years ago, treated successfully with an antidepressant and psychotherapy for 10 weeks, no recurrence
- Seasonal allergic rhinitis, chronic for 4 years

### ■ FH

- Both parents living: mother 58 yo with HTN, father 64 yo with COPD
- One brother 35 yo apparently in good health
- No family history of cancer or familial atypical multiple mole syndrome

### ■ SH

- Drinks 6-pack of beer on weekends, 2 beers nightly during the week
- Denies tobacco use and IVDA
- Has been married for 14 years, second marriage, going well
- Has been an engineer for Union Pacific Railroad for 11 years
- History of several blistering sunburns as a child
- Works out 2×/week at the gym (weights and treadmill)

## ■■■ Meds

- Uses an OTC antihistamine April–September for seasonal allergic rhinitis
- No other medications

## ■■■ All

- Aspirin (hives and wheezing)
- Cats (wheezing, watery eyes, runny nose)

## ■■■ ROS

- No changes in vision, smell, or hearing
- No headaches, cough, fever, chills, night sweats, nausea, or vomiting
- No changes in bowel or bladder habits
- No fatigue or weakness

*Patient Case Question 1.* Why is the lack of clinical manifestations in the ROS above significant?

## ■■■ PE and Lab Tests

### General

- Fair complexion and healthy-looking white male in no apparent discomfort
- Red hair with green eyes
- Appears pleasant, alert, and conversant but anxious

*Patient Case Question 2.* Identify *two* risk factors for melanoma that this patient has.

### VS

BP 125/80, P 82, RR 15, T 98.2°F; Wt 175 lbs, Ht 5′9″

*Patient Case Question 3.* Is this patient considered *underweight, overweight, obese,* or is this patient's weight considered *healthy*?

### Skin

- Fair complexion with multiple scattered nevi on the back
- Negative for rashes and other lesions
- Warm to the touch and slightly diaphoretic
- Normal distribution of body hair

## HEENT

- 7-mm nodule on scalp above the right ear, dome-shaped, symmetric, dark brown in color, no variegations
- PERRLA
- EOMI
- Funduscopy WNL
- Normal sclera
- TMs intact
- Mucous membranes moist
- Throat without lesions, edema, exudates, or erythema
- Poor dentition, several fractured teeth

*Patient Case Question 4.* Based on this rather limited information, which subtype of melanoma is most likely?

## Neck/LN

- Neck supple
- Significant cervical lymphadenopathy, bilateral, >2 cm
- No thyromegaly, carotid bruits, or JVD

*Patient Case Question 5.* Why is the information directly above especially critical to the prognosis of this patient?

*Patient Case Question 6.* Identify *two* possible pathophysiologic causes of lymphadenopathy in this patient.

## Chest

- Lungs CTA & P bilaterally without wheezing, rales, or rhonchi
- A well-healed surgical incision is visible on the left anterior chest wall

## Cardiac

- RRR
- $S_1$, $S_2$ normal
- No m/r/g

## Abd

- Soft, NT/ND
- (+) BS
- No rebound or guarding
- No HSM
- No masses or bruits

## Rect/Genit

- Normal sphincter tone
- Rectum negative for masses
- Heme (−)

- Prostate normal size without nodules
- Normal male genitalia

## MS/Ext

- Normal strength and ROM
- No CCE
- Distal pulses 2+ bilaterally

## Neuro

- A & O × 3 (self, location, and year)
- CNs II–XII intact
- Normal DTRs bilaterally
- Sensory levels intact
- Speech clear and language normal
- Gait normal

## Biopsy

An excisional biopsy of the mole showed cells consistent with that of a *nodular melanoma*. Tumor thickness was 3.8 mm. Cervical nodes were enlarged and measured 2.3 and 2.7 cm. A CT scan of the thorax was negative. With the exception of questionable shadows in the liver, the abdominal CT scan was also negative. A CT scan of the brain was clearly positive for 3 lesions.

## Laboratory Blood Test Results

See Patient Case Table 83.1

| Patient Case Table 83.1 Laboratory Blood Test Results | | | | | | | |
|---|---|---|---|---|---|---|---|
| Na | 142 meq/L | Cr | 0.6 mg/dL | WBC | 7,200/mm³ | AST | 115 IU/L |
| K | 4.5 meq/L | Glu, fasting | 103 mg/dL | RBC | 5.3 million/mm³ | ALT | 145 IU/L |
| Cl | 103 meq/L | Hb | 16.3 g/dL | Ca | 10.3 mg/dL | Alk phos | 278 IU/L |
| HCO₃ | 31 meq/L | Hct | 43% | Mg | 2.7 mg/dL | Bilirubin, total | 1.7 mg/dL |
| BUN | 14 mg/dL | Plt | 239,000/mm³ | PO₄ | 4.4 mg/dL | Alb | 3.5 g/dL |

*Patient Case Question 7.* Are any of the laboratory blood test results above abnormal and, if so, what is suggested by the abnormality?

*Patient Case Question 8.* How might this patient be best treated?

*Patient Case Question 9.* What is the current probability that this patient will be alive in 10 years?

# CASE STUDY

# 84

## PSORIASIS

 *For the Disease Summary for this case study, see the CD-ROM.*

## PATIENT CASE

### History of Present Illness

K.B. is a 40-year-old white female with a 5-year history of psoriasis. She has scheduled an appointment with her dermatologist due to another relapse of psoriasis. This is her third flare-up since a definitive diagnosis was made. This outbreak of plaque psoriasis is generalized and involves large regions on the arms, legs, elbows, knees, abdomen, scalp, and groin.

K.B. was diagnosed with limited plaque-type psoriasis at age 35 and initially responded well to topical treatment with high-potency corticosteroids. She has been in remission for 18 months. Until now, lesions have been confined to small regions on the elbows and lower legs.

### Past Medical History

K.B. suffered a major episode of rheumatic fever at age 14 that has lead to complications associated with rheumatic heart disease. She has no other chronic medical conditions and no other acute or recent illnesses.

### Family History

Her father is alive and well. Her mother recently passed away from ovarian cancer after a long illness. She has three sisters and two brothers. Except for a younger sister who has also recently developed signs of heart disease from a bout of rheumatic fever many years ago, all of her siblings are well. There is no family history of psoriasis or immune disease in her family.

### Social History

K.B. has been a purchasing agent for a large national insurance company for 13 years. She smokes 4–5 cigarettes each day, uses alcohol only socially, does not use illicit drugs, is married, and has one son (age 15) in high school. There have been increasing tensions and anxiety at work recently because rumors have been circulating of possible downsizing and layoffs. K.B. has also been stressed at home due to "bitter words" exchanged between her father and siblings.

## ■ Medications

She is taking ibuprofen for occasional headaches and Rolaids for occasional "heartburn."

## ■ Allergies

K.B. has no known drug allergies, but was counseled recently by her primary care provider about stomach cramps from eating lettuce.

## ■ Additional History

The patient's skin "itches terribly despite using a non-medicated moisturizer several times a day." She has no joint stiffness or pain. She has been feeling nervous and stressed lately because of tensions at work, in the family, and due to the recent death of her mother.

## ■ Physical Examination and Laboratory Tests

### General

K.B. is a white female who is alert, mildly anxious, but in no apparent distress.

### Vital Signs

BP = 145/90; P = 75; RR = 14; T = 98.5°F; Ht = 5′2″; Wt = 165 lbs.

### Skin

- Confluent plaque-type psoriasis with extensive lesions on the patient's upper and lower extremities, scalp, abdomen, and groin; approximately 40% of total body surface area is involved
- Lesions are bright red in color with sharply defined borders except where confluent and are covered with loose, silvery-white scales
- No pustules or vesicles present
- Lesions on the arms, legs, and abdomen consistent with scratching (i.e., *excoriations*)

### Head, Eyes, Ears, Nose, and Throat

- Extensive scaly lesions on scalp
- PERRLA
- EOMI
- Fundi normal
- TMs intact
- Pharynx clear

### Neck

No lymphadenopathy, bruits, or thyromegaly

### Chest

Clear to auscultation anteriorly and posteriorly

### Heart

- RRR with no rubs or gallops
- A murmur can be distinctly heard

## Abdomen

- Positive bowel sounds
- Soft and non-tender with no masses
- Extensive scaly lesions and excoriations on skin

## Genitalia

Normal

## Rectal

Deferred exam

## Breasts

No masses, dimpling, discharge, or discoloration

## Musculoskeletal, Extremities

- No swelling, warmth, redness, or tenderness of joints
- Psoriatic lesions on elbows, knees, forearms, and calves
- Yellow spots in nail plates on fingers
- Peripheral pulses 2+ throughout

## Neurologic

- Alert and oriented × 3
- Cranial nerves II–XII intact
- DTRs (biceps and patella) 2+
- Gait steady

## Laboratory Blood Test Results

See Patient Case Table 84.1

### Patient Case Table 84.1 Laboratory Blood Test Results

| Na | 144 meq/L | HCO₃ | 26 meq/L | Hb | 11 g/dL | RBC | 4.0 million/mm³ | Bilirubin, total | 1.1 mg/dL |
|---|---|---|---|---|---|---|---|---|---|
| K | 4.0 meq/L | BUN | 15 mg/dL | Hct | 32% | AST | 23 IU/L | Alb | 3.8 g/dL |
| Cl | 102 meq/L | Cr | 1.1 mg/dL | Plt | 260,000/mm³ | ALT | 39 IU/L | Protein, total | 7.3 g/dL |
| Ca | 6.9 mg/dL | Glu, fasting | 94 mg/dL | WBC | 7,500/mm³ | Alk phos | 114 IU/L | Cholesterol | 289 mg/dL |

*Patient Case Question 1.* Is this patient technically *underweight, overweight, obese,* or is this patient's weight considered *healthy and normal* for her height?

*Patient Case Question 2.* What has possibly triggered this patient's current outbreak of psoriasis?

*Patient Case Question 3.* Why should a topical medication not be considered an option for this patient?

*Patient Case Question 4.* What is the preferred treatment for this patient?

***Patient Case Question 5.*** Other than widespread plaques and scales, does this patient have any abnormal clinical signs or laboratory tests that are consistent with a diagnosis of psoriasis?

***Patient Case Question 6.*** From the physical examination and laboratory tests, identify *seven* clinical manifestations unrelated to psoriasis that should concern the primary care provider.

***Patient Case Question 7.*** Why is it important that the primary care provider know that the only medications that K.B. has been taking are ibuprofen and Rolaids?

PART

# 14

# DISEASES
# OF THE
# BLOOD

# 85

# ACUTE LYMPHOBLASTIC LEUKEMIA

 *For the Disease Summary for this case study,*
*see the CD-ROM.*

## PATIENT CASE

### ▬ HPI

J.O. is a 5 yo girl who is brought to the pediatric clinic by her mother. Mrs. O. reports that, for the past week, her daughter has been very tired, lacks energy, sleeps more than usual, and has not had much of an appetite. Furthermore, there are unexplained bruises on her arms and legs.

### ▬ PMH

J.O. was a full-term infant from an uncomplicated pregnancy and delivery. All immunizations are current. She has had only one childhood disease—measles, at age 2 years.

### ▬ FH

The patient has one brother, age 3 years, who is in apparent good health. The family history is unremarkable with one exception: The paternal grandmother died at age 62 from gastric cancer. J.O. has not been exposed to ionizing radiation.

### ▬ SH

The patient's developmental milestones are on target. She can tie her shoes, print her own name, and likes to help with household tasks.

### ▬ ROS

Deferred

### ▬ Meds

None

# ■■■ All

NKDA

# ■■■ PE and Lab Tests

## Gen

- Alert, interactive, but ill-appearing white child
- Patient's height and weight seem normal for a 5-year-old

## VS

See Patient Case Table 85.1

| Patient Case Table 85.1 Vital Signs* |
| --- |
| Systolic blood pressure = 109 mm (94–109 mm) |
| Diastolic blood pressure = 67 mm (56–69 mm) |
| HR = 130/min (70–115/min awake) |
| RR = 20/min (17–27/min) |
| T = 98.6°F (98.3–98.6°F) |
| HT = 41 inches (41–43 inches) |
| WT = 37 lbs (40–50 lbs) |

*Reference vital signs appropriate for a 5-year-old girl are provided in parentheses.

***Patient Case Question 1.*** Suggest a reasonable cause of tachycardia in this patient.

## Skin

- Very pale, warm, and dry
- Ecchymoses on extremities, over the buttocks, and lower left flank area
- No rashes

## HEENT

- Head is normocephalic and atraumatic
- Pupils equal at 3 mm, round, and reactive to light and accommodation
- Extra-ocular muscles intact
- Tympanic membranes clear and intact
- Nares are clear bilaterally
- Throat is without redness or soreness
- Petechiae of mucous membranes in oral cavity
- Dental development consistent with age: has incisors, cuspids, and 1st and 2nd molars; no signs of maxillary or mandibular shedding

## Neck/LN

- Neck supple and non-tender
- Mild cervical adenopathy
- Three palpable, non-tender, 2-cm lymph nodes in the submaxillary chain

> *Patient Case Question 2.* Explain the enlarged lymph nodes in this patient.

## Lungs/Chest

- Clear to auscultation bilaterally without crackles or wheezes
- Good ventilation throughout

## Cardiac

Heart rate and rhythm normal and without murmurs

## Abd

- Soft and non-tender without distension
- Good bowel sounds
- No masses
- Liver and spleen are enlarged

> *Patient Case Question 3.* Explain the patient's enlarged liver and spleen.

## Genit/Rect

No tenderness, bruising, or blood observed

## MS/Ext

- Mild adenopathy in the inguinal region bilaterally
- Femoral pulses are 2+ bilaterally
- Extremities show no cyanosis, clubbing, or edema
- No bone or joint pain elicited by palpation

## Neuro

- No dysmorphic features
- Fixes and follows well with conjugate eye movements
- Hearing is within normal limits
- Motor exam shows 5/5 muscle tone in all extremities
- Gait is normal
- Cranial nerves intact
- Deep tendon reflexes present and equal at 2+
- Facial muscles symmetric and normal

## Laboratory Blood Test Results

See Patient Case Table 85.2

**Patient Case Table 85.2 Laboratory Blood Test Results**

| | | | |
|---|---|---|---|
| Hb | 7.1 g/dL | AST | 80 IU/L |
| Hct | 21% | ALT | 103 IU/L |
| RBC | 2.9 million/mm³ | Total bilirubin | 0.8 mg/dL |
| WBC | 12,800/mm³ | Total protein | 6.9 g/dL |
| • Neutrophils | 59% | Alb | 3.5 g/dL |
| • Lymphocytes | 26% | Ca | 9.2 mg/dL |
| • Monocytes | 3% | Phos | 4.0 mg/dL |
| • Eosinophils | 1% | Uric acid | 4.3 mg/dL |
| • Basophils | 1% | PT | 13 sec |
| • Blasts | 10% | PTT | 25 sec |
| Plt | 28,000/mm³ | Glucose, fasting | 90 mg/dL |

**Patient Case Question 4.** Why might this patient's AST and ALT concentrations be abnormal?

## Other Tests

J.O. was immediately referred to a pediatric oncologist and admitted to the children's hospital for further workup.

## Bone Marrow Aspirate

- 93% blasts, 3% erythroblasts, 4% all other cells
- RT-PCR: (+) for TEL-AML1 fusion gene with no other cytogenetic abnormalities

## Chest X-Ray

Normal with no mediastinal mass

## Lumbar Puncture

- Spinal fluid clear and colorless
- Opening pressure 90 mm $H_2O$
- Glucose 50 mg/dL
- Total protein 18 mg/dL
- No blasts present

## Immunology

(+) for cytoplasmic μ heavy-chain proteins

**Patient Case Question 5.** What is the significance of this patient's spinal tap?

**Patient Case Question 6.** Which type of acute lymphoblastic leukemia does this patient have?

**Patient Case Question 7.** Can this patient's prognosis be characterized as *very favorable, fair,* or *poor*?

## ■ Clinical Course

On the 2nd day following admission, J.O. was treated with irradiated/filtered platelets, packed red blood cells, and allopurinol.

**Patient Question 8.** Why was the patient treated with allopurinol prior to intensive chemotherapy?

## ■ Day 3 Remission Induction Therapy Orders

- Prednisone 1 mg IV Q wk × 4
- Vincristine 1 mg IV Q wk × 4
- Asparaginase 3,600 units IM on chemotherapy days 3, 6, 9, 13, 16, 20
- Intrathecal therapy with methotrexate on chemotherapy days 3 and 17

**Patient Case Question 9.** Why was intrathecal therapy begun when the patient had no clinical signs of leukemia in the central nervous system?

# 86

# CHRONIC MYELOGENOUS LEUKEMIA

 *For the Disease Summary for this case study, see the CD-ROM.*

## PATIENT CASE

### ■ Patient's Chief Complaints

"I have some pain on my left side that won't seem to go away. I've also been really tired lately and my exercise tolerance is nearly zero."

### ■ HPI

B.K. is a 54 yo woman who complains of DOE, an unintentional weight loss of 15 lbs, and fatigue that began approximately 3½ months ago. She also reports fullness with mild discomfort (3/10 on the pain scale) in her LUQ, early satiety, and a generally poor appetite.

### ■ PMH

- Hepatitis B carrier
- Gout × 25 years
- H/O kidney stones
- Fibromyalgia
- S/P tubal ligation
- Chronic pancreatitis (S/P stent placement in pancreatic duct)
- Alcoholic hepatitis
- Pneumonia 6 months ago (hospitalization required)
- Menopausal hot flashes diagnosed at age 47
- Osteoporosis × 1 year
- Vaccinations unknown

### ■ FH

- Father is living with Alzheimer disease and DM type 2 at age 82
- Mother died at age 29 from "heart failure"
- Brother, age 51, alive and well

- Sister, age 56, has depression
- No family history of cancer

## ■ SH

- Married and lives with husband of 16 years
- Has worked full-time as a hospital x-ray technician for 24 years
- Son murdered 3 years ago, no other children
- H/O alcohol abuse, currently 2 drinks whiskey/week
- 10 pack-year cigarette smoker (½ pack/year × 20 years)
- Had been walking 1–1½ miles every day but "has not had the energy lately"

## ■ ROS

- Progressive weakness and tiredness
- Occasional chills and night sweats
- Unaware of any fevers
- Shortness of breath with exertion
- Denies bleeding, easy bruising, headaches, nausea, vomiting, chest pain, urinary symptoms

## ■ Meds

- Allopurinol 300 mg po QD
- Pancrelipase 2 capsules (16,000 USP units lipase activity + 60,000 USP units amylase activity + 60,000 USP units protease activity) po TID with meals
- MVI 1 po QD
- Conjugated estrogens 0.3 mg/day for 25 days, followed by 5 days off
- Alendronate sodium 10 mg po QD
- Denies taking any herbal products
- Amitriptyline 40 mg po HS PRN for fibromyalgia symptoms

## ■ All

Fexofenadine → occasional palpitations

*Patient Case Question 1.* Why is the patient taking alendronate sodium?

*Patient Case Question 2.* Why is the patient taking allopurinol?

*Patient Case Question 3.* Why is the patient taking pancrelipase?

*Patient Case Question 4.* Why is the patient taking conjugated estrogens?

## ■ PE and Lab Tests

### Gen

- Thin, white female in mild pain and is rubbing her left side below the ribcage
- Appears fatigued, anxious, and uncomfortable
- Pleasant and cooperative

- Appears A & O
- Wears glasses and appears to be her stated age

## VS

See Patient Case Table 86.1

| Patient Case Table 86.1 Vital Signs | | | |
|---|---|---|---|
| BP | 130/88 right arm, sitting | HT | 5'5½" |
| P | 58 and regular | WT current | 103 lbs |
| RR | 15 and unlabored | BMI | 17.0 |
| T | 99.4°F | WT 4 months ago | 119 lbs |

## Skin

- Warm and dry with normal turgor
- Negative for rash, ecchymoses, petechiae, cyanosis, tumors, and nevi
- Marked "crow's feet" wrinkling around the eyes

## HEENT

- PERRLA
- EOM intact and full
- Fundi intact, clear disc margins without arteriolar narrowing, hemorrhages, exudates, or papilledema
- Sclerae anicteric
- No strabismus, nystagmus, or conjunctivitis
- Normal pink conjunctiva
- TMs WNL bilaterally
- Nares patent
- No sinus discharge or tenderness
- Throat not erythematous
- Mucous membranes pink, moist, and intact
- Wears dentures

## Neck/LN

- Supple without stiffness
- No carotid bruits auscultated
- No goiter or JVD observed
- Approximately 2-cm, non-tender palpable right cervical node
- 2-cm non-tender left supraclavicular lymph node palpable

## Chest

- Clear to A & P bilaterally
- No crackles or wheezes noted upon auscultation
- No CVAT or spinal tenderness

## Cardiac

- NSR
- Normal $S_1$ and $S_2$
- No murmur, rub, or gallop
- No $S_3$ or $S_4$

## Abd

- Soft and symmetric
- Splenomegaly prominent with exquisite LUQ tenderness to light palpation
- Normoactive BS in all four quadrants
- No hepatomegaly noted
- No fluid wave

## GU/Rect

- Normal female genitalia
- Pelvic exam normal and uterus intact
- No abnormal vaginal discharge
- Normal sphincter tone, no masses, and guaiac-negative stool
- No polyps or hemorrhoids

## MS/Ext

- No joint deformities, active synovitis, arthritis, or peripheral edema
- ROM WNL
- Muscle strength 5/5 and symmetric throughout
- 2+ dorsalis pedis and posterior tibial pulses bilaterally
- No hematomas
- No swelling, tenderness, or clubbing
- Capillary refill normal at < 2 sec

## Neuro

- CNs II–XII intact
- DTRs 2+ throughout
- Gait steady and coordination normal
- Oriented to person, place, and time
- Memory intact
- Sensory and motor levels normal
- Negative Babinski
- No focal neurologic deficits

## Laboratory Blood Test Results (Fasting)

See Patient Case Table 86.2

| Patient Case Table 86.2 Laboratory Blood Test Results (Fasting) | | | | | |
|---|---|---|---|---|---|
| Na | 139 meq/L | Plt | 498,000/mm$^3$ | ALT | 55 IU/L |
| K | 4.6 meq/L | WBC | 98,000/mm$^3$ | Alk Phos | 105 IU/L |
| Cl | 103 meq/L | • Neutros | 60% | T bilirubin | 1.0 mg/dL |
| HCO$_3$ | 23 meq/L | • Myeloblasts | 17% | T protein | 6.3 g/dL |
| BUN | 20 mg/dL | • Lymphs | 4% | Alb | 3.7 g/dL |
| Cr | 1.2 mg/dL | • Monos | 1% | Ca | 8.3 mg/dL |
| Glu | 95 mg/dL | • Basos | 10% | Mg | 3.0 mg/dL |
| Hb | 10.9 g/dL | • Eos | 8% | Phos | 4.2 mg/dL |
| Hct | 29% | AST | 34 IU/L | Uric acid | 9.8 mg/dL |

## Peripheral Blood Smear

- (+) normochromic normocytic RBC
- Excessive numbers of neutrophils and myeloblasts

## UA

SG 1.017, pH 6.1; no protein, glucose, ketones, WBC, or RBC

## Bone Marrow Biopsy

Cytogenetic studies revealed a translocation involving the long arms of chromosome 9 and 22 with 98% of malignant cells Philadelphia chromosome-positive. Trisomy of chromosome 9 was also observed. The marrow was hypercellular and consisted of an excessive number of myeloblasts.

## Polymerase Chain Reaction

(+) for abl-bcr oncogene

*Patient Case Question 5.* List a minimum of *20* clinical manifestations in this patient that are consistent with a diagnosis of chronic myelogenous leukemia.

*Patient Case Question 6.* Identify *two* potential risk factors for chronic myelogenous leukemia in this case study.

*Patient Case Question 7.* Which phase of chronic myelogenous leukemia has developed in this patient?

*Patient Case Question 8.* Provide a strong rationale for your answer to Question 7 directly above.

*Patient Case Question 9.* Neither the patient's brother nor sister will consent to donating their bone marrow to the patient. What type of approach to treatment would you suggest for this patient?

*Patient Case Question 10.* Which *two* of this patient's pre-existing health conditions may be promoted by the onset and development of chronic myelogenous leukemia?

# CASE STUDY

## 87

# FOLIC ACID DEFICIENCY ANEMIA

 *For the Disease Summary for this case study, see the CD-ROM.*

## PATIENT CASE

### ■ Patient's Chief Complaints

"I've been feeling really lousy lately. I have no energy whatsoever and I'm always cranky."

### ■ HPI

W.L. is an 80 yo man who presents to the Veterans Administration Hospital for a routine checkup. Upon questioning, he states that he "has been feeling weak and terrible" for nearly six months now but has not experienced any loss in weight.

### ■ PMH

- Multiple DVT with chronic venous insufficiency
- Type 2 DM
- HTN
- Hyperlipidemia
- Prostate cancer S/P prostatectomy
- S/P CVA
- DJD; hip fracture 7 years ago; chronic pain in lower back and right buttock
- Mild memory loss
- Chronic allergic rhinitis
- Seizure disorder × 17 years; no seizures with medication in 3 years
- COPD × 11 years

### ■ FH

- Father and brother were coal mine workers and died at ages 62 and 68 from complications of anthracosis ("black lung disease")
- No information available for mother
- One brother at age 73 is alive with HTN and DM

416

## ▬ SH

- Retired at age 62 after 42 years as a coal miner
- Long-term history of cigarette use, which continues at 10 cigarettes/day
- Heavy EtOH use (mostly beer) on and off × 15 years, which continues
- Very little physical activity
- Married for 51 years
- Wife is 75 yo and in relatively good health

## ▬ Meds

- Docusate sodium 100 mg po BID
- Triamterene 25 mg po QD
- Loratadine 10 mg po QD
- Cyclobenzaprine 10 mg po BID PRN
- Acetaminophen 325 mg po Q 4–6h PRN
- Glipizide 20 mg po BID
- HCTZ 12.5 mg po QD
- Pravastatin 40 mg po HS
- Warfarin sodium 5 mg po QD
- Ipratropium bromide MDI 2 puffs QID
- Phenytoin 100 mg po TID

*Patient Case Question 1.* Why is this patient taking docusate sodium?

*Patient Case Question 2.* For which pre-existing condition is this patient taking triamterene?

*Patient Case Question 3.* For which pre-existing condition is this patient taking loratadine?

*Patient Case Question 4.* For which pre-existing condition is this patient taking cyclobenzaprine?

*Patient Case Question 5.* For which pre-existing condition is this patient taking glipizide?

*Patient Case Question 6.* For which pre-existing condition is this patient taking HCTZ?

*Patient Case Question 7.* For which pre-existing condition is this patient taking pravastatin?

*Patient Case Question 8.* For which pre-existing condition is this patient taking warfarin sodium?

*Patient Case Question 9.* For which pre-existing condition is this patient taking ipratropium bromide?

*Patient Case Question 10.* For which pre-existing condition is this patient taking phenytoin?

*Patient Case Question 11.* Identify *five* risk factors that have placed this patient at risk for folic acid deficiency anemia.

## ▬ All

- Codeine (rash)
- Morphine (hallucinations)

## ■ ROS

- (–) SOB, headache, swelling of ankles, chest pain, anorexia, sore mouth/tongue, lightheadedness, pain with swallowing, muscle/abdominal pain, and diarrhea
- (+) some difficulty focusing attention
- (–) paresthesias
- (–) bruising and bleeding

## ■ PE and Lab Tests

### Gen

The patient is a pleasant, elderly white man in NAD that appears to be his stated age of 80. He is cooperative and oriented. Speech is slightly rambling but easily directed.

### VS

See Patient Case Table 87.1

| Patient Case Table 87.1 Vital Signs | | | | | |
|---|---|---|---|---|---|
| BP | 130/85 sitting, right arm | RR | 18 | BMI | 28.1 |
| P | 110 | T | 97.8°F | O$_2$ saturation | 95.5% |

**Patient Case Question 12.** Briefly comment on the patient's vital signs.

### Skin

- Actinic keratosis on face and upper extremities
- Cool with normal turgor
- Pallor is prominent
- (–) for jaundice

**Patient Case Question 13.** What is the primary cause of actinic keratosis?

### HEENT

- NC/AT
- Patient wears glasses
- PERRLA
- EOMI
- Funduscopic exam reveals mild arteriolar narrowing without hemorrhages, exudates, or papilledema
- Slightly pale conjunctiva
- Subnormal hearing bilaterally
- Dentures present
- Deviated nasal septum with little airflow through right nostril
- (–) glossitis
- Significant pallor of oral mucosa was noted

# Neck

- Supple without masses
- Normal thyroid
- (–) JVD, lymphadenopathy, and bruits
- Trachea mid-line

# Lungs

Decreased breath sounds bilaterally with diffuse inspiratory and expiratory wheezes bilaterally

# Cardiac

- Tachycardia with NSR
- Systolic murmur heard best at the right sternal border
- No rubs

# Abd

- Soft, non-tender, and non-distended
- Normal and reactive BS
- No masses, bruits, splenomegaly, or hepatomegaly
- No guarding, rebound, or rigidity

# Ext

- No lower leg edema
- No warmth or pain
- Negative for paresthesias, clubbing, and cyanosis
- Age-appropriate strength and range of motion throughout
- Capillary refill WNL
- Radial and pedal pulses 3+ bilaterally

# Rect/GU

- Good sphincter tone
- Stool heme-negative
- (–) hemorrhoids
- Normal testes and penis

# Neuro

- A & O × 3 (day, place, president)
- Slight left facial weakness from CVA
- Proprioception intact bilaterally
- Coordination intact
- Vibratory sensation intact
- Negative for ataxia
- DTRs WNL

***Patient Case Question 14.*** What is the significance of the *absence* of SOB, JVD, ankle/leg swelling, hepatomegaly, and splenomegaly in this patient?

*Patient Case Question 15.* What is the significance of the *absence* of paresthesias and ataxia and the *presence* of intact vibratory sensation in this patient?

## Laboratory Blood Test Results

See Patient Case Table 87.2

| Patient Case Table 87.2 Laboratory Blood Test Results | | | | | |
|---|---|---|---|---|---|
| Na | 137 meq/L | RBC | $3.0 \times 10^6/mm^3$ | AST | 17 IU/L |
| K | 4.6 meq/L | Plt | $139 \times 10^3/mm^3$ | ALT | 49 IU/L |
| Cl | 104 meq/L | WBC | $4.4 \times 10^3/mm^3$ | Alk phos | 126 IU/L |
| $HCO_3$ | 22 meq/L | MCV | 103 fL | Bilirubin | 1.2 mg/dL |
| BUN | 20 mg/dL | MCHC | 33.5 g/dL | Albumin | 3.5 g/dL |
| Cr | 1.1 mg/dL | Fe | 67 µg/dL | TSH | 3.97 µU/mL |
| Ca | 9.5 mg/dL | TIBC | 312 µg/dL | $HbA_{1c}$ | 9.3% |
| Mg | 2.4 mg/dL | Transferrin saturation | 39% | Cholesterol | 194 mg/dL |
| Glu, fasting | 185 mg/dL | Ferritin | 124 ng/mL | LDL | 99 mg/dL |
| Hb | 8.8 g/dL | Vitamin $B_{12}$ | 230 pg/mL | HDL | 30 mg/dL |
| Hct | 19.7% | Folate | 1.7 ng/mL | INR | 2.5 |

## Peripheral Blood Smear

- Anisocytosis + poikilocytosis
- Large neutrophils with 6–7 segments
- Macrocytic, normochromic RBCs

*Patient Case Question 16.* Identify a minimum of *fifteen* clinical manifestations (including laboratory blood test results) that are consistent with and relevant to a diagnosis of folic acid deficiency anemia.

*Patient Case Question 17.* Is this patient's diabetes mellitus under control?

*Patient Case Question 18.* Is this patient's hyperlipidemia under control?

*Patient Case Question 19.* Is this patient's drug-induced anticoagulation under control?

*Patient Case Question 20.* Hypothyroid disease is a risk factor for folic acid deficiency anemia. Does the patient have any clinical signs that he has become hypothyroid?

*Patient Case Question 21.* Would you consider this patient *high risk* for the development of infections *at this time?*

*Patient Case Question 22.* Do you think that the bone marrow in this patient is *acellular, hypocellular, normocellular,* or *hypercellular?*

# 88  IRON DEFICIENCY ANEMIA

 *For the Disease Summary for this case study,*
*see the CD-ROM.*

# PATIENT CASE

## ■ Patient's Chief Complaints

"I've been having some bleeding between periods and some rather heavy bleeding with mild cramping during my last two periods. I've also been extremely weak and tired lately, and I've been going to the bathroom more often lately."

## ■ HPI

J.D. is a 37 yo white woman who presents to her gynecologist complaining of a 2-month history of intermenstrual bleeding, menorrhagia, increased urinary frequency, mild incontinence, extreme fatigue, and weakness. Her menstrual period occurs every 28 days and lately there have been 6 days of heavy flow and cramping. She denies abdominal distension, backache, and constipation. She has not had her usual energy levels since before her last pregnancy.

## ■ PMH

Upon reviewing her past medical history, the gynecologist notes that her patient is a $G_5P_5$ with four pregnancies within four years, the last infant having been delivered vaginally four months ago. All five pregnancies were unremarkable and without delivery complications. All infants were born healthy.

Patient history also reveals a 3-year history of osteoarthritis in the left knee, probably the result of sustaining significant trauma to her knee in an MVA when she was 9 yo. When asked what OTC medications she is currently taking for her pain and for how long she has been taking them, she reveals that she started taking ibuprofen, three tablets each day, about 2½ years ago for her left knee. Due to a slowly progressive increase in pain and a loss of adequate relief with three tablets, she doubled the daily dose of ibuprofen. Upon the recommendation from her nurse practitioner and because long-term ibuprofen use can cause peptic ulcers, she began taking OTC omeprazole on a regular basis to prevent gastrointestinal bleeding.

Patient history also reveals a 3-year history of HTN for which she is now being treated with a diuretic and a centrally acting antihypertensive drug. She has had no previous surgeries.

## FH

- Father alive, age 66, with angina
- Mother alive, age 62, with arthritis
- One brother, age 35, alive with DM and hyperlipidemia
- One sister, age 34, with history of depression and hypothyroid disease
- Both paternal grandparents had heart disease
- Five children, ages 4 months to 9 years, alive and well

## SH

- Born in the United States of Greek parents
- Married homemaker, lives with husband
- Non-smoker and non-drinker
- (–) illicit drug use
- Strict vegetarian × 5 years
- Admits to lacking a regularly scheduled exercise program, "although the kids keep me running all the time"

## ROS

- Reveals a craving for cold celery for the past 3 weeks
- (+) mild urinary urgency with incontinence
- (–) hematuria, hematemesis, hemoptysis, melena
- (+) recent mild SOB with exertion, progressive irritability with difficulty concentrating
- (–) palpitations
- (–) abnormal nail bed changes, sore tongue and lips, headaches, restless legs, chest pain, cold intolerance, dysphagia, cold hands and feet, dizziness, lightheadedness
- (–) history of cardiac or pulmonary disease

## Meds

- 35 μg ethinyl estradiol with 0.5 mg norethindrone (10 tablets) and 35 ∝g ethinyl estradiol with 1.0 mg norethindrone (11 tablets) monthly
- OTC ibuprofen 200 mg po 6×/day PRN
- OTC omeprazole 20 mg po QD
- Hydrochlorothiazide 30 mg and methyldopa 500 mg po BID
- (–) for multivitamins, calcium supplements, and iron supplements

## All

- Erythromycin → upset stomach
- Aspirin → upset stomach

## PE and Lab Tests

### Gen

- Tired- and pale-looking, overweight white female in NAD
- Appears her stated age
- Pleasant, cooperative, alert, and oriented × 3

### VS

See Patient Case Table 88.1

| Patient Case Table 88.1 Vital Signs | | | | | |
|---|---|---|---|---|---|
| BP | 100/40 sitting, right arm | RR | 17 and unlabored | HT | 5'6" |
| P | 140 and regular | T | 98.0°F | WT | 173 lbs |

## Skin

- Pale and cool with normal turgor
- (–) rash
- Seborrheic keratosis over upper back

## HEENT

- NC/AT
- PERRLA
- EOMI
- Normal funduscopic exam
- Bluish sclerae
- Slightly pale conjunctiva
- Ear canals clear and eardrums negative
- Nares normal
- (–) swelling or tenderness above maxillary and ethmoid sinuses
- Teeth intact
- Tongue mid-line and negative for glossitis
- Tonsils intact and normal
- Oral mucous membranes pale but moist
- Pharynx unremarkable
- (–) angular stomatitis

## Neck/LN

- Normal motion of neck
- Trachea mid-line
- No lymphadenopathy or thyromegaly
- No bruits, masses, or other abnormalities

## Lungs/Thorax

- Bilateral breath sounds
- No wheezes or crackles
- (–) CVAT

## Breasts

- Symmetric bilaterally
- Without masses, discoloration, dimpling, or discharge
- Normal axilla

## Cardiac

- Tachycardia
- Systolic murmur heard best at right sternal border
- (–) rubs

## Abd

- Slightly obese, soft, and tender to palpation
- No masses
- (+) bowel sounds
- (–) hepatomegaly and splenomegaly

## Genit/Rect

- Good anal sphincter tone
- Guaiac-negative stool
- Normal external female genitalia
- Irregular, non-tender nodularity of uterus on bimanual examination

## MS/Ext

- Joint enlargement and limited ROM of left knee, consistent with DJD
- (–) paresthesias, clubbing, or cyanosis
- Pulses 2+ bilaterally
- No edema or ulcers

## Neuro

- A & O × 3
- Good auditory acuity
- Proprioception intact bilaterally
- Coordination intact
- (–) ataxia and nystagmus
- CNs II–XII grossly intact
- Muscle strength in UE and LE equal bilaterally
- Vibratory sense intact
- Reflexes intact at 2+
- Mental status intact
- Plantars downgoing

## Laboratory Blood Test Results

See Patient Case Table 88.2

| Patient Case Table 88.2 Laboratory Blood Test Results | | | | | |
|---|---|---|---|---|---|
| Na | 141 meq/L | MCV | 71 fL | Alb | 4.4 g/dL |
| K | 4.2 meq/L | MCH | 19 pg | Cholesterol | 273 mg/dL |
| Cl | 99 meq/L | MCHC | 27 g/dL | Ca | 9.1 mg/dL |
| $HCO_3$ | 27 meq/L | WBC | $7.9 \times 10^3/mm^3$ | Iron | 35 µg/dL |
| BUN | 20 mg/dL | Plt | $623 \times 10^3/mm^3$ | TIBC | 706 µg/dL |
| Cr | 1.0 mg/dL | AST | 36 IU/L | Transferrin sat | 5.0% |
| Glu, fasting | 97 mg/dL | ALT | 43 IU/L | Ferritin | 9.7 ng/mL |
| Hb | 9.1 g/dL | Bilirubin | 1.2 mg/dL | FEP | 54 µg/dL |
| Hct | 27.5% | LDH | 114 IU/L | Vitamin B12 | 680 pg/mL |
| RBC | $3.3 \times 10^6/mm^3$ | Protein | 7.1 g/dL | Folic acid | 420 ng/mL |

# Urinalysis

See Patient Case Table 88.3

| Patient Case Table 88.3 Urinalysis | | | | | |
|---|---|---|---|---|---|
| Color | *Yellow* | Protein | (–) | Ketones | (–) |
| Appearance | *Hazy* | Glucose | (–) | Bacteria | (–) |
| pH | 6.4 | Hemoglobin | (+) | RBC | 2/HPF |
| SG | 1.017 | Bilirubin | (–) | WBC | 2/HPF |

# Peripheral Blood Smear

- (+) significant number of hypochromic, microcytic RBC
- (+) mild anisocytosis and poikilocytosis

# Pelvic Ultrasonography

- Irregularly enlarged uterus with 5 distinct uterine masses visible
- 3 masses submucous in location (½–1″ in diameter)
- 1 mass subserous in location (2″ in diameter)
- 1 mass intramural in location (¾″ in diameter)
- Findings are consistent with a diagnosis of uterine fibroids/leiomyomas

*Patient Case Question 1.* The patient in this case study has *seven* potential contributing factors for the development of iron deficiency anemia. What are they?

*Patient Case Question 2.* What is causing increased urinary frequency, urinary urgency, and mild incontinence in this patient?

*Patient Case Question 3.* What is causing intermenstrual bleeding and menorrhagia in this patient?

*Patient Case Question 4.* Why did the gynecologist question the patient about constipation?

*Patient Case Question 5.* Why is this patient taking ethinyl estradiol and norethindrone tablets?

*Patient Case Question 6.* Why were serum vitamin B12 and folic acid concentrations tested?

*Patient Case Question 7.* What is the potential significance that the patient was born of Greek parents?

*Patient Case Question 8.* *Symptoms* are subjective clinical manifestations of an illness that can only be reported by the patient. Identify *seven* clinical symptoms in this case study that are consistent with a diagnosis of iron deficiency anemia.

*Patient Case Question 9.* *Signs* are objective clinical manifestations of an illness that can be observed by someone other than the patient. Identify a minimum of *twenty* clinical signs in this case study that are consistent with a diagnosis of iron deficiency anemia.

*Patient Case Question 10.* Provide *five* different treatment modalities that will help resolve iron deficiency anemia in this patient.

*Patient Case Question 11.* To which stage of iron deficiency has the patient in this case progressed?

*For the Disease Summary for this case study,*
*see the CD-ROM.*

## PATIENT CASE

### ■■■ Patient's Chief Complaints

"My arms and legs hurt a lot more than usual today. The ibuprofen has stopped working and I need something stronger. I may have overdone it at the gym."

### ■■■ History of Present Illness

I.T. is an 18-year-old African American male with sickle cell anemia who presents with a one-day history of increasing pain localized to his arms and legs. His pain has not been relieved with 400-mg ibuprofen every 6 hours for the past 24 hours. He rates his current pain intensity level as 8 out of 10. He reports that he always seems to have some pain in his arms, legs, and back, but the pain intensified approximately 36 hours after a workout at the gym that was more vigorous than usual. "I know that I shouldn't have done that," he confesses, "but the guys needed a 6th player for a game of 3-on-3. And, on top of that, I forgot to take my water bottle to the gym."

### ■■■ Past Medical History

The patient was diagnosed with homozygous HbS disease at age 11 months. He first presented with a severe case of dactylitis at 10½ months with significant swelling and pain in both hands and feet. Electrophoresis revealed a hemoglobin proportion of 86.5% HbS, 11.3% HbF, and 2.2% HbA$_2$.

At age 16 months, the patient was hospitalized with acute sequestration syndrome and splenomegaly, treated, and released. At age 30 months and again at age 34 months, the patient was hospitalized for *Streptococcus pneumoniae* pneumonia, treated with IV antibiotics, and released. He also experienced one episode of acute staphylococcal osteomyelitis of the left knee at age 13. Since the age of 3 years, the patient has averaged three painful crises per year but has had as many as 10 attacks in a year. He has experienced chronic low-grade pain in his arms, legs, and back since becoming a teenager but has been able to cope by taking ibuprofen when needed.

Other medical conditions and surgeries of note include:

• Born with hypospadias, which was surgically corrected at 8 months of age
• Tonsillectomy as a child

- Childhood asthma that resolved at puberty
- Chronic sinus drainage/rhinitis × 2 years

# Family History

- Mother and father are both alive and well; both tested positive for sickle cell trait
- One brother, age 17, with sickle cell trait

# Social History

- Parents are divorced
- Single male who lives at home with his mother and brother during the summer and will reside in a college dormitory during the next academic year
- Recently graduated from high school with honors and hopes to pursue a college education and major in business
- Works part-time as a cashier at JC Penney's
- Does not smoke, drink alcohol, or use illicit drugs "except for one trial of pot 2 years ago"
- Reports being sexually active last year with one sexual partner; not currently sexually active
- Gets as much exercise daily as he can tolerate
- Tries to maintain a healthy and balanced diet
- Does not drink coffee but consumes 2–3 caffeinated soft drinks/day

# Review of Systems

- Denies headache, cough, fever, chills, dizziness, lightheadedness, nausea, vomiting, diarrhea, shortness of breath, blurred vision, chest pain, blood in the urine, abdominal pain, and painful urination
- Admits to feeling tired much of the time but has generally been able to tolerate it

# Medications

- Folic acid 1 mg po QD
- Ibuprofen 400 mg po TID PRN
- Flunisolide 2 sprays each nostril QD

# Allergies

- Aspirin → diarrhea
- Allergic to poison sumac

# Physical Examination and Laboratory Tests

## General Appearance

The patient is a tall, thin, African American male in moderate-to-severe pain

## Vital Signs

See Patient Case Table 89.1

| **Patient Case Table 89.1 Vital Signs** | | | | | |
|---|---|---|---|---|---|
| BP | 95/60 | RR | 18 | BMI | 18.7 |
| P | 58 | T | 98.5°F | Pulse ox | 96% on room air |

## Skin and Hair

- Warm and dry with poor turgor/some tenting
- (–) rashes, bruises, or lesions
- Hair quantity, distribution, and texture unremarkable

## Head, Eyes, Ears, Nose, and Throat

- Normocephalic and atraumatic
- Pupils equal at 3 mm, round, and reactive to light
- Extra-ocular muscles intact without nystagmus
- Normal sclerae
- Funduscopic exam revealed sharp optic disc margins with no arteriolar narrowing or hemorrhages
- External auricular canals clear
- Tympanic membranes gray and reveal good cone of light bilaterally
- Nasal mucous membranes dry
- Oral mucosa dry and without erythema
- No oropharyngeal lesions
- Lips dry

## Neck and Lymph Nodes

- Neck supple
- (–) cervical, axillary, and inguinal nodes bilaterally
- (–) thyromegaly, nodules, carotid bruits, and jugular vein distension

## Lungs and Thorax

- Clear to auscultation throughout with good breath sounds
- No costovertebral angle tenderness or spinal tenderness

## Heart

- Regular rate and rhythm
- (–) rubs and gallops
- Systolic ejection murmur is prominent

## Abdomen

- Normoactive bowel sounds in all four quadrants
- Soft, non-tender, and non-distended without guarding
- (–) organomegaly, masses, and bruits

## Rectum/Genitalia

- Guaiac negative
- Normal penis

- Minimal scarring on penis post-surgically from repair of hypospadias
- Testicles in scrotum bilaterally

## Musculoskeletal and Extremities

- 2+ peripheral pulses in dorsalis pedis and tibialis pedis bilaterally
- (–) edema, ulcers, and clubbing
- Normal strength
- Limited range of motion in elbows, wrists, knees, and ankles

## Neurological

- Alert and oriented × 3
- Cranial nerves II–XII intact
- Deep tendon reflexes intact throughout
- Sensory and motor levels intact
- (–) focal abnormalities
- Negative Babinski sign

## Laboratory Blood Test Results

See Patient Case Table 89.2

| Patient Case Table 89.2 Laboratory Blood Test Results | | | | | |
|---|---|---|---|---|---|
| Na | 141 meq/L | Hct | 28.1% | Bilirubin—total | 1.4 mg/dL |
| K | 3.6 meq/L | Plt | $225 \times 10^3/mm^3$ | Bilirubin—indirect | 0.9 mg/dL |
| Cl | 101 meq/L | WBC | $7.0 \times 10^3/mm^3$ | Alb | 3.7 g/dL |
| $HCO_3$ | 22 meq/L | MCV | 82.1 fL | Protein—total | 6.3 g/dL |
| BUN | 13 mg/dL | Retic | 6.4% | Ca | 9.3 mg/dL |
| Cr | 1.2 mg/dL | AST | 25 IU/L | Mg | 1.9 mg/dL |
| Glu, fasting | 87 mg/dL | ALT | 22 IU/L | $PO_4$ | 4.0 mg/dL |
| Hb | 10.9 g/dL | Alk phos | 75 IU/L | Folic acid | 515 ng/mL |

## Peripheral Blood Smear

(+) sickled and crescent forms and target cells

## Chest X-Rays

Clear

## Electrocardiogram

Normal sinus rhythm

## Echocardiogram

Normal left ventricular function, normal left ventricular wall thickness, mild dilation of right ventricle

## Urinalysis

(–) blood and protein

***Patient Case Question 1.*** What precipitating factors probably triggered this painful crisis?

***Patient Case Question 2.*** What specifically is causing this patient's current pain crisis?

***Patient Case Question 3.*** Identify this patient's *two* major risk factors for sickle cell anemia.

***Patient Case Question 4.*** Which *single* clinical finding provided a definitive diagnosis of sickle cell anemia in this patient?

***Patient Case Question 5.*** Excluding laboratory test results, list a minimum of *eight* clinical manifestations or complications from this case that are consistent with a diagnosis of sickle cell anemia.

***Patient Case Question 6.*** Identify *two subnormal* clinical values from the laboratory blood test results in Table 89.2 and briefly explain why they are abnormal.

***Patient Case Question 7.*** Identify *three* clinical blood test results from Table 89.2 that were elevated and briefly explain why they are elevated.

***Patient Case Question 8.*** Does this patient require an adjustment in his daily dose of folate?

***Patient Case Question 9.*** Why is this patient taking flunisolide?

***Patient Case Question 10.*** List a minimum of *four* laboratory blood test results that indicate that hepatic injury has not yet occurred from sickle cell anemia.

***Patient Case Question 11.*** If both parents are carriers of the HbS mutation, what is the probability that their child will . . .

a. have sickle cell anemia?

b. be a carrier of the HbS mutation?

***Patient Case Question 12.*** If one parent has all of the clinical manifestations of sickle cell anemia and the other parent does not have sickle cell anemia nor is a carrier of the HbS mutation, what is the probability that their child will . . .

a. have sickle cell anemia?

b. be a carrier of the HbS mutation?

# CASE STUDY 90

# VITAMIN B12 DEFICIENCY ANEMIA

 *For the Disease Summary for this case study, see the CD-ROM.*

## PATIENT CASE

### ■ Patient's Chief Complaints

"I've been feeling terrible for nearly six months. Lately, I've been having problems talking and some difficulty with concentration and remembering things that I did yesterday. I've also had some numbness in both of my legs and, sometimes, I have trouble walking. I think all that booze and all those 8-balls have finally taken a toll on me. I'm feeling old and I know that I have to change before it kills me."

### ■ History of Present Illness

J.K. is a 26-year-old male who presented with pallor and fatigue. He complains of a two-day history of difficulty expressing his thoughts and problems with both concentration and short-term memory. In addition, he describes a three-month history of bilateral lower extremity numbness and weakness that has been progressing upwards and gait difficulty.

Onset of his symptoms was gradual and included numbness and intermittent tingling sensations in both hands and both feet. He described his gait difficulty as "unsteadiness that is worse in the dark." He also reported an episodic shooting pain that begins in his neck and passes down his back and into both arms. He denied any history of previous trauma.

### ■ Past Medical History

- No prior history of serious medical diseases or infections
- Questionable compliance with medications in the past
- Hospitalized at ages 17 and 20 for detoxification from alcohol and cocaine plus psychiatric evaluation
- History of genital herpes infections

### ■ Family History

- Family history is negative for genetic, neurologic, endocrine, and autoimmune diseases
- Father has history of alcohol abuse

431

- Mother developed bacterial thyroiditis and hypothyroid disease at age 34
- Both parents are alive; mother has re-married but father has not and lives alone

## ■■■■ Social History

- Did not graduate from high school but received GED at age 19
- Parents divorced when he was 14 years old
- Single and lives alone; has three daughters with different mothers
- Has worked various jobs of construction, cement work, and brick-laying for the past 5 years
- No tobacco use
- Excessive use of alcohol and cocaine since age 17
- Long history of poor nutrition: meals have consisted mainly of donuts, grilled cheese, and peanut butter and jelly sandwiches, French fries, potato chips, and beer for the past 4 years; very few meats, dairy products, fresh fruits, or vegetables

## ■■■■ Review of Systems

- Denies double-vision and vision loss, difficulty swallowing, dizziness and vertigo, hearing loss, loss of smell or taste, loss of consciousness, shortness of breath, chest pain, abdominal pain, nausea and vomiting, hallucinations, depression, and symptoms of bowel or bladder dysfunction
- Reports significant weight loss in last 3 months of 15–20 lbs
- Mild-to-moderate "burning" of tongue for about 3 days
- (+) paresthesias, upper and lower extremities bilaterally

## ■■■■ Medications

- Occasional OTC anti-inflammatory drugs for neck pain
- Has used OTC famotidine "almost every day" for the past 2 years for heartburn

## ■■■■ Allergies

- No known drug allergies

---

***Patient Case Question 1.*** Identify *three* major risk factors that have likely contributed to a vitamin B12 deficiency state in this patient.

## ■■■■ Physical Examination and Laboratory Tests

### General

- Patient is an apparently undernourished white adult male in mild distress
- Reports feeling unwell overall; 2–3 on a scale of 10 for general well-being
- Strong smell of cigarette smoke and alcohol but does not appear intoxicated
- Pleasant and cooperative but slow to answer questions
- Unkempt and unshaven and appears tired and underweight
- Appears noticeably restless

## Vital Signs

See Patient Case Table 90.1

| **Patient Case Table 90.1 Vital Signs** | | | | | |
|---|---|---|---|---|---|
| BP | 165/82, sitting | RR | 18, regular and not labored | HT | 5′9″ |
| P | 84, regular | T | 98.2°F | WT | 121 lbs |

## Skin

- Pallor with mild jaundice
- Turgor normal
- Negative for rash or other lesions

## Head, Eyes, Ears, Nose, and Throat

- Normocephalic and atraumatic
- Sclera mildly icteric
- Tympanic membranes intact
- Beefy-red tongue consistent with glossitis
- Pallor of mucous membranes; otherwise, oropharynx unremarkable

## Neck and Lymph Nodes

- Significant discomfort of neck with flexion
- Trachea mid-line
- No lymphadenopathy, audible bruits, thyromegaly, masses, or other abnormalities

## Chest and Lungs

- Bilateral breath sounds
- No wheezes or crackles

## Back

No spinal or costovertebral angle tenderness

## Heart

- Regular rate and rhythm
- Systolic murmur heard best at right sternal border
- No rubs

## Abdomen

- Soft, non-tender, and non-distended
- No masses, bruits, or organomegaly
- Positive bowel sounds

## Genitalia and Rectum

- Normal male genitalia
- Normal anal sphincter tone
- Stool guaiac-negative

## Musculoskeletal and Extremities

- No clubbing, cyanosis, or edema of extremities bilaterally
- No warmth or pain
- Normal range of motion

## Neurologic

### Mental Status

- Cooperative, alert, attentive, and oriented × 3
- Response time was somewhat slowed
- Mini-mental exam 25/30 (missed four points on serial 9 subtraction; recent memory was mildly impaired recalling 3 of 4 items at 5 minutes)

### Cranial Nerve Function

| | |
|---|---|
| II | Visual acuity 20/20 bilaterally |
| | Normal funduscopic exam |
| | Pupils equal at 3 mm, round, and reactive to light with no pupillary defect |
| | Visual fields intact |
| III, IV, VI | Extra-ocular movements intact |
| | Intact facial sensation |
| | Intact masseter motor strength |
| VII–XI | Intact |
| XII | Tongue protruded mid-line |

### Motor Examination

Mild 4/5 weakness of iliopsoas muscle on right side; otherwise normal

### Reflexes

- Deep tendon reflexes were 2+ in the biceps, triceps, brachioradialis, and patellar but absent at the ankles
- Plantar responses were upgoing bilaterally (+ Babinski sign)

### Sensory Examination

- Diminished pinprick and temperature sensations in stocking-and-glove distribution (to ankles and wrists)
- Sense of vibration lost in both lower extremities from knees down
- Romberg test showed patient able to stand with feet together when eyes open, but unsteady with eyes closed

### Cerebellar

Normal finger-to-nose, heel-to-shin and rapid alternating movements

### Gait

- Slow, cautious, unsteady, and wide based
- With each step, the foot was thrust outwards and made an audible "slapping" sound as it struck the floor

***Patient Case Question 2.*** Clinical *symptoms* are subjective expressions of disease that can only be reported by the patient. Identify a minimum of *eight* symptoms in the case study above that are consistent with a diagnosis of vitamin B12 deficiency.

*Patient Case Question 3.* Clinical *signs* are objective expressions of disease that can be detected by someone other than the patient. Identify a minimum of *fifteen* signs in the case study above that are consistent with a diagnosis of vitamin B12 deficiency.

## Laboratory Blood Test Results

See Patient Case Table 90.2

| Patient Case Table 90.2 Laboratory Blood Test Results | | | | | | | |
|---|---|---|---|---|---|
| Na | 142 meq/L | WBC | $4.1 \times 10^3/mm^3$ | Bilirubin, indirect | 1.4 mg/dL |
| K | 4.0 meq/L | Reticulocytes | $21 \times 10^3/mm^3$ | Alb | 3.0 g/dL |
| Cl | 106 meq/L | MCV | 123.4 fL | T Protein | 5.4 g/dL |
| $HCO_3$ | 24 meq/L | MCH | 37.6 pg | T Chol | 192 mg/dL |
| BUN | 13 mg/dL | MCHC | 33.5 g/dL | HDL | 29 mg/dL |
| Cr | 1.1 mg/dL | Vitamin B12 | 87 pg/mL | LDL | 132 mg/dL |
| Glu, fasting | 93 mg/dL | Folic acid | 8 ng/mL | Trig | 147 mg/dL |
| Hb | 10.9 g/dL | AST | 16 IU/L | TSH | 3.26 μU/mL |
| Hct | 28.4% | ALT | 7 IU/L | Iron | 73 μg/dL |
| RBC | $3.44 \times 10^6/mm^3$ | Alk phos | 87 IU/L | MMA | 2.51 mg/L |
| Plt | $110 \times 10^3/mm^3$ | T Bilirubin | 1.9 mg/dL | Homocys | 520 μmol/L |

*Patient Case Question 4.* Identify a minimum of *twelve* laboratory blood test findings that are consistent with a diagnosis of vitamin B12 deficiency.

*Patient Case Question 5.* Identify *all* abnormal laboratory blood test findings in Table 90.2 that are not necessarily specific for a vitamin B12 deficiency.

*Patient Case Question 6.* Is the patient's renal function *normal* or *abnormal*?

*Patient Case Question 7.* Is the patient's hepatic function *normal* or *abnormal*?

*Patient Case Question 8.* Is the patient's lipid profile *normal* or *abnormal*?

## Peripheral Blood Smear

- Anisocytosis
- Poikilocytosis
- Giant platelets
- Hypersegmented neutrophils, some with 6 lobes
- Macrocytic RBC

## Serum Antibodies

- (–) IF
- (–) parietal cells

*Patient Case Question 9.* Does this patient have pernicious anemia? Briefly explain your answer.

*Patient Case Question 10.* The patient in this case study has . . .

a. megaloblastic anemia

b. neurologic abnormalities

c. both a and b

d. none of the above

***Patient Case Question 11.*** What is the medical terminology that is used for "neck pain shooting down the back and into the arms" and what is the significance of this patient complaint?

***Patient Case Question 12.*** What is causing this patient's so-called *slapping gait?*

***Patient Case Question 13.*** What is the significance of the Romberg test in this patient?

# ■■ Clinical Course

The patient was started on intramuscular vitamin B12 injections. He was initially given 1000 μg vitamin B12 with potassium every other day for two weeks. Then the patient was treated with a dose of 1000 μg vitamin B12 every month thereafter. Almost immediately after initiation of the injections, he reported improvement with concentration. He also underwent detoxification for alcohol and drug use and joined Alcoholics Anonymous. Within two weeks, he noticed an improvement in gait. Six months later, he showed mild difficulty with gait, but there were no paresthesias or episodes of shooting pain in the neck and back. With rehabilitation, the prognosis is good and J.K. should be able to recover completely.

# PART 5

# DISORDERS OF THE EYES, EARS, NOSE, AND THROAT

# CASE STUDY

## 91

# ACUTE OTITIS MEDIA

 *For the Disease Summary for this case study, see the CD-ROM.*

## PATIENT CASE

### ■■■ Mother's Chief Complaints

"Our daughter's ear infection seemed to be getting better but then suddenly got worse. It's strange that K. has been having so many ear infections, because I breast-fed her for the first six months."

### ■■■ History of Present Illness

K.J. is a 17-month-old Winnebago Indian female who is brought to her pediatrician by both parents. The patient has had a 24-hour history of fever, irritability, crying, tugging at both ears, and significantly decreased appetite. Her mother reports that K.'s temperature last evening was 101°F and that she had difficulty sleeping despite taking ibuprofen. Mom also reports taking the child to the nurse practitioner nine days ago with cough, runny nose, and apparent earache and receiving a prescription for Pediazole. "There have been colds going around the daycare center," she informs the doctor. She has been very conscientious about giving K. her Pediazole three times a day for the past nine days.

### ■■■ Past Medical History

- Former 40-week 8 lb-1 oz infant delivered vaginally; uncomplicated prenatal course; Apgar scores WNL; was breast-fed and supplemented with formula
- No surgeries or hospitalizations
- Immunizations are current
- One episode of pneumonia at age 14 weeks
- Recurrent AOM × 5 during the past 14 months; most recent episode 9 days ago and currently receiving treatment with Pediazole
- Patient has previously received both cephalosporins and macrolides for AOM; only adverse effect has been significant diarrhea with Augmentin

*Patient Case Question 1.* Which *five* characteristics/functions are assessed in determining an Apgar score for a newborn infant?

*Patient Case Question 2.* Why is Prevnar an important vaccine for this patient?

*Patient Case Question 3.* Which two antibacterial medications are combined in Pediazole and why is this drug appropriate for treating acute otitis media?

*Patient Case Question 4.* Which two antibacterial medications are combined in Augmentin and why is this drug appropriate for treating acute otitis media?

## ■ Developmental Milestones

- Within normal limits for 1- to 2-year-old toddler
- Child can pull self up to stand and walk a few steps without support, use exclamations, say "dada" and "mama," try to imitate words, respond to "no," wave bye-bye, and use objects correctly

## ■ Family History

- Parents are both in good health
- One sister, age 3½ years, has had a recent upper respiratory infection

## ■ Social History

- K. lives at home with her parents, who are both employed outside the home
- She attends a daycare facility every week day
- Father is a smoker; mother is a former smoker who quit 6 years ago
- There is a pet gerbil in the home

## ■ Medications

- Pediazole 100 mg po Q6h
- Ibuprofen 15 mg po Q6h

## ■ Allergies

No known drug allergies

*Patient Case Question 5.* Identify *seven* risk factors that are consistent with a diagnosis of acute otitis media in this patient.

*Patient Case Question 6.* Which *three* of the risk factors that you have identified in Question 5 above are probably most significant for triggering this patient's current bout of acute otitis media?

## ■ Physical Examination and Laboratory Tests

### General

- Patient lying supine
- WDWN young female
- Now crying with intermittent screaming

## Vital Signs

See Patient Case Table 91.1

| Patient Case Table 91.1 Vital Signs | | | | | |
|---|---|---|---|---|---|
| BP | 105/65 | RR | 35 | WT | 20 lbs* |
| HR | 145 | T | 102°F w/ibuprofen | HT | 30 in* |

*Normal growth-development feature for 17 months

## Head, Eyes, Ears, Nose, and Throat

- Pupils equal at 3 mm, round, responsive to light and accommodation
- (+) tears
- Both TMs bulging with no mobility
- Left TM is yellow and opaque and there appears to be some purulent fluid behind it
- Right TM is erythematous
- No otorrhea present
- Nares patent with no discharge
- Throat shows significant erythema

## Neck/Lymph Nodes

- Neck supple with no apparent pain or stiffness with movement
- No lymphadenopathy present

*Patient Case Question 7.* What is the significance of the neck examination with respect to the patient's earache?

## Chest

- Clear to auscultation bilaterally without crackles or wheezes
- Chest wall rise is symmetric

## Cardiac

Regular rate and rhythm with no murmurs, rubs, or gallops

## Abdomen

- Soft, non-tender, and non-distended
- (+) bowel sounds
- (−) hepatosplenomegaly and masses

## Genitalia

Normal-appearing external genitalia

## Extremities

- 20 digits
- No cyanosis, clubbing, or edema

- Brachial pulses palpable
- Capillary refill WNL
- Moves all extremities well
- Skin is warm and pink with no rashes or lesions

## Neurologic

- Responsive to stimulation
- Deep tendon reflexes 2+ throughout
- Cranial nerves intact
- Hearing appears intact
- Motor exam shows normal muscle tone and bulk
- Facial strength appears symmetric and normal

## Laboratory Blood Test Results

See Patient Case Table 91.2

| Patient Case Table 91.2 Laboratory Blood Test Results | | | | | | | |
|---|---|---|---|---|---|---|---|
| WBC | 12,100/mm³ | Lymphs | 21% | Eos | 1% | Plt | 270,000/mm³ |
| Neutros | 75% | Monos | 3% | RBC | 5.0 million/mm³ | ESR | 18 mm/hr |

*Patient Case Question 8.* What *subjective* clinical information supports a diagnosis of acute otitis media?

*Patient Case Question 9.* What *objective* clinical data support a diagnosis of acute otitis media?

*Patient Case Question 10.* What information indicates the *severity* of acute otitis media in this patient?

*Patient Case Question 11.* Does the patient's white blood cell differential suggest a *bacterial* or *viral* infection?

*Patient Case Question 12.* Describe a scenario in which it would be appropriate to use clarithromycin to treat this patient's AOM.

*Patient Case Question 13.* In addition to antibiotics, which non-drug therapies may be beneficial for this patient?

*Patient Case Question 14.* Would prophylactic antibiotics be appropriate for this patient?

*For the Disease Summary for this case study,*
*see the CD-ROM.*

# PATIENT CASE

## ■■■ Patient's Chief Complaints

"My throat hurts and it's hard to swallow. I'm cold, too."

## ■■■ History of Present Illness

S.J. is an 11-year-old girl who has been ill for three days with a sore throat, a temperature of 102.3°F, chills, and pain with swallowing. She presents to the hospital emergency room today with her mother. The patient's appetite has been poor for 48 hours, but fluid intake has been steady. There has been no headache, rash, vomiting, stomach pain, difficulty breathing, joint pain, or cold symptoms. No one else in the family has been recently ill, although her mother notes that "strep has been going around at her school for the past two weeks."

## ■■■ Past Medical History

- (−) for surgeries and hospitalizations
- (−) for serious injuries and bone fractures
- Viral-like URI at age 9
- Chickenpox at age 6
- Ear infections at ages 3 and 4
- No previous episodes of streptococcal pharyngitis or rheumatic fever
- Immunizations are up to date

## ■■■ Family History

Non-contributory

## ■■■ Social History

- Patient lives with her mother, her stepfather, and two siblings
- Attends 6th grade, gets As and Bs in school, and enjoys baseball and working on arts and crafts projects

- The Denver Broncos are her favorite football team
- Both mother and mother's boyfriend smoke in the home
- There are no pets in the home
- Biological father's whereabouts unknown; S.J. has not seen him for years but receives occasional letters

## Review of Systems

- (+) for tiredness
- (−) for muscle aches

## Medications

None

## Allergies

PCN → hives and difficulty breathing

## Limited Physical Examination and Laboratory Tests

### General

The patient is a pleasant, alert, oriented, intelligent, and cooperative 11-year-old white female who appears ill, pale, and is shivering noticeably. She is tightly wrapped in two warm blankets that the ER nurse has provided.

### Vital Signs

BP = 110/70 (sitting, left arm)
HR = 104 and regular
RR = 17 and unlabored
T (oral) = 103.1°F
WT = 88 lbs
HT = 4'11"
$SaO_2$ = 97%

### Skin

Very warm and pale with no rash

### Head, Eyes, Ears, Nose, and Throat

- PERRLA
- (−) for conjunctivitis
- TMs translucent
- (−) for nasal drainage
- Tonsillar edema and erythema with yellow-white exudate
- Soft palate erythema
- Prominent "strawberry" tongue

## Neck

Several small, mobile anterior lymph nodes that are tender with palpation

## Chest

CTA

## Cardiac

- RRR
- $S_1$ and $S_2$ normal
- (−) for murmur

## Abdomen

- Soft and non-tender with normal BS
- (−) for HSM

## Musculoskeletal/Extremities

- Muscle strength and tone 5/5 throughout
- Peripheral pulses normal throughout

## Neurologic

- Cranial nerves II–XII intact
- DTRs 2+

## Laboratory Blood Test Results

See Patient Case Table 92.1

| Patient Case Table 92.1 Laboratory Blood Test Results | | | | | |
|---|---|---|---|---|---|
| Hb | 13.2 g/dL | • Neutrophils | 72% | • Basophils | 1% |
| Hct | 43.9% | • Lymphocytes | 21% | ESR | 18 mm/hr |
| Plt | 390,000/mm³ | • Monocytes | 5% | CRP | 2.3 mg/dL |
| WBC | 15,500/mm³ | • Eosinophils | 1% | (+) Rapid streptococcal antigen test | |

*Patient Case Question 1.* List *eighteen* patient-specific clinical features including signs and symptoms, medical history, findings on physical examination, and laboratory blood test results that support a diagnosis of group A β-hemolytic streptococcal pharyngitis.

*Patient Case Question 2.* What is the *single major risk factor* for acute streptococcal pharyngitis in this case study?

*Patient Case Question 3.* What are the drugs of choice for this patient?

*Patient Case Question 4.* For which type of heart disease is this patient at risk if treatment is not started?

*For the Disease Summary for this case study, see the CD-ROM.*

# PATIENT CASE

## Patient's Chief Complaints

"My eyes and nose have been itching all the time. I've been sneezing a lot and I have some drainage down the back of my throat that has made it sore. I've had difficulty sleeping at night because I've had a stuffy nose. I'm starting to get cranky during the day. It is all beginning to take a toll on my performance at work and my relationships at home."

## History of Present Illness

D.R. Sr. is a 33-year-old man who presents at the infirmary on the military base stating that he has had a long history of nasal allergies. Post-nasal drainage began several days prior to soreness in his throat and has continued now for five days. The patient denies fever, chills, earache, headache, and facial pain/tenderness. He also states that he has had an occasional non-productive cough. The patient denies that he has been exposed to any new pets.

Today's allergy counts in the area are: trees 0 (low), pollens 5 (low), weeds 120 (high), ragweed 40 (moderate).

## Past Medical History

• Perennial rhinitis since age 13
• Eczema since age 27
• GERD with recurrent symptoms since age 30
• Athlete's foot 3 months ago

## Family History

• Father died at age 65 from CHF
• Mother alive in Colorado with asthma and hypothyroid disease; has remarried
• Has one male child, age 4, born 3 months prematurely, who has asthma and nasal allergies
• Maternal grandmother had "severe skin disorder" and a seizure disorder secondary to head trauma sustained in MVA

## ■ Social History

- Divorced; remarried for 5 years with one child
- U.S. Air Force communications specialist for 10 years
- Recently moved into a newly built home on the prairie in southeastern Wyoming
- Denies use of tobacco and alcohol
- There are no pets in the home

## ■ Medications

- Loratadine 10 mg po QD × 2½ years
- Hydrocortisone cream 1% PRN (eczema)
- Ranitidine 150 mg po BID
- Hydrocortisone cream 0.5% applied TID PRN (itchy feet)
- Tolnaftate cream applied BID PRN

***Patient Case Question 1.*** For which condition is this patient probably taking ranitidine?

***Patient Case Question 2.*** For which condition is this patient probably applying tolnaftate cream?

## ■ Allergies

- Cats
- Pollen (type unknown)
- States that "it seems I'm allergic to everything"

## ■ Review of Systems

(−) for wheezing, SOB, chest pain, abdominal discomfort, bowel and bladder symptoms, dysuria, and focal weakness

## ■ Limited Physical Examination and Laboratory Tests

### General Appearance

The patient is a WDWN white male who appears tired, has a "husky" voice, and sounds congested. He is alert, in NAD, and appears to be his stated age.

### Vital Signs

See Patient Case Table 93.1

| Patient Case Table 93.1 Vital Signs | | | | | |
|---|---|---|---|---|---|
| BP | 130/82 (L arm, sitting) | RR | 12 | HT | 5′11″ |
| P | 62 | T | 98.5°F | WT | 186 lbs |

## Skin

Several small, red, scaly, weeping or shiny patches on the neck, upper trunk, and bends of the knees representing acute flares of eczema

## Head, Eyes, Ears, Nose, and Throat

- NC/AT
- PERRLA
- EOMI
- Red conjunctiva
- TMs intact
- (−) epistaxis and nasal discharge
- Prominent transverse crease on lower external nose
- Mucous membranes moist
- Oropharynx without lesions
- Significant erythema over anterior tonsillar pillars
- (−) exudate, posterior pharyngeal swelling, and masses

## Neck

Supple without lymphadenopathy, thyromegaly, JVD, or carotid bruits

## Chest

- CTA bilaterally
- No wheezes or crackles
- Diaphragmatic excursions normal

## Heart

RRR without rubs, gallops, or murmurs

## Abdomen

- Soft, non-tender, non-distended with normal BS
- Several small areas of rough, red skin noted

## Extremities

- (−) CCE
- Pulses 2+ throughout

## Neurologic

- A & O × 3
- DTRs 2+ throughout
- Motor strength 5/5 throughout
- CNs I–XII intact

*Patient Case Question 3.* Which part of the physical examination suggests that this patient does not have anosmia, a clinical symptom that is consistent with a diagnosis of allergic rhinitis?

*Patient Case Question 4.* Identify *five* risk factors that predispose this person to allergic rhinitis *at this time*.

*Patient Case Question 5.* Identify *nine* clinical manifestations, both objective and subjective, that are consistent with a diagnosis of allergic rhinitis.

## Laboratory Blood Test Results

See Patient Case Table 93.2

| Patient Case Table 93.2 Laboratory Blood Test Results | | | | | |
|---|---|---|---|---|---|
| Hb | 17.1 g/dL | WBC | 9,275/mm³ | • Basos | 1% |
| Hct | 43.1% | • PMNs | 57% | • Lymphs | 25% |
| Plt | 375,000/mm³ | • Eos | 14% | • Monos | 3% |

*Patient Case Question 6.* Identify *one* abnormal finding in the patient's complete blood count that is consistent with allergic rhinitis.

## Nasal Cytology

Eosinophilia pronounced in nasal smear

*Patient Case Question 7.* What is the significance behind the results of the patient's chest examination?

*Patient Case Question 8.* What is the single best pharmacotherapeutic approach that might be beneficial for this patient?

# 94

## CATARACTS

 *For the Disease Summary for this case study, see the CD-ROM.*

# PATIENT CASE

## ■ Patient's Chief Complaints

"My vision is getting worse in both eyes. Brighter lamps and the drops that were prescribed three months ago aren't working anymore and I think that I am finally going to need eye surgery."

## ■ HPI

Dr. EGB is a 71 yo white woman who has made an appointment with her ophthalmologist for further evaluation of her cataracts. She has a five-year history of gradual and progressive deterioration of vision in both eyes. The right eye is worse than the left. She reports that, even with a change in prescription for eyeglasses less than five months ago, "objects keep getting fuzzier. Far-vision is still relatively good in my left eye but near-vision has gotten noticeably worse. Near-vision is good in my right eye but far-vision is getting bad. My left eye is also susceptible to glare and I see halos around lights with it." The patient has been followed for some time for chronic renal insufficiency related to membranous nephropathy and is being treated with dialysis. She recently reported for her annual physical exam and was found to have gained 23 pounds in the last 12 months. She has a history of refractory hypertension that required multiple medications before BP was adequately regulated. She has a home BP monitor, but often forgets to perform her BP checks. Earlier today, her home BP measurement was 165/96 mm Hg.

## ■ PMH

- ESRD (chronic membranous glomerulonephritis)
- IV access difficulties
- Anemia secondary to CRF
- HTN
- Hyperlipidemia
- Type 2 DM—diet-controlled
- AMI × 2; coronary artery angioplasty 9 years ago
- Rheumatoid arthritis
- S/P appendectomy

- S/P cholecystectomy
- S/P hysterectomy
- 5-year history of bilateral cataracts, second sight in right eye for 9 months last year

## ■■ FH

- Father had HTN and died from AMI at age 69; (+) for cataracts
- No information available for mother
- One brother at age 64 is alive with HTN and DM
- Has four daughters from previous marriage (all alive and healthy) and one son who committed suicide

## ■■ SH

- Divorced and remarried, lives with husband
- Retired university professor and surgical pathologist; still writes textbooks
- Smoker, quit 5 years ago, previously 2 ppd
- Occasional glass of wine with dinner
- No history of illicit drug use

## ■■ ROS

- States that overall she is "doing okay and holding her own, albeit not the best"
- Unremarkable, except for vision problems at this time

## ■■ Meds

- Diltiazem CD 120 mg po BID
- Atorvastatin 20 mg po QD
- Furosemide 160 mg po QD
- EC ASA 325 mg po QD
- Prochlorperazine 10 mg po TID PRN
- Nitroglycerin 0.4 mg SL PRN
- Calcium acetate 667 mg 2 gel caps po PC
- Nitroglycerin transdermal patch 0.4 mg QD at night with removal in AM
- Acetaminophen 650 mg po QID PRN
- Clonidine 0.2 mg po TID but not before dialysis
- Nabumetone 750 mg 2 tabs Q HS
- Prednisone 5 mg ½ tab po Q AM
- Methotrexate 2.5 mg 6 tabs po once a week
- Folic acid 1 mg po QD

## ■■ All

- IV dye → worsened renal function (4 years ago)
- Codeine intolerance → nausea and vomiting

*Patient Case Question 1.* Identify *seven* contributing factors that have increased susceptibility to cataract formation in this patient.

*Patient Case Question 2.* Which of the seven risk factors that you listed above is the single greatest risk factor for cataracts?

*Patient Case Question 3.* Match the pharmacotherapeutic agents in the left-hand column directly below with the medical conditions in the right-hand column.

a. diltiazem + furosemide + clonidine     _____ coronary artery disease

b. ASA + nitroglycerin     _____ rheumatoid arthritis

c. nabumetone + prednisone + methotrexate + folic acid     _____ hyperlipidemia

d. atorvastatin     _____ hypertension

*Patient Case Question 4.* Why is the patient taking folic acid?

# ■■■ PE and Lab Tests

## Snellen Visual Acuity Examination

- Right eye > 20/200
- Left eye = 20/60

## Swinging Flashlight Test

(−) each eye

## Slit-Lamp Examination

- Lid margins were without inflammation, each eye
- Cornea clear and smooth, each eye
- Lenses: opacity noted in center of right lens + opacity noted in back of left lens under the capsule
- Iris round and without neovascularization or abnormality, each eye
- Vitreous examination: clear, each eye
- Color vision: WNL, each eye
- Lens position: (−) for subluxation, each eye

## Gen

Obese white woman who appears her stated age and is in NAD

## VS

See Patient Case Table 94.1

| Patient Case Table 94.1 Vital Signs | | | | | | |
|---|---|---|---|---|---|---|
| BP | 170/105 right arm, sitting | P | | 86 | HT | 5'5" |
| BP | 165/103 left arm, sitting | T | | 98.4°F | WT | 194 lbs |

## Skin

- Warm and dry
- Good turgor

## HEENT

- Eyes are negative for pain and redness
- PERRLA
- EOMI
- Arteriolar narrowing on funduscopic exam
- Negative for hemorrhages, exudates, or papilledema
- Oropharynx clear
- Oral mucosa pink and moist

## Chest

CTA bilaterally

## Cardiac

- RRR
- $S_1$ and $S_2$ normal
- Negative for $S_3$ and $S_4$
- Negative for murmurs and rubs

## Abd

- Obese, soft, and non-tender with no guarding
- (+) BS
- (−) HSM, masses, and bruits

## Genit/Rect

Stool heme (−)

## MS/Ext

- Negative for CCE
- Capillary refill <2 sec
- Age-appropriate strength and ROM

## Neuro

- A & O × 3
- Moderately subnormal sensation in lower legs
- CNs II–XII intact

## Laboratory Blood Test Results

See Patient Case Table 94.2

| Patient Case Table 94.2 Laboratory Blood Test Results | | | | | |
|---|---|---|---|---|---|
| Na | 135 meq/L | Cr | 9.1 mg/dL | WBC | $6.9 \times 10^3/mm^3$ |
| K | 3.8 meq/L | Glu, fasting | 109 mg/dL | Ca | 8.7 mg/dL |
| Cl | 102 meq/L | Hb | 9.1 g/dL | Mg | 2.4 mg/dL |
| $HCO_3$ | 23 meq/L | Hct | 27% | Phos | 2.6 mg/dL |
| BUN | 72 mg/dL | Plt | $229 \times 10^3/mm^3$ | Alb | 3.4 g/dL |

***Patient Case Question 5.*** Identify *four* abnormal laboratory blood test results that are consistent with a diagnosis of chronic renal failure.

***Patient Case Question 6.*** Account for the "moderately subnormal sensation in the lower legs."

***Patient Case Question 7.*** Is the cataract in the left eye more likely to be *subcapsular, nuclear,* or *cortical?*

***Patient Case Question 8.*** Is the cataract in the right eye more likely to be *subcapsular, nuclear,* or *cortical?*

***Patient Case Question 9.*** Is the cataract in the left eye more likely to be *mature, immature,* or *incipient?*

***Patient Case Question 10.*** Is the cataract in the right eye more likely to be *mature, immature,* or *incipient?*

***Patient Case Question 11.*** What probably caused the "arteriolar narrowing" that was observed with funduscopy?

***Patient Case Question 12.*** Is hypertension in this patient well regulated?

# ■■■ Clinical Course

Phacoemulsification and intra-ocular lens implantation were performed on both eyes. After a three-week recovery period, the patient's visual acuity was 20/30 in the right eye and 20/20 in the left eye. There were no complications.

# CASE STUDY

# 95

# OPEN-ANGLE GLAUCOMA

 *For the Disease Summary for this case study, see the CD-ROM.*

# PATIENT CASE

## ■ Patient's Chief Complaint

"I think that my glaucoma is getting worse. I can't see nearly as well as I could a month ago."

## ■ History of Present Illness

Mr. B.L. is a pleasant, 45-year-old African American man with a four-year history of open-angle glaucoma. Today, he presents to his ophthalmologist complaining of a recent loss of peripheral vision in both eyes and occasional blurriness centrally in the right eye.

The patient had experienced reasonably good health until he developed uveitis secondary to a herpes simplex infection. Intra-ocular inflammation responded well to short-term use of topical corticosteroids. However, shortly after treatment, B.L. complained of blurred vision. A brain MRI revealed no abnormalities. An ophthalmology consult was sought and the patient was ultimately diagnosed with open-angle glaucoma.

For several years, B.L. was managed by a general ophthalmologist, who prescribed timolol (0.5%) in both eyes BID. Successful bilateral laser trabeculoplasty was also performed 20 months ago with reductions of IOP in the left eye from 24 to 17 mm Hg and in the right eye from 27 to 20 mm Hg. However, within 4 months, IOP in both eyes was significantly elevated again. Trials of latanoprost (0.005%) once daily at night and brimonidine (2%) TID were added to timolol, but were ineffective. Dorzolamide (2%) TID was then added and IOP in both eyes was reduced to a normal range. Other ocular history includes myopia since childhood and an occasional episode of dry eyes.

## ■ Past Medical History

- Migraine headache, 1–2/month
- Bipolar disorder, has been successfully treated with lithium in the past
- Status post-tonsillectomy as a child

## ■ Social History

- Married and lives with his wife of 18 years
- Works full-time in the maintenance department of a local beef packaging company

454

- Patient has 4 brothers, all in good health
- Has one daughter and one son, both in good health
- Father and mother both have hypertension and glaucoma; mother also has chronic renal insufficiency
- Patient smoked 1 pack cigarettes/day for 20 years until he quit 5 years ago
- Denies alcohol or illicit drug use

## ■ Allergies

Codeine and penicillin (rash and hives)

## ■ Review of Systems

- Non-contributory
- No heart, lung, gastrointestinal, genitourinary, or circulatory problems

**Patient Case Question 1.** Identify *six* risk factors that predispose this patient to glaucoma.

## ■ Physical Examination and Laboratory Tests

### Vital Signs

- BP 123/78
- P 75
- RR 17
- T 98.5°F
- BMI 22.8

**Patient Case Question 2.** Are any of this patient's vital signs considered abnormal?

### Eyes

- No evidence of macular edema or cataracts
- Visual acuity: left eye—hand motion at 5 inches with corrective eyeglasses; right eye—20/40
- Intra-ocular pressure: left eye—24 mm; right eye—20 mm
- Vitreous exam: clear in both eyes
- Color vision: right eye—unable to see; left eye—unable to see
- Visual fields: left eye—unable to see Amsler grid, can only see hand motion at 5 inches away; right eye—20/40, diurnal curve of IOP reveals IOP WNL
- Discs: right eye—the disc appeared whitish with significant cupping and marked pallor, CD ratio = 0.70; left eye—the disc appeared whitish with significant cupping and marked pallor, CD ratio = 0.89
- Slit-lamp exam:
  –Lid margins without inflammation in both eyes
  –Cornea clear and smooth in both eyes

–Lenses clear in both eyes

–Irises round in both eyes and without neovascularization or other abnormalities

–No masses or nodules

*Patient Case Question 3.* Is glaucoma more advanced in the right or left eye?

## Cardiovascular

* Regular rate and rhythm with no murmurs, rubs, or gallops
* Carotid pulses are brisk and equal bilaterally

## Neurologic

* Smell (cranial nerve I) and corneal sensation are intact bilaterally
* Facial symmetry, muscle tone, and sensation are intact bilaterally
* Gait was intact
* Cranial nerves II–XII were intact
* Finger-to-nose test was WNL
* Reflexes were normal and symmetric
* Sensation was intact and symmetric to pinprick, proprioception, and light touch
* Motor strength of all extremities was 5/5

## Laboratory Blood Test Results

See Patient Case Table 95.1

| Patient Case Table 95.1 Laboratory Blood Test Results | | | | | | | |
|---|---|---|---|---|---|---|---|
| Hb | 16.9 g/dL | Plt | 330,000/mm³ | Cl | 110 meq/L | Glu, fasting | 93 mg/dL |
| Hct | 46.9% | Na | 141 meq/L | HCO₃ | 29 meq/L | BUN | 18 mg/dL |
| WBC | 6,500/mm³ | K | 3.9 meq/L | Ca | 10.3 mg/dL | Cr | 0.6 mg/dL |

*Patient Case Question 4.* Are any of this patient's laboratory test results abnormal?

## ■■■ Clinical Course

The patient underwent repeat bilateral laser trabeculoplasty with mitomycin C.

*Patient Case Question 5.* Why are two anti-cancer medications, mitomycin C and 5-fluorouracil, used intraoperatively in the treatment of glaucoma?

*Patient Case Question 6.* Is the type of open-angle glaucoma in this case study considered *primary* or *secondary*?

*Patient Case Question 7.* Can glaucoma be prevented?

*Patient Case Question 8.* An herbal supplement known as *bilberry* has been promoted as a remedy for glaucoma. Is it acceptable to take bilberry for glaucoma?

# NUTRITIONAL DISORDERS

# 96

## ANOREXIA NERVOSA

 *For the Disease Summary for this case study, see the CD-ROM.*

# PATIENT CASE

## ■ History of Present Illness

Jenny is a 16-year-old girl who is in the 11th grade. This is her first visit to the Eating Disorders Clinic. Physicians at the emergency room had referred her to the clinic. She had fainted at school during gymnastics class and sustained several minor bruises on her arms and legs and a laceration on her forehead.

When she was younger, Jenny was of normal weight and height and ate freely. Her father owns a construction business, spends a significant amount of time traveling, and drinks excessively when he is at home. He is also violent and quick to anger when he drinks. He shouts, uses abusive language, and has thrown plates and books at Jenny's mother and the children. Jenny never knows what to expect from him and is terrified of him. Her mother always defends her father's poor behavior and violent actions. "Your father works very hard and needs a few drinks to relax."

Jenny has felt totally neglected in the family during the last several years. She is the only female and her father tends to get involved more in the activities of his two sons because "they can play sports." Jenny has taken a part-time job at the ice cream shop, has become very involved in her studies and closest friendships, and rarely comes home before 10 PM.

One year ago, she decided that she needed to lose several pounds but would not say exactly how many. She began to exercise by walking 45 minutes each day during lunchtime and tried out for both the girls' track and volleyball teams. She started reading articles in *Cosmopolitan* magazine about weight loss, being thin, and being beautiful like the Hollywood actresses and supermodels. She experimented with Lasix for several weeks, but decided that it was not helping her lose weight as she desired. She began skipping breakfast and lunch completely. For dinner, she would have a large bowl of cereal and would feel filled up. Several months ago, she bought online and began taking Metabo-Speed XXX, advertised as the "Diet Pill of the Stars, the Appetite Killer, Metabolism Booster, and Fat Blaster." She denies using any laxatives or ipecac. She denies any forced vomiting.

Her mother informs the eating disorders specialist that "Jenny has not been herself lately. She has been losing too much weight and has been very touchy and argumentative lately. She is always a good girl, works hard on her schoolwork and job, and always does what's expected of her."

Jenny confides in her healthcare provider that she "has one very good friend who also comes from a dysfunctional family. We understand one another and we support one another, but we have both grown up too fast." She admits to feeling "very sad, ignored, and worried for almost two years." She cries frequently at night and wakes up around 4 AM unable to go back to sleep. She often lies awake at night when she goes to bed, crying and tossing and turning for hours before falling asleep. She occasionally experiences nightmares about her father chasing her with a knife.

Jenny admits to having suicidal thoughts but no plan. "I probably wouldn't be able to go through with it." More recently, she has had thoughts that she wishes she could "just go to sleep and wake up in heaven." She denies any history of sexual abuse.

***Patient Case Question 1.*** Identify *one* major risk factor for anorexia nervosa from this patient's history of present illness.

## ■ Past Medical History

- No previous psychiatric history or major medical problems or hospitalizations
- Measles as a young child
- History of urinary tract infections
- One episode of iron deficiency anemia last year
- Menarche began at age 12
- Occasional headaches

## ■ Family History

Jenny is the middle child of three children. She has an older brother and a younger brother. Father and paternal grandfather are alcoholics and smokers. Mother is in good health.

## ■ Social History

- Straight "A" student who would like to go to college
- Enjoys reading and writing
- Very active in various student activities, including track and volleyball; a member of the student council and journal club; also, a class officer
- Denies use of tobacco, alcohol, or illicit drugs

## ■ Review of Systems

- States that overall she is doing okay
- Trying to lose weight so that she will be more attractive
- Doesn't like her size and shape
- Doesn't believe that she has lost too much weight
- Complains of weakness and always feeling cold
- Denies chest pain, but occasionally feels "heart flutters"
- No history of seizures
- Reports a decrease in both appetite and energy and has felt fatigued for the last 3 weeks
- Has had no abdominal pain
- Usually has one bowel movement daily, but admits that she has not had one in the past 3 days
- Last menses was 6 months ago
- Denies nausea, vomiting, diarrhea, shortness of breath, and hemoptysis
- No blood in the stool

*Patient Case Question 2.* Identify a minimum of *seven* clinical manifestations from the review of systems above that are consistent with a diagnosis of anorexia nervosa.

# Medications

No prescribed medications but she has been taking Metabo-Speed XXX for weight loss and used furosemide from her parents' medicine cabinet

# Allergies

No known drug allergy

# Physical Examination and Laboratory Tests

## General

- The patient is a cooperative, pleasant, young female in no apparent distress
- She is appropriately dressed with regard to clothing size
- She is extremely thin
- Easily engaged in conversation
- She is not guarded with her answers and makes good eye contact
- Answers all questions with a soft voice
- No odd or inappropriate motor behavior

## Vital Signs

See Patient Case Table 96.1

| Patient Case Table 96.1 Vital Signs | | | | | |
|---|---|---|---|---|---|
| BP | 125/80* | RR | 15 | Ht | 62 in |
| P | 52 | T | 95.3°F | Wt | 89 lbs |

*A normal blood pressure for a 15–17-year-old female is <128/82.

*Patient Case Question 3.* Identify *three* vital signs that are consistent with a diagnosis of anorexia nervosa.

*Patient Case Question 4.* Calculate this patient's body mass index to confirm that the patient is technically underweight.

## Skin

- Cool to touch
- Dry with some scaling
- Negative for rashes or lesions
- Skin tone normal in color
- Decreased turgor

## Head, Eyes, Ears, Nose, and Throat

- Pupils equal at 3 mm, round, and reactive to light and accommodation
- Extra-ocular movements intact
- Sclera without icterus
- Fundi benign
- Tympanic membranes clear throughout without drainage
- Teeth show no signs of erosion
- Dry mucous membranes
- Throat without erythema or soreness
- Hair is thin and dry

*Patient Case Question 5.* Identify *three* clinical manifestations from the skin and HEENT examinations above that suggest Jenny is dehydrated.

*Patient Case Question 6.* Why did the eating disorders specialist examine the patient's teeth, a procedure that is not common in a physical examination?

## Neck/Lymph Nodes

- Neck supple without lymphadenopathy or thyromegaly
- No jugular vein distension or carotid bruits

## Breasts

Normal without masses, discoloration, discharge, or dimpling

## Lungs

- Clear to auscultation bilaterally
- No wheezing or crackles

## Cardiac

- Regular rate and rhythm, slow beat
- No murmurs, rubs, or gallops
- $S_1$ and $S_2$ normal; no additional cardiac sounds

## Abdomen

- Soft and non-tender
- Hypoactive bowel sounds
- No hepatosplenomegaly
- No masses or bruits
- No guarding or rebound tenderness

*Patient Case Question 7.* Which negative abdominal clinical sign parallels a single clinical symptom reported by the patient during the review of systems?

## Genitalia/Rectum

Stool heme-negative

---

> **Patient Case Question 8.** What is the significance of the rectal examination?

## Musculoskeletal/Extremities

- Extremities are slightly cool to touch
- No cyanosis or clubbing but mild-to-moderate (1+ level) peripheral edema
- Range of motion within normal limits
- Good peripheral pulses bilaterally
- Age-appropriate strength

## Neurologic

- Alert and oriented to time, place, and person
- Cranial nerves II–XII intact
- Deep tendon reflexes 2+ throughout
- Negative Babinski sign
- No gross motor-sensory deficits present

## Laboratory Blood Test Results

See Patient Case Table 96.2

| Patient Case Table 96.2 Laboratory Blood Test Results | | | | | |
|---|---|---|---|---|---|
| Na | 148 meq/L | Hb | 14.8 g/dL | AST | 30 IU/L |
| K | 2.9 meq/L | Hct | 47% | ALT | 38 IU/L |
| Cl | 111 meq/L | Plt | 170,000/mm$^3$ | Alk phos | 123 IU/L |
| HCO$_3$ | 22 meq/L | WBC | 3,900/mm$^3$ | T protein | 4.9 g/dL |
| BUN | 30 mg/dL | Ca | 8.3 mg/dL | TSH | 2.1 µU/mL |
| Cr | 1.1 mg/dL | Mg | 1.7 mg/dL | T cholesterol | 190 mg/dL |
| Glu, fasting | 60 mg/dL | Phos | 2.3 mg/dL | FSH | 0.2 mU/mL |

## Urinalysis

The patient's urine was clear in appearance, but amber in color. Complete urinalysis is pending.

## Electrocardiogram

Except for bradycardia, no abnormalities were observed.

---

> **Patient Case Question 9.** Which *four* laboratory blood test results in Table 96.2 are consistent with dehydration?
>
> **Patient Case Question 10.** Do any of the laboratory data in Table 96.2 support a diagnosis of anemia?

***Patient Case Question 11.*** Is this patient at risk for developing infections?

***Patient Case Question 12.*** This patient has many clinical manifestations that are associated with hypothyroid disease. Is this patient hypothyroid?

***Patient Case Question 13.*** Based on the patient's laboratory blood test results, provide *one* reasonable explanation for the observed level 1+ peripheral edema.

***Patient Case Question 14.*** Can the patient's recent amenorrhea be explained by any of the laboratory blood test results shown in Table 96.2?

***Patient Case Question 15.*** Which of the following findings from the laboratory blood tests has to be of greatest concern and why: hypernatremia, hypokalemia, hypoglycemia, hypomagnesemia, hypocalcemia, or hypophosphatemia?

***Patient Case Question 16.*** Some patients with anorexia nervosa are hypercholesterolemic. Does the patient in this case study have a markedly elevated serum cholesterol concentration?

*For the Disease Summary for this case study,*
*see the CD-ROM.*

## PATIENT CASE

### ■ Patient's Chief Complaints

"I feel bloated and I have no energy. I've had some swelling around my ankles and my throat has been a little sore for the last few days. I really don't want to be here, but my mother insisted upon it."

> ***Patient Case Question 1.*** Identify *four* clinical manifestations in this patient (3 symptoms and 1 sign) that are consistent with a diagnosis of bulimia.

### ■ Mother's Comments

"I'm worried. I believe that my daughter has an eating disorder, but she vehemently denies it."

### ■ HPI

B.B. is a 17 yo female who is in the 12th grade. Today, she presents to the medical clinic complaining of a three-week history of bloating, tiredness, muscular weakness, and ankle edema. Her throat has been sore for the past three days. After noticing significant changes in her daughter's behavior, her mother has persuaded her to see the family pediatrician. When she was younger, B.B. was of normal height and weight and ate freely from all food groups. Her parents divorced when she was 12 yo and she began living with her mother and younger sister. At age 13 she was 5'4" tall, weighed 125–130 pounds, and entered menarche. She felt that she could lose some weight but did not feel overweight. "My uncle and mother called it baby fat." B.B. began to exercise by jogging 30 minutes three times a week and tried out for the girls' basketball and golf teams. At age 14, she weighed 138 pounds and also began running the 400-meter in track. She still participated in basketball and golf, but team sports did not bring her the satisfaction of self-accomplishment.

Two years ago (at age 15), she began reading magazine articles about Hollywood starlets and the sacrifices that they had made to stay thin and maintain an attractive body shape. "I wish that I looked like them," she had told her mother. It was at this same time that B.B. moved in with her father because she could not deal with her younger sister's "problem" anymore. Her sister has ADHD and B.B. reported that her sister would hit and bite her. Within 6 months, however, B.B. moved back to live with her mother. Her father always seemed to be working and was dating a woman whom B.B. did not like. Her father's girlfriend was always very critical and constantly nagged her about working harder in school, choosing better friends, and losing some weight.

Soon after returning to live with her mother, B.B. began missing family meals. The apartment building where she was living had a weight room. B.B. would lift weights for an hour a day, jog on the treadmill, and then do 100 sit-ups. This activity was in addition to the conditioning she did at school as part of track and basketball.

She denies using laxatives, ipecac, diuretics, and drugs that increase basal metabolic rate. She also denies any forced vomiting and suicidal thoughts, but affirms that she has been "feeling very sad lately" and "doesn't like her body."

## ▰▬ PMH

- (–) for surgeries and hospitalizations
- (–) for serious injuries
- Measles at age 7

## ▰▬ FH

- Oldest of two female children
- Has a 13 yo sister diagnosed with ADHD
- Parents have been divorced for 5 years; father is a businessman; mother is a fashion designer
- Mother was treated for anorexia nervosa as a teenager and for a major depressive episode for 18 months immediately following her divorce
- Maternal grandmother has been diagnosed with depression
- Paternal grandfather died from a ruptured esophageal varix secondary to chronic alcoholism

## ▰▬ SH

- Straight "A" student
- Would like to go to Providence University "like dad, so that he would be proud of me"
- Enjoys playing viola
- Very active in various student activities, including basketball and track; is also senior class secretary
- Denies use of tobacco, alcohol, or illicit drugs
- Denies sexual activity

## ▰▬ ROS

- Denies dizziness and abdominal pain
- States that she has felt her heart "flutter" from time to time but denies chest pain
- Positive for fatigue during the past 2–3 weeks
- Reports appetite as being "good" and both bowel movements and menstrual periods as "regular"

## ▰▬ Meds

- No prescribed or OTC medicines currently
- Has taken Metabolife in the past because "it is a natural way to maintain a healthy weight"

## ■ All

NKDA

## ■ PE and Lab Tests

### Gen

The patient is a young, white female from a well-to-do family. Although her body language suggests some degree of agitation, she is cooperative. The patient is also attractive, appears mildly anxious, well groomed, and is appropriately dressed. Speech is normal in both rate and volume. There are no definitive signs of mania or psychosis. Affect is depressed, but she does not appear to be delusional or hallucinating. She denies suicidal ideation. She appears alert and has a good attention span and ability to concentrate. She often avoids eye contact.

**Patient Case Question 2.** Identify a minimum of *seven* risk factors that may have predisposed this patient to bulimia.

### VS

See Patient Case Table 97.1

| Patient Case Table 97.1 Vital Signs | | | | | |
|---|---|---|---|---|---|
| BP | 115/80 | RR | 20 | HT | 5′7″ |
| P | 110 | T | 98.4°F | WT | 135 lbs |

**Patient Case Question 3.** Is this patient technically *underweight, overweight, obese,* or is weight considered *healthy and normal*?

### Skin

• Warm and moist with no rashes or bruising
• Normal turgor
• Significant Russell sign on index finger and long finger of right hand

### HEENT

• PERRLA
• EOMI
• Fundi sharp and well visualized
• Mucous membranes moist

### Neck

Supple and (−) for thyromegaly and lymphadenopathy

# Heart

- Tachycardia with regular rhythm
- $S_1$ and $S_2$ normal with no additional heart sounds
- No m/r/g

# Lungs

Rapid, clear breath sounds

# Abd

- Non-tender and non-distended
- (−) for rebound and guarding
- (−) for HSM, masses, or bruits

# Genit/Rect

- (−) for hemorrhoids
- Remainder of exam deferred

# Neuro

- A & O
- CNs II–XII normal
- DTRs 2+ bilaterally
- Sensory and motor function intact

# ECG

- NSR
- Mild tachycardia

***Patient Case Question 4.*** Provide *two* abnormal findings from this patient's physical examination that are consistent with a diagnosis of bulimia.

# Laboratory Blood Test Results

See Patient Case Table 97.2

| Patient Case Table 97.2 Laboratory Blood Test Results | | | | | |
|---|---|---|---|---|---|
| Na | 135 meq/L | Glu, fasting | 65 mg/dL | Plt | 290,000/mm³ |
| K | 3.1 meq/L | Ca | 8.7 mg/dL | WBC | 6,300/mm³ |
| Cl | 100 meq/L | Mg | 0.9 mg/dL | AST | 19 IU/L |
| HCO₃ | 25 meq/L | Alb | 2.8 g/dL | ALT | 44 IU/L |
| BUN | 16 mg/dL | Hb | 10.9 g/dL | Bilirubin, total | 0.3 mg/dL |
| Cr | 1.0 mg/dL | Hct | 29% | Amylase | 240 IU/L |

## ABG

- pH 7.48
- $PaO_2$ 90 mm Hg
- $PaCO_2$ 33 mm Hg
- $SaO_2$ 97%

---

***Patient Case Question 5.*** Identify *six* clinical manifestations that indicate dehydration is not a concern in this patient at this time.

***Patient Case Question 6.*** Identify *seven* abnormal laboratory test results.

***Patient Case Question 7.*** What is a likely cause of this patient's tachycardia?

***Patient Case Question 8.*** Which *two* abnormal laboratory blood test results are consistent with the patient's report of tiredness and fatigue?

***Patient Case Question 9.*** Which important *mineral deficiency* explains the abnormal laboratory blood test results identified in Question 8?

***Patient Case Question 10.*** Does the clinical data support a *purging* or *non-purging* type of bulimia?

***Patient Case Question 11.*** There are at least *five* definitive signs that support a correct response to Question 10 above. What are they?

***Patient Case Question 12.*** How can parents make an impact to prevent the development of bulimia nervosa in their children?

# CASE STUDY
# 98

## OBESITY

 *For the Disease Summary for this case study, see the CD-ROM.*

## PATIENT CASE

### Patient's Chief Complaints

"I need to lose some weight and I can't do it by myself. I'm always tired and out of breath and my back and knees are killing me. I'd like to have stomach staples, if possible."

### HPI

B.L. is a 57 yo Hispanic woman of Puerto Rican heritage who states that she maintained her ideal weight, which she believes is about 115 lbs, until she was divorced 15 years ago. "I was in the military years ago and I was very trim at that time." She has been continually gaining weight, mostly through "comfort eating" after her divorce. She also admits to nibbling on snacks at work—mostly high-calorie foods like brownies and Twinkies. She has previously tried OTC diet pills, multiple fad diets (South Beach and Sugar Busters), meal replacement diets (Slim-Fast), "water pills," and most recently a combination of herbal products (chitosan and Garcinia). "I lose a bunch of weight over one or two months and then I gain it all back plus some." She is tearful as she talks about her weight struggles. "I realize that my weight is affecting my health and I want to finally get some help to lose some and then keep it off for good."

### PMH

- HTN × 8 years
- Gallstones 5 years ago, treated with lithotripsy and ursodeoxycholic acid
- Hypothyroidism × 5 years
- Bilateral osteoarthritis of knees and lower back
- Depression × 4 years

### PSH

- TAH 20 years ago
- Carpal tunnel release surgery in both wrists 3 years ago

## FH

- Father died at age 65 from complications after a traumatic fall; had "heart trouble" and HTN
- Mother died at age 80 from hip fracture and pneumonia
- Her only sibling is a brother who died at age 67 from bladder cancer
- One son and one daughter, both thin, alive, and well
- She states that her "mother and grandmother were heavy, but not obese"
- No other family members have a significant medical history

## SH

- The patient is a divorced woman who lives with her 30 yo daughter
- She has never smoked and denies IVDA
- She has been a data entry clerk for the past 11 years and has been limited to sedentary work because of her weight
- She feels insecure at work, because she is "the only employee working there without a college degree and I always have to prove myself"
- Before her divorce, she enjoyed walking for exercise. Now she is limited by her knee and back pain, limited mobility, and breathlessness.
- Except for her daughter, she is socially isolated and rarely has friends or family over to her house
- She watches a lot of television and feeds the birds and squirrels for enjoyment

## Diet

B.L. met with a nutritionist several years ago and learned about the benefits of a low-fat, low-carbohydrate diet, but soon became bored and frustrated with her food plan and stopped dieting. In her current attempt to lose weight, she has cut down her number of meals to one daily each evening that includes larger portion sizes and usually a baked dessert. Upon further probing, she admits to some snacking throughout the evening.

## Meds

- Levothyroxine 0.15 µg po QD
- Acetaminophen 500 mg po PRN
- HCTZ 12.5 mg po QD
- Benazepril 10 mg po QD
- Doxazosin 4 mg po Q HS
- Imipramine 100 mg po QD

***Patient Case Question 1.*** Which *three* medications is the patient taking for hypertension?

## PE and Lab Tests

### Gen

The patient is a pleasant, but tearful, extremely overweight Hispanic female in NAD.

## VS

See Patient Case Table 98.1

| Patient Case Table 98.1 Vital Signs | | | | | |
|---|---|---|---|---|---|
| BP | 138/88 | T | 97.5°F | Waist | 48 in |
| P | 85 and regular | HT | 5 ft-1 in | Hips | 39 in |
| RR | 30 | WT | 290 lbs | SaO$_2$ | 96% |

## Skin

- Warm with normal distribution of body hair
- No rashes or moles noted

## HEENT

- Funduscopic exam normal
- Ears, nose and throat all WNL

## Cardiac

- RRR
- S$_1$ and S$_2$ normal with no m/r/g

## Lungs

CTA & P bilaterally

## Breasts

Exam deferred

## Abd

- Severely obese with multiple striae
- NT/ND
- (+) BS
- No palpable masses or bruits
- (−) HSM
- Hysterectomy scar well healed

## Genit/Rect

Exam deferred

## Ext

- (+) for lower extremity varicosities
- Palpation of knees reveals limited ROM, bony crepitus, and patient discomfort bilaterally
- Pedal pulses 2+ bilaterally

## Neuro

- A & O × 3
- CNs II–XII intact
- Sensory and motor levels intact
- DTRs 2+
- (−) Babinski

## Laboratory Blood Test Results

See Patient Case Table 98.2

| Patient Case Table 98.2 Laboratory Blood Test Results | | | | | |
|---|---|---|---|---|---|
| Na | 140 meq/L | Ins | 190 μU/mL | PLT | 190,000/mm³ |
| K | 3.9 meq/L | AST | 14 IU/L | Cholesterol | 314 mg/dL |
| Cl | 107 meq/L | ALT | 29 IU/L | LDL | 195 mg/dL |
| HCO₃ | 29 meq/L | Bilirubin, total | 0.9 mg/dL | HDL | 14 mg/dL |
| BUN | 15 mg/dL | Hct | 49% | Triglycerides | 219 mg/dL |
| Cr | 0.8 mg/dL | Hb | 17.4 g/dL | TSH | 3.7 μU/mL |
| Glu, fasting | 118 mg/dL | WBC | 6,700/mm³ | Uric acid | 1.7 mg/dL |

## Arterial Blood Gases

$PaO_2$ = 90 mm Hg; $PaCO_2$ = 33 mm Hg; pH = 7.35

## Spirometry Tests

- VC = 4000 mL
- TLC = 5000 mL
- ERV = 1000 mL

## Chest X-Ray

WNL

*Patient Case Question 2.* Identify *ten* risk factors for obesity in this case study.

*Patient Case Question 3.* Identify *ten* health consequences that may have developed in this patient from obesity.

*Patient Case Question 4.* Does the patient have any signs of liver dysfunction?

*Patient Case Question 5.* Other than the patient's complaint of "always being out of breath," does she have any signs of abnormal pulmonary function at this time?

*Patient Case Question 6.* Does the patient's hypothyroid condition need a drug dosage adjustment at this time?

*Patient Case Question 7.* Into which class of obesity can this patient be categorized: I, II, or III?

*Patient Case Question 8.* What is the risk for this patient to develop disease if she continues at this weight?

*Patient Case Question 9.* Calculate the body fat percentage in this patient.

# SEXUALLY TRANSMITTED DISEASES

**CASE STUDY**

# 99

# GENITAL HERPES

*For the Disease Summary for this case study, see the CD-ROM.*

## PATIENT CASE

### Patient's Chief Complaints

"I have some very painful blisters near my vagina and I think there may be some inside, too. I felt a strange stinging sensation for a couple days and then broke out. I've also had several horrific headaches and muscle aches the past few days—almost like the flu."

### HPI

DJB is a 43 yo nulligravida woman who presents to her OB-GYN specialist for evaluation of genital lesions that have been present for five days. She is single, sexually active with one partner currently, and admits to frequent unprotected vaginal sex. She denies IV drug use, is heterosexual, and, other than high blood pressure and cholesterol, she is aware of no active medical problems. She denies both oral and anal intercourse.

### PMH

- Turner syndrome with primary amenorrhea, infertility, and hypoestrogenism secondary to ovarian dysgenesis
- Recurrent UTIs, most recent 4 months ago
- Recurrent vaginal candidiasis, most recent 1 year ago
- Hypercholesterolemia × 3½ years
- Gonorrhea × 2, most recent episode 6 years ago
- Chlamydia × 2, most recent episode 6 years ago
- Trichomonas vaginalis, 7 years ago
- HTN × 10 years
- No previous history of cold sores, fever blisters, or genital herpes simplex

### FH

- Mother alive with hypothyroidism for approximately 25 years
- Father alive with HTN for approximately 35 years
- No history of cancer, heart disease, diabetes, or stroke

## ■ SH

- Graduated from high school
- Never married
- Lives with boyfriend (who has a bipolar disorder) of 6 years
- Works as a bookkeeper for pediatrician
- Admits to occasional use of alcohol (wine only)
- Denies cigarette smoking, use of marijuana, cocaine, and methamphetamines
- Admits to having 10–15 different sexual partners in the past 20 years

## ■ Meds

- Multivitamin 1 tablet po QD
- Ibuprofen for headache and myalgias 200 mg po PRN
- Simvastatin 20 mg po QD
- Conjugated estrogens 0.625 mg po QD (3 weeks on medication + 1 week off)

---

***Patient Case Question 1.*** Distinguish between *primary* and *secondary* amenorrhea.

***Patient Case Question 2.*** Why is this patient taking simvastatin?

***Patient Case Question 3.*** Why is this patient taking conjugated estrogens?

---

## ■ All

PCN (rash, 25 years ago)

## ■ ROS

- (–) cough, night sweats, weight loss, dysuria, urinary frequency, anorectal pain, vaginal discharge
- (+) some malaise with moderately depressed appetite, headaches, and myalgias

## ■ PE and Lab Tests

### Gen

The patient is an unmarried, middle-aged, white woman of extremely short stature. She appears moderately overweight and is apprehensive but in NAD.

### VS

See Patient Case Table 99.1

| Patient Case Table 99.1 Vital Signs | | | | | |
|---|---|---|---|---|---|
| BP (rt arm, sitting) | 155/95 | RR | 15 rpm and unlabored | HT | 4′8″ |
| P | 75 bpm | T | 99.2°F | WT | 128 lbs |

> ***Patient Case Question 4.*** Is this patient technically considered *overweight* or *obese*?
>
> ***Patient Case Question 5.*** What important question regarding the patient's vital signs, past medical history, and medication profile needs to be asked?

## Skin

- Patches of dry skin on the arms and legs
- Multiple brown-black nevi on chest, abdomen, back, and extremities
- Normal color and turgor but warmer than expected
- (–) rashes

## HEENT

- Small mandible
- PERRLA
- EOMI
- (–) nystagmus
- Eyes without corneal lesions, normal fundi
- TMs intact
- High arched palate
- Throat and pharynx clear
- Nose without discharge or congestion
- Moist mucous membranes

> ***Patient Case Question 6.*** Is PERRLA a *positive* or *negative* sign?
>
> ***Patient Case Question 7.*** Is EOMI a *positive* or *negative* sign?

## Neck

- Supple without stiffness
- Significant webbing bilaterally
- (–) adenopathy, JVD, carotid bruits, and thyromegaly

## Chest and Lungs

- Air entry equal
- Normal breath sounds with auscultation
- No crackles or wheezing
- Unusually broad chest with widely spaced nipples

## Cardiac

- RRR
- Normal $S_1$ and $S_2$
- (–) for $S_3$ and $S_4$
- (–) for murmurs and rubs

## Abd

- Soft and protuberant without ascites and negative for tenderness to palpation
- (+) BS

- (–) HSM
- (–) guarding

## Genit/Rect

- Tender inguinal lymphadenopathy
- Sparse pubic hair growth
- External exam (–) for lice and nits
- Clusters of small vesicular lesions over vulva and labia
- Several ruptured vesicles → erythematous and weeping erosions interspersed
- Cervix WNL, no cervical motion tenderness
- Corpus, non-tender with no palpable masses
- Adnexa with no palpable masses or tenderness
- Rectum with no external or internal lesions
- Sphincter tone WNL
- Guaiac-negative stool

## Breasts

- Small breasts
- (–) for masses, discharge, retraction, edema, ulcerations, or discoloration
- (–) for palpable axillary nodes

## Spine

(–) tenderness to percussion

## Ext

- Peripheral pulses 2+ bilaterally
- Muscle mass WNL
- DTRs 2+
- (–) for joint swelling, redness, or tenderness
- (–) for cyanosis or clubbing
- ROM WNL
- Grip strength 5/5 in both upper extremities

## Neuro

- Alert and oriented
- CNs II–XII intact
- (–) for cerebellar, motor, and sensorial abnormalities
- Normal plantar flexion

## Laboratory Blood Test Results

See Patient Case Table 99.2

| Patient Case Table 99.2 Laboratory Blood Test Results | | | | | |
|---|---|---|---|---|---|
| Na | 138 meq/L | Cr | 1.2 mg/dL | WBC | 9,300/mm³ |
| K | 4.3 meq/L | Glu, fasting | 75 mg/dL | • Neutros | 67% |
| Cl | 105 meq/L | Hb | 15.4 g/dL | • Eos | 1% |
| HCO₃ | 27 meq/L | Hct | 40.3% | • Lymphs | 25% |
| BUN | 14 mg/dL | Plt | 258,000/mm³ | • Monos | 7% |

## Specialized Tests

- Viral culture of genital vesicular fluid: (+) for HSV-2
- Vulval swab monoclonal stain: (+) for HSV-2
- Rectal and cervical cultures: (–) for *Neisseria gonorrhoeae* and *Chlamydia trachomatis*

---

***Patient Case Question 8.*** What *subjective* clinical data (i.e., clinical symptoms) are consistent with a primary genital herpes infection? There are *six* distinct clinical symptoms in this case study.

***Patient Case Question 9.*** What *objective* clinical data (i.e., clinical signs) are consistent with a primary genital herpes infection? There are *six* distinct clinical signs in this case study.

***Patient Case Question 10.*** Identify *three* major risk factors for genital herpes in this patient.

***Patient Case Question 11.*** Six months later, the patient called the OB-GYN specialist again complaining of genital lesions that looked and felt the same as the lesions she had experienced 6 months earlier when seen and treated in the clinic. Is daily suppressive therapy indicated because she had a recurrent episode?

# 100 GONORRHEA

 *For the Disease Summary for this case study, see the CD-ROM.*

# PATIENT CASE

## ■ Patient's Chief Complaints

"I probably have done something that I shouldn't have on prom night and now it hurts when I go to the bathroom."

## ■ HPI

J.L. is a 17 yo junior in high school who presents to her pediatrician's office. She has been in reasonably good health for the past 17 years but has recently developed urinary tract manifestations—urgency to urinate, more frequent urination, and increasingly severe urethral burning during urination that has persisted for three days. She awoke from sleep with urgency last night and noticed an abnormal discharge from her vagina. She describes the discharge as "yellow and kind of thick." She reported this to her mother who kept her out of school today and immediately made a doctor's appointment. She also reports mild anal itching, but denies chills, fever, nausea, vomiting, and abdominal pain. When questioned further, she reported that she "had sex for the very first time with my prom date two weeks ago." They did not use a condom, but she has been taking the pill for six months. She denies oral and anal intercourse. Her LMP occurred four days ago. She denies any recent travel other than to local volleyball games on the school bus.

## ■ PMH

- (–) previous history of urinary or female reproductive tract infections
- (–) previous pregnancies
- Asthma × 11 years
- Immunizations are up to date and patient receives annual physical examinations and routine follow-up care for asthma

## ■ FH

- Father died last year from sudden cardiac death at age 45
- Mother has a heart murmur
- Younger brother, age 15, is in good physical health

- Older brother, age 19, is having "muscle problems in his hands and arms, but the doctors don't know yet what is causing them"
- Maternal grandmother has "high blood pressure"

## SH

J.L. is very popular at school and is well liked by her teachers and classmates. She has dated a few boys from school, but claims not to have been sexually active before prom night. She comes from an upper socioeconomic background. She does not drink alcohol, smoke, or use any recreational drugs. She claims that it is "very uncool" with her friends to engage in any activities like that. She is on the varsity volleyball team and practices most days after school. Her home life has been difficult during the past 10 months due to the death of her father, with whom she was very close. J.L. claims that, for the most part, she has a very caring and close family.

## Meds

- Ethinyl estradiol 35 μg with norethindrone 0.5 mg (7 tablets) + ethinyl estradiol 35 μg with norethindrone 0.75 mg (7 tablets) + ethinyl estradiol 35 μg with norethindrone 1 mg (7 tablets)
- Albuterol 90 μg MDI 2 puffs PRN
- Beclomethasone 42 μg MDI 2 puffs TID
- Salmeterol 21 μg 2 puffs Q 12 h
- Albuterol 2.5 mg with ipratropium bromide 0.5 mg per 3 mL for nebulization PRN

## All

NKDA

*Patient Case Question 1.* Why is the patient taking ethinyl estradiol and norethindrone?

*Patient Case Question 2.* Why is the patient taking albuterol and beclomethasone?

*Patient Case Question 3.* Briefly describe the mechanisms of drug action for albuterol and beclomethasone that make them uniquely different but important.

## ROS

- (+) increased frequency of urination and urgent urination with mild incontinence
- (–) rectal discharge and bleeding
- (–) rectal pain, tenesmus, and constipation
- (–) rash and other skin manifestations
- (–) joint/tendon pain and swelling
- (–) recent onset headache, neck pain, and stiffness
- (–) chest pain, cough, SOB, and palpitations
- (–) sore throat and dysphagia

## PE and Lab Tests

### Gen

- WDWN young, white female in NAD
- Pleasant and trim but appears mildly fatigued

## VS

See Patient Case Table 100.1

| Patient Case Table 100.1 Vital Signs | | | | | |
|---|---|---|---|---|---|
| BP | 114/64 mm Hg, sitting | RR | 16 not labored | WT | 114 lbs |
| P | 120 BPM regular | T | 98.7°F | HT | 65 in |

## Skin

- Intact, warm, and dry with good turgor
- (–) rashes, bruises, papules, and pustules

## HEENT

- PERRLA
- (–) photophobia
- EOMI
- No hemorrhages, exudates, or papilledema on funduscopic exam
- Sclerae white without icterus
- (–) conjunctival erythema, edema, and exudate
- TMs clear throughout with no drainage
- (–) erythema, swelling, and exudate within pharynx

## Neck/LN

- Neck supple without masses
- (–) lymphadenopathy, JVD, bruits, and thyromegaly

## Chest

- Normal breath sounds without wheezes
- Good air entry
- (–) breast lesions or discoloration

## Cardiac

- RRR
- (–) murmurs and rubs
- $S_1$ and $S_2$ normal
- No $S_3$ and $S_4$

## Abd

- (–) for rebound tenderness and guarding in all 4 quadrants with palpation
- Soft and non-distended
- (+) BS
- (–) HSM
- (–) masses and bruits

## Genit/Rect

- (–) vulval erythema and edema
- Vagina with thick yellow-white discharge and mild erythema

- Cervix is friable and shows yellow-white discharge from os
- (–) masses on bimanual exam
- (+) cervical motion tenderness
- (–) adnexal tenderness
- (–) stool heme
- (+) mild anal erythema and edema

## MS/Ext

- (–) adenopathy, lesions, and rashes
- (–) arthritis and tenosynovitis
- Capillary refill WNL at < 2 sec
- (–) femoral bruits
- (–) CCE
- Pulses 2+ throughout
- Normal ROM and muscle strength at 5/5 throughout

## Neuro

- A & O × 3
- CNs II–XII intact
- DTRs 2+ and symmetric bilaterally
- No gross motor-sensory deficits present
- (–) Babinski

## Laboratory Blood Test Results

See Patient Case Table 100.2

| Patient Case Table 100.2 Laboratory Blood Test Results | | | | | |
|---|---|---|---|---|---|
| Na | 134 meq/L | Glu, fasting | 98 mg/dL | WBC | $13.5 \times 10^3/mm^3$ |
| K | 4.4 meq/L | Mg | 1.9 mg/dL | • Neutros | 70% |
| Cl | 101 meq/L | Phos | 4.2 mg/dL | • Bands | 8% |
| $HCO_3$ | 27 meq/L | Hb | 13.4 g/dL | • Lymphs | 17% |
| BUN | 12 mg/dL | Hct | 43.1% | • Monos | 4% |
| Cr | 1.1 mg/dL | Plt | $225 \times 10^3/mm^3$ | • Eos | 1% |

## UA

- Color: dark yellow
- Appearance: slightly cloudy
- SG: 1.022
- pH 5.0
- 10 WBC/HPF
- 10 RBC/HPF
- (+) gram-negative diplococci

## Nucleic Acid Amplification Test

- PCR of cervical swab specimen: (+) *Neisseria gonorrhoeae* and *Chlamydia trachomatis*
- PCR of urine specimen: (+) *Neisseria gonorrhoeae* and *Chlamydia trachomatis*

***Patient Case Question 4.*** Identify the *single most important* risk factor in this case study.

***Patient Case Question 5.*** Identify the *two most definitive signs* of gonorrhea in this patient.

***Patient Case Question 6.*** Provide a *specific* assessment/diagnosis of this patient's condition.

***Patient Case Question 7.*** Briefly cite the clinical evidence that *supports* or *excludes* a diagnosis of gonococcal proctitis.

***Patient Case Question 8.*** Briefly cite the clinical evidence that *supports* or *excludes* a diagnosis of gonococcal urethritis.

***Patient Case Question 9.*** Briefly cite the clinical evidence that *supports* or *excludes* a diagnosis of gonococcal cervicitis.

***Patient Case Question 10.*** Briefly cite the clinical evidence that *supports* or *excludes* a diagnosis of gonococcal pharyngitis.

***Patient Case Question 11.*** Briefly cite the clinical evidence that *supports* or *excludes* a diagnosis of gonococcal conjunctivitis.

***Patient Case Question 12.*** Briefly cite the clinical evidence that *supports* or *excludes* a diagnosis of gonococcal perihepatitis.

***Patient Case Question 13.*** Briefly cite the clinical evidence that *supports* or *excludes* a diagnosis of gonococcal pelvic inflammatory disease.

***Patient Case Question 14.*** Briefly cite the clinical evidence that *supports* or *excludes* a diagnosis of gonococcal meningitis.

***Patient Case Question 15.*** Briefly cite the clinical evidence that *supports* or *excludes* a diagnosis of gonococcal endocarditis.

***Patient Case Question 16.*** Which *three* blood test findings are consistent with a diagnosis of gonococcal infection?

***Patient Case Question 17.*** Briefly cite the clinical evidence that *supports* or *excludes* a diagnosis of disseminated gonococcal infection.

PART

18

APPENDICES

# APPENDIX A. TABLE OF CLINICAL REFERENCE VALUES

## CLINICAL REFERENCE VALUES FOR CASE STUDY PROBLEM-SOLVING*

| COMPLETE BLOOD COUNT (CBC) | |
|---|---|
| Hematocrit (Hct), whole blood | Males: 39–49%<br>Females: 35–45% |
| Hemoglobin, total (Hb), whole blood | Males: 13.6–17.5 g/dL<br>Females: 12.0–15.5 g/dL<br>**Panic: <7.1 g/dL** |
| Mean corpuscular hemoglobin (MCH), whole blood | 26–34 pg |
| Mean corpuscular hemoglobin concentration (MCHC), whole blood | 31–36 g/dL |
| Mean corpuscular volume (MCV), whole blood | 80–100 fL |
| Basophil count, whole blood | 10–120/cu mm |
| Eosinophil count, whole blood | 40–500/cu mm |
| Lymphocyte count, whole blood | 800–3,500/cu mm |
| Monocyte count, whole blood | 200–800/cu mm |
| Platelet (Plt) count, whole blood | 150,000–450,000/cu mm<br>**Panic: <25,000/cu mm** |
| Red blood cell (RBC) count, whole blood | 4.7–6.1 million/cu mm |
| Reticulocyte count, whole blood | 33,000–137,000/cu mm |
| White blood cell (WBC) count, whole blood | 4,800–10,800/cu mm<br>**Panic: <1,500/cu mm** |
| White blood cell differential, whole blood | Neutrophils (segs), 57–67%<br>Lymphocytes, 25–33%<br>Monocytes/macrophages: 3–7%<br>Eosinophils: 1–4%<br>Basophils: 0–1% |
| ELECTROLYTES | |
| Bicarbonate ($HCO_3^-$), carbon dioxide total, serum | 22–32 meq/L<br>**Panic: <15 or >40 meq/L** |
| Calcium ($Ca^{+2}$), serum | 8.5–10.5 mg/dL<br>**Panic: <6.5 or >13.5 mg/dL** |
| Chloride ($Cl^-$), serum | 101–112 meq/L |
| Magnesium ($Mg^{+2}$), serum | 1.8–3.0 mg/dL<br>**Panic: <0.5 or >4.5 mg/dL** |
| Phosphate ($PO_4^{-3}$), serum | 2.5–4.5 mg/dL<br>**Panic: <1.0 mg/dL** |
| Potassium ($K^+$), serum | 3.5–5.0 meq/L<br>**Panic: <3.0 or >6.0 meq/L** |
| Sodium ($Na^+$), serum | 135–145 meq/L<br>**Panic: <125 or >155 meq/L** |

*(Continued)*

| RENAL FUNCTION TESTS | |
|---|---|
| Blood urea nitrogen (BUN), serum | 8–20 mg/dL |
| Creatinine (Cr), serum | 0.6–1.2 mg/dL |

| LIVER FUNCTION TESTS | |
|---|---|
| Alanine aminotransferase (ALT), serum | 7–56 IU/L |
| Alkaline phosphatase (Alk Phos), serum | 41–133 IU/L |
| Aspartate aminotransferase (AST), serum | 0–35 IU/L |
| Gamma-glutamyl transferase (GGT), serum | 9–85 IU/L |
| Bilirubin, total, serum | 0.1–1.2 mg/dL |
| Bilirubin, direct or conjugated, serum | 0.1–0.5 mg/dL |
| Bilirubin, indirect or unconjugated, serum | 0.1–0.7 mg/dL |

| THYROID FUNCTION TESTS | |
|---|---|
| Thyroid-stimulating hormone (TSH), serum | 0.4–6 μU/mL |
| Thyroxine, free (FT$_4$), serum | 9–24 pmol/L |
| Thyroxine, total (T$_4$), serum | 5–11 μg/dL |
| Triiodothyronine, total (T$_3$), serum | 95–190 ng/dL |
| Radioactive iodine (I$^{123}$) uptake | − 12–20% uptake by thyroid gland in 6 hrs<br>− 5–25% uptake by thyroid gland in 24 hrs |

| TESTS FOR IRON IN THE BLOOD | |
|---|---|
| Ferritin, serum | Males: 16–300 ng/mL<br>Females: 4–161 ng/mL |
| Free erythrocyte protoporphyrin (FEP), whole blood | <35 μg/dL |
| Iron (Fe$^{2+}$), serum | 50–175 μg/dL |
| Iron-binding capacity, total (TIBC), serum | 250–460 μg/dL |
| Transferrin saturation | 30–50% |

| ARTERIAL BLOOD GAS ASSESSMENT | |
|---|---|
| Carbon dioxide, partial pressure (PaCO$_2$ or PCO$_2$), arterial whole blood | 32–48 mm Hg<br>**Panic: >50 mm Hg** |
| Oxygen, partial pressure (PaO$_2$ or PO$_2$), arterial whole blood | 83–108 mm Hg<br>**Panic: <60 mm Hg** |
| Oxygen saturation (SaO$_2$), room air | ≥95% |
| pH arterial, whole blood | 7.35–7.45 |
| Effect of altitude on PaO$_2$, pH 7.40/38.0°C<br><br>• Sea level<br>• 2,000 feet<br>• 4,000 feet<br>• 6,000 feet<br>• 8,000 feet<br>• 10,000 feet<br>• 15,000 feet | PaO$_2$<br>• 99 mm Hg<br>• 88 mm Hg<br>• 77 mm Hg<br>• 68 mm Hg<br>• 58 mm Hg<br>• 50 mm Hg<br>• 30 mm Hg |

*(Continued)*

## ARTERIAL BLOOD GAS ASSESSMENT (*Continued*)

| Effect of PaO$_2$ on % saturation of hemoglobin, SaO$_2$ | % saturation of hemoglobin, SaO$_2$ |
|---|---|
| • 100 mm Hg | • 97.5% |
| • 90 mm Hg | • 96.5% |
| • 80 mm Hg | • 94.5% |
| • 70 mm Hg | • 92.7% |
| • 60 mm Hg **critical** | • 89.0% |
| • 50 mm Hg | • 83.5% |
| • 40 mm Hg | • 75.0% |
| • 30 mm Hg | • 57.0% |
| • 20 mm Hg | • 35.0% |
| • 10 mm Hg | • 13.5% |

## HORMONE ASSAYS

| | |
|---|---|
| Adrenocorticotropic hormone (ACTH), plasma | 9–52 pg/mL |
| Calcitonin, plasma | Males: 0–11.5 pg/mL<br>Females: 0–4.6 pg/mL |
| Cortisol, serum | 8 AM: 5–20 µg/dL |
| Dehydroepiandrosterone sulfate (DHEAS), serum | 1–12 µmol/L |
| Follicle-stimulating hormone (FSH), serum | **Female**<br>Follicular phase:  4–13 mU/mL<br>Luteal phase:  2–13 mU/mL<br>Midcycle:  5–22 mU/mL<br>Postmenopause:  30–138 mU/mL<br>**Male:**  1–10 mU/mL |
| Human chorionic gonadotropin, β subunit (β-HCG), serum | 0–4 mU/mL |
| Insulin (Ins), serum | 6–35 µU/mL |
| Luteinizing hormone (LH), serum | **Female**<br>Follicular phase:  1–18 mU/mL<br>Luteal phase:  0.4–20 mU/mL<br>Midcycle:  24–105 mU/mL<br>Postmenopause:  15–62 mU/mL<br>**Male:**  1–10 mU/mL |
| Parathyroid hormone (PTH), serum | 11–54 pg/mL |
| Prolactin (PRL), serum | <20 ng/mL |
| Testosterone, serum | Males: 175–781 ng/dL<br>Females: 10–75 ng/dL |

## LIPID PANEL

| | |
|---|---|
| Cholesterol, serum | **Desirable:** <200 mg/dL<br>**Borderline:** 200–239 mg/dL<br>**High risk:** >240 mg/dL |
| High-density lipoprotein (HDL) cholesterol, serum | **Desirable: >40 mg/dL in men and >50 mg/dL in women** |
| Low-density lipoprotein (LDL) cholesterol, serum | <130 mg/dL<br>**Desirable**<br>**Very high risk (has both cardiovascular disease and diabetes mellitus) <70 mg/dL**<br>**High risk (has cardiovascular disease) <100 mg/dL**<br>**Moderate risk (2 or more risk factors) <130 mg/dL**<br>**Low risk (0–1 risk factors) <160 mg/dL** |
| Triglycerides (Trig), serum | <165 mg/dL |

*(Continued)*

| CARDIAC MARKERS | |
|---|---|
| Creatine kinase (CK), serum | 32–267 IU/L |
| Creatine kinase MB (CK-MB), serum | <16 IU/L |
| Troponin I, serum | <0.05 ng/mL |

| VITAMINS | |
|---|---|
| Folic acid, whole blood | 165–760 ng/mL |
| Vitamin A, serum | 30–65 mg/dL |
| Vitamin B12, serum | 140–820 pg/mL |
| Vitamin D, 25OH, serum | 10–50 ng/mL |
| Vitamin D, 1,25OH, serum | 20–76 pg/mL |
| Vitamin E, serum | 0.5–0.7 mg/dL |

| BLOOD CLOTTING ASSESSMENT | |
|---|---|
| International normalized ratio (INR) | Approximately 1.0 in healthy patients not receiving anti-coagulant therapy; INR >2.0 suggests liver dysfunction<br><br>Ideal target for warfarin prophylaxis and treatment of DVT = **2.5 (range 2.0–3.0)**<br><br>Ideal target for patients with prosthetic cardiac valves = **2.5–3.5**<br><br>INR = (PT$^{Patient}$/PT$^{Control}$)$^{ISI}$<br>ISR = International Sensitivity Index (Each manufactured thromboplastin reagent has an ISI that should be used to calculate the INR.) |
| Partial thromboplastin time, activated (PTT), plasma | 25–35 seconds<br>**Panic: ≥60 seconds** |
| Prothrombin time (PT), whole blood | 11–15 seconds<br>**Panic: ≥30 seconds** |

| MISCELLANEOUS BLOOD TESTS | |
|---|---|
| Albumin (Alb), serum | 3.4–4.7 g/dL |
| Alpha-1-Antitrypsin (AAT), serum | 110–270 mg/dL |
| α-Fetoprotein (AFP), serum | 0–15 ng/mL |
| Ammonia ($NH_3$), plasma | 18–60 µg/dL |
| Amylase, serum | 20–110 IU/L |
| Anion gap | 6–12 meq/L |
| Carcinoembryonic antigen (CEA), serum | 0–5 ng/mL |
| Ceruloplasmin, serum | 20–60 mg/dL |
| C-reactive protein (CRP), plasma | 0–0.5 mg/dL |
| Erythrocyte sedimentation rate (ESR), whole blood | Males: <10 mm/hr<br>Females: <15 mm/hr |
| Glucose (Glu), serum, fasting | 60–110 mg/dL<br>**Panic: <40 or >500 mg/dL** |
| Glucose, 2-hr post-prandial blood (PPBG) | <150 mg/dL<br>**>200 mg/dL suggests diabetes mellitus** |
| Glycosylated hemoglobin (HbA$_{1c}$), serum | 3.9–6.9% |
| Homocysteine (Homocys), serum | 3.3–10.4 µmol/L |
| Lactate dehydrogenase (LDH), serum | 88–230 IU/L |
| Methylmalonic acid (MMA), serum | 0–0.05 mg/L |
| Osmolality, serum | 273–293 mmol/kg $H_2O$<br>Panic: <240 or >320 mmol/kg $H_2O$ |

*(Continued)*

## MISCELLANEOUS BLOOD TESTS (*Continued*)

| | |
|---|---|
| Prostate-specific antigen (PSA), serum | Ages 40–49: 0–2.4 ng/mL<br>Ages 50–59: 0–3.4 ng/mL<br>Ages 60–69: 0–4.4 ng/mL<br>Ages 70–79: 0–5.4 ng/mL |
| Protein, total, serum | 6.0–8.0 g/dL |
| Uric acid, serum | Males: 2.4–7.4 mg/dL<br>Females: 1.4–5.8 mg/dL |

### CEREBROSPINAL FLUID ANALYSIS

| | |
|---|---|
| Glucose | 50–70% of patient's serum glucose concentration |
| Lumbar puncture CSF appearance | Clear and colorless |
| Lumbar puncture opening pressure | 70–180 mm $H_2O$ |
| Protein | 15–45 mg/dL |
| Red blood cell (RBC) count | 0/cu mm |
| White blood cell (WBC) count | 0–6/cu mm |
| Lymphocyte count | 0–5/cu mm |

### KNEE JOINT FLUID ANALYSIS

| | |
|---|---|
| Volume | <3.5 mL |
| Clarity | Transparent |
| Color | Colorless |
| White blood cell count | 200–300/cu mm |
| Neutrophils and macrophages | <25% |
| Culture | Negative |
| Glucose | Approximately equal to serum glucose concentration |

### URINALYSIS

| | |
|---|---|
| pH | 5.0–6.5 |
| Specific gravity (SG) | 1.016–1.022 |
| Red blood cells (RBC) | 0–5 RBC/high power field (HPF) |
| White blood cells (WBC) | 0–5 WBC/HPF |
| Acetone (ketones) | Negative |
| Amylase | 4–400 IU/L |
| Calcium excreted per 24 hrs | 100–300 mg/24 hrs |
| Chloride | Depends on diet |
| Citrate excreted per 24 hrs | 287–708 mg/24 hrs |
| Cortisol (free) excreted per 24 hrs | 10–110 µg/24 hrs |
| Creatinine excreted per 24 hrs | 15–25 mg/kg/24 hrs |
| Dopamine excreted per 24 hours | 52–480 µg/24 hrs |
| Epinephrine excreted per 24 hrs | 2–24 µg/24 hrs |
| Glucose | <0.05 g/dL |
| Microalbumin | <20 µg/mL |
| Norepinephrine excreted per 24 hrs | 15–100 µg/24 hrs |
| Osmolality | 100–900 mOsm/kg $H_2O$ |
| Phosphorus excreted per 24 hrs | 1 g/24 hrs |
| Potassium | Depends on diet |
| Protein, total, excreted per 24 hrs | <165 mg/24 hrs |

(*Continued*)

| **URINALYSIS (*Continued*)** | |
|---|---|
| Sodium | Depends on diet |
| Urea nitrogen excreted per 24 hrs | 6–17 g/24 hrs |
| Urine volume per 24 hrs | 1–2 L/24 hrs |

| **VITAL SIGNS** | |
|---|---|
| Heart rate | 60–90 bpm |
| Heart rate, during sleep | 50–60 bpm |
| Heart rate, conditioned athlete | 40–60 bpm |
| Bradycardia | <60 bpm in non-athletes |
| Tachycardia | >100 bpm |
| Body mass index (BMI) = weight in kilograms/ (height in meters)$^2$ <br> 1 kg = 2.2 lb <br> 1 m = 39.37 in | <18.5 = underweight <br> 18.5–24.9 = healthy weight <br> 25.0–29.9 = overweight <br> 30.0–34.9 = obesity, class I <br> 35.0–39.9 = obesity, class II <br> >40.0 = obesity, class III |
| Respiratory rate, at rest | 12–14/min |
| Tachypnea | >16/min |
| Systolic blood pressure | 90–130 mm |
| Diastolic blood pressure | <85 mm |
| Hypotension | Systolic BP <90 mm |
| Potentially hypertensive | ≥140/90 mm |
| High-normal blood pressure | 130–139/85–89 mm |
| Stage 1 hypertension | 140–159/90–99 mm |
| Stage 2 hypertension | ≥160/100 mm |

| **PHYSICAL EXAMINATION TESTS** | |
|---|---|
| *Auscultation of the Heart* | |
| Normal Heart Sounds: <br> $S_1$ = normal heart sound with closure of the AV valves, esp. mitral <br> $S_2$ = normal heart sound with closure of semilunar valves, esp. aortic | Abnormal Heart Sounds: <br> $S_3$ = normal heart sound in children and young adults but suggests ventricular dysfunction in middle-aged and older adults ("ventricular gallop") <br> $S_4$ = rarely heard in absence of cardiac disease, suggests an overfilled ventricle, and is consistent with high blood pressure, aortic stenosis, fluid overload and post-heart attack ("atrial gallop") |
| Maximum vertical distance from sternal angle high in sternum to an observable right internal jugular vein | <3 cm is normal <br> >3 cm indicates jugular venous distension due to increased central venous pressure |
| *Auscultation and Percussion of the Lungs* | |
| Normal Lung Sounds with Auscultation: <br> Described as **vesicular** (in lung periphery) or **bronchial** (when substernal) | Abnormal Lung Sounds with Auscultation: <br> **Wheezes** (high-pitched, whistling), **rhonchi** (low-pitched and gurgling), and **crackles** (popping quality) |
| Normal Lung Sounds with Percussion: <br> Described as **resonant** | Abnormal Lung Sounds with Percussion: <br> **Dull:** Suggests lack of air, such as from a tumor or organizing pneumonia <br> **Hyper-resonant:** Suggests too much air, such as from emphysema |
| *Cranial Nerve (CN) Examination* | |
| | CN I = smell <br> CN II = vision <br> CN III, IV, VI = pupils, lids, eye movements |

*(Continued)*

| *Cranial Nerve (CN) Examination (Continued)* | |
|---|---|
| | CN V = jaw muscles<br>CN VII = lower and upper facial muscles<br>CN VIII = hearing<br>CN IX, X = uvula, palate, tonsils, tongue, vocal cords<br>CN XI = shoulder and neck muscles (shoulder shrug and head rotation)<br>CN XII = anatomy and physiology of the tongue |
| *Deep Tendon Reflexes (DTRs)* | |
| | 0 = no response<br>1 = diminished response<br>2 = normal response<br>3 = moderately exaggerated response<br>4 = hyperreflexia (suggests upper motor neuron disease) |
| Patellar reflex | Sudden contraction of the anterior muscles of the thigh caused by a sharp tap on the patellar tendon while the leg hangs loosely at a right angle with the thigh. Synonymous with **knee-jerk reflex, quadriceps reflex.** |
| Plantar reflex | Tactile stimulation of the ball of the foot causes plantar flexion (i.e., toes bend or curve downward)<br>**Babinski sign (abnormal):** great toe extends upward and other toes fan out, indicates pyramidal tract dysfunction |
| Triceps reflex | Sudden contraction of the triceps muscle caused by a sharp tap on its tendon when the forearm hangs loosely at a right angle with the upper arm |
| *Edema, Grading* | |
| | 0 = no swelling<br>1 = mild edema<br>2 = moderate edema<br>3 = severe edema<br>4 = very severe edema |
| *Glasgow Coma Scale* | |
| Eyes Opening Response<br>4 Spontaneous<br>3 To command<br>2 To pain stimulus<br>1 No response<br>Best Motor Response<br>6 Obedience to verbal commands<br>5 Localization of pain<br>4 Withdrawal in response to pain<br>3 Abnormal flexion<br>2 Extensor response<br>1 Flaccidity<br>Verbal<br>5 Appropriate orientation<br>4 Confused conversation<br>3 Inappropriate words<br>2 Incomprehensible sounds<br>1 No response | **3–15  total score**<br><br>**15: completely normal brain function**<br>**13–14: mild brain injury**<br><br>**9–12:  moderate brain injury**<br><br>**3–8: severe brain injury** |

*(Continued)*

| Muscle Tone | |
|---|---|
| | 0 = no contraction/movement<br>1 = trace of contraction but no movement<br>2 = movement with gravity eliminated (e.g., movement while resting on a table)<br>3 = movement against gravity but not resistance (e.g., raising the arm)<br>4 = movement against resistance<br>5 = full power |
| *Pupillary Examination* | |
| Pupillary reflex | Pupil constricts with light |
| Pupillary size and function | 3 mm, equal, and reactive to light and accommodation<br>**Panic: Pupils that are pinpointed (1 mm), small (1.5–2.0 mm), dilated (4–5 mm), and fixed to light are abnormal.** |
| *Specialized Cardiac Function Testing* | |
| Cardiac output at rest | 4–8 L/min |
| Stroke volume at rest | 60–100 mL/beat |
| End diastolic volume | ≈ 120 mL |
| End systolic volume | ≈ 50 mL |
| Stroke volume | ≈ 70 mL |
| Ejection fraction | 60–75%<br><60% indicates ventricular dysfunction |
| *Specialized Pulmonary Function Testing (Spirometry)* | |
| 1) TLC = IRV + TV + ERV + RV<br>2) VC = TLC − RV<br>3) VC = IRV + TV + ERV | –Total lung capacity (TLC) ~ 5700–6200 mL<br>–Inspiratory reserve volume (IRV) ~ 3000–3300 mL<br>–Expiratory reserve volume (ERV) ~ 1000–1200 mL<br>–Vital capacity (VC) ~ 4500–5000 mL<br>–Residual volume (RV) ~ 1200 mL<br>–Tidal volume (TV) ~ 500 mL |

*All values apply to adolescents and adults only; IU, International Units

# APPENDIX B. TABLE OF NORMAL HEIGHT AND WEIGHT IN CHILDREN AGES 1–18 YEARS

**THE FOLLOWING TABLE IS BASED ON GROWTH CHARTS DEVELOPED BY THE CENTERS FOR DISEASE CONTROL AND PREVENTION (CDC) THAT SHOW THE AVERAGE RANGES OF WEIGHT AND HEIGHT.**

| AGE (YRS) | NORMAL HEIGHT—FEMALES (INCHES) | NORMAL HEIGHT—MALES (INCHES) | NORMAL WEIGHT—FEMALES (POUNDS) | NORMAL WEIGHT—MALES (POUNDS) |
|---|---|---|---|---|
| 1 | 27 to 31 | 28 to 32 | 15 to 20 | 17 to 21 |
| 2 | 31.5 to 36 | 32 to 37 | 22 to 32 | 24 to 34 |
| 3 | 34.5 to 40 | 35.5 to 40.5 | 26 to 38 | 26 to 38 |
| 4 | 37 to 42.5 | 37.5 to 43 | 28 to 44 | 30 to 44 |
| 6 | 42 to 49 | 42 to 49 | 36 to 60 | 36 to 60 |
| 8 | 47 to 54 | 47 to 54 | 44 to 80 | 46 to 78 |
| 10 | 50 to 59 | 50.5 to 59 | 54 to 106 | 54 to 102 |
| 12 | 55 to 64 | 54 to 63.5 | 68 to 136 | 66 to 130 |
| 14 | 59 to 67.5 | 59 to 69.5 | 84 to 160 | 84 to 160 |
| 16 | 60 to 68 | 63 to 73 | 94 to 172 | 104 to 186 |
| 18 | 60 to 68.5 | 65 to 74 | 100 to 178 | 116 to 202 |

# APPENDIX C. TABLE OF BLOOD PRESSURE IN CHILDREN BY GENDER AND AGE

| AGE (YEARS) | BOYS, NORMAL BLOOD PRESSURE (mm Hg) | BOYS, HIGH BLOOD PRESSURE (mm Hg) | GIRLS, NORMAL BLOOD PRESSURE (mm Hg) | GIRLS, HIGH BLOOD PRESSURE (mm Hg) |
|---|---|---|---|---|
| 1 | <103/54 | ≥106/58 | <103/56 | ≥107/60 |
| 2 to 3 | <109/63 | ≥113/67 | <106/65 | ≥110/69 |
| 4 to 5 | <112/70 | ≥116/74 | <109/70 | ≥113/74 |
| 6 to 7 | <115/74 | ≥119/78 | <113/73 | ≥116/77 |
| 8 to 10 | <119/78 | ≥123/82 | <118/76 | ≥122/80 |
| 11 to 12 | <123/79 | ≥127/83 | <122/78 | ≥133/90 |
| 13 to 14 | <128/80 | ≥132/84 | <125/80 | ≥136/92 |
| 15 to 17 | <136/84 | ≥140/89 | <128/82 | ≥132/86 |

(Source: National Heart, Lung and Blood Institute, National Institutes of Health, The Fourth Report on the Diagnosis, Evaluation and Treatment of High Blood Pressure in Children and Adolescents, NIH Publication No. 05-5267, May 2005.)

# APPENDIX D. TABLE OF KARNOFSKY PERFORMANCE STATUS

## KARNOFSKY PERFORMANCE STATUS

| SCORE | |
|---|---|
| 100 | Normal: no complaints, no evidence of disease |
| 90 | Able to carry on normal activities; minor symptoms |
| 80 | Normal activities with effort; some symptoms |
| 70 | Cares for self; unable to carry on normal activities |
| 60 | Requires occasional assistance; cares for most needs |
| 50 | Requires considerable assistance and frequent care |
| 40 | Disabled: requires special care and assistance |
| 30 | Severely disabled: hospitalized but death not imminent |
| 20 | Very sick: active supportive care needed |
| 10 | Moribund: fatal processes are progressing rapidly |
| 0 | Patient expired |

(Adapted with permission from Karnofsky DA, Burchenal JH. The clinical evaluation of chemotherapeutic agents in cancer. In: MacLeod CM, ed. Evaluation of Chemotherapeutic Agents. New York: Columbia University Press, 1949:196.)

| A | |
|---|---|
| A & O | alert and oriented |
| A & P | auscultation and percussion |
| A & W | alive and well |
| AA | aplastic anemia |
| AAA | abdominal aortic aneurysm |
| AAO | awake, alert, and oriented |
| Abd | abdomen |
| ABG | arterial blood gases |
| ABW | actual body weight |
| AC | before meals (*ante cibos*) |
| ACEI | angiotensin-converting enzyme inhibitor |
| ACTH | adrenocorticotropic hormone |
| AD | Alzheimer disease, right ear (*auris dextra*) |
| ADH | antidiuretic hormone |
| ADHD | attention-deficit hyperactivity disorder |
| ADL | activities of daily living |
| AF | atrial fibrillation |
| AFP | a-fetoprotein |
| AI | aortic insufficiency |
| AIDS | acquired immunodeficiency syndrome |
| AKA | above-knee amputation |
| ALD | alcoholic liver disease |
| All | allergies |
| ALL | acute lymphocytic leukemia, acute lymphoblastic leukemia |
| ALP | alkaline phosphatase |
| ALS | amyotrophic lateral sclerosis |
| ALT | alanine aminotransferase |
| AMI | acute myocardial infarction (heart attack) |
| AML | acute myelogenous leukemia, acute myelocytic leukemia |
| ANA | antinuclear antibody |
| AOM | acute otitis media |
| AP | anteroposterior |
| APAP | acetaminophen (acetyl-p-aminophenol) |
| aPTT | activated partial thromboplastin time |
| ARDS | adult respiratory distress syndrome |
| ARF | acute renal failure |
| AS | left ear (*auris sinistra*) |

| ASA | aspirin (acetylsalicylic acid) |
| ASCVD | arteriosclerotic cardiovascular disease |
| ASD | atrial septal defect |
| AST | aspartate aminotransferase |
| AT | atraumatic |
| ATN | acute tubular necrosis |
| AU | each ear (*auris uterque*) |
| AV | arteriovenous, atrioventricular |
| AVM | arteriovenous malformation |
| AVR | aortic valve replacement |
| **B** | |
| Basos | basophils |
| BBB | blood–brain barrier |
| BC | blood culture |
| BE | barium enema |
| BID | twice daily (*bis in die*) |
| BKA | below-knee amputation |
| BM | bone marrow, bowel movement |
| BMD | bone mineral density |
| BMI | body mass index |
| BMR | basal metabolic rate |
| BMT | bone marrow transplantation |
| BP | blood pressure |
| BPH | benign prostatic hyperplasia |
| bpm, BPM | beats per minute |
| BR | bedrest |
| BRBPR | bright red blood per rectum |
| BS | bowel sounds, breath sounds |
| BSO | bilateral salpingo-oophorectomy |
| BUN | blood urea nitrogen |
| Bx | biopsy |
| **C** | |
| CA | carcinoma (or cancer) |
| CABG | coronary artery bypass graft |
| CAD | coronary artery disease |
| CAH | chronic active hepatitis |
| CAPD | continuous ambulatory peritoneal dialysis |
| CBC | complete blood count |
| CBD | common bile duct |
| CC | chief complaint |
| CCA | calcium channel antagonist |
| CCB | calcium channel blocker |
| CCE | clubbing, cyanosis, edema |
| CCPD | continuous cycling peritoneal dialysis |
| CCU | coronary care unit |
| CEA | carcinoembryonic antigen |

| CECT | contrast-enhanced computed tomography |
|------|----------------------------------------|
| CF | cystic fibrosis |
| CHF | congestive heart failure |
| CHOP | cyclophosphamide, hydroxydaunomycin (doxorubicin), Oncovin (vincristine), prednisone |
| CK | creatine kinase |
| CLL | chronic lymphocytic leukemia |
| CML | chronic myelogenous leukemia, chronic myelocytic leukemia |
| CMV | cytomegalovirus |
| CN | cranial nerve |
| CNS | central nervous system |
| C/O | complains of |
| CO | cardiac output, carbon monoxide |
| COLD | chronic obstructive lung disease |
| COPD | chronic obstructive pulmonary disease |
| CP | chest pain, cerebral palsy |
| CPK | creatine phosphokinase |
| CPR | cardiopulmonary resuscitation |
| Cr | creatinine |
| CRF | chronic renal failure, corticotropin-releasing factor |
| CRH | corticotropin-releasing hormone |
| CRI | catheter-related infection |
| CSA | cyclosporine |
| CSF | cerebrospinal fluid |
| CTA | clear to auscultation |
| CTA & P | clear to auscultation and percussion |
| CTP | clear to percussion |
| CT | computed tomography |
| CTZ | chemoreceptor trigger zone |
| CV | cardiovascular |
| CVA | cerebrovascular accident (stroke) |
| CVAT | costovertebral angle tenderness |
| CVC | central venous catheter |
| CVP | central venous pressure |
| Cx | culture |
| CXR | chest x-ray |
| **D** | |
| $D_5W$ | 5% dextrose in water |
| DBP | diastolic blood pressure |
| D/C | discontinue, discharge |
| DCC | direct current cardioversion |
| DEXA | dual-energy x-ray absorptiometry |
| DI | diabetes insipidus |
| DIC | disseminated intravascular coagulation |
| Diff | differential |
| DIP | distal interphalangeal |
| DJD | degenerative joint disease |

| DKA | diabetic ketoacidosis |
| dL | deciliter |
| DM | diabetes mellitus |
| DNA | deoxyribonucleic acid |
| DOA | dead on arrival |
| DOB | date of birth |
| DOE | dyspnea on exertion |
| DP | dorsalis pedis |
| DRE | digital rectal examination |
| DTP | diphtheria-tetanus-pertussis |
| DTR | deep tendon reflex |
| DVT | deep vein thrombosis |
| Dx | diagnosis |
| **E** | |
| EBV | Epstein-Barr virus |
| EC | enteric-coated |
| ECF | extended care facility |
| ECG | electrocardiogram |
| ECHO | echocardiography |
| ECT | electroconvulsive therapy |
| ED | emergency department |
| EEG | electroencephalogram |
| EENT | eyes, ears, nose, throat |
| EF | ejection fraction |
| Endo | endoscopy |
| EOM | extra-ocular movements (or muscles) |
| EOMI | extra-ocular movements (or muscles) intact |
| Eos | eosinophils |
| EPO | erythropoietin |
| ER | emergency room, estrogen receptor |
| ERT | estrogen replacement therapy |
| ERV | expiratory reserve volume |
| ESR | erythrocyte sedimentation rate |
| ESRD | end-stage renal disease |
| ESWL | extracorporeal shockwave lithotripsy |
| EtOH | ethanol |
| Ext | extremities |
| **F** | |
| FBS | fasting blood sugar |
| $FEV_1$ | forced expiratory volume in one second |
| FFP | fresh frozen plasma |
| FH | family history |
| fl | femtoliter |
| FM | face mask |
| FOC | fronto-occipital circumference |
| FPG | fasting plasma glucose |

| FSH | follicle-stimulating hormone |
|---|---|
| F/U | follow-up |
| FUO | fever of unknown origin |
| FVC | forced vital capacity |
| Fx | fracture |
| **G** | |
| GAD | generalized anxiety disorder |
| GB | gallbladder |
| GBS | group B *Streptococcus* |
| GC | *Gonococcus* |
| GDM | gestational diabetes mellitus |
| GE | gastroesophageal, gastroenterology |
| Genit | genitalia |
| Genit/Rect | genitalia/rectum |
| GERD | gastroesophageal reflux disease |
| GFR | glomerular filtration rate |
| GGT | γ-glutamyl transferase |
| GI | gastrointestinal |
| GN | glomerulonephritis |
| GP | gravida para |
| GPA | gravida para abortions |
| GSW | gunshot wound |
| gtt | drops (*guttae*) |
| GTT | glucose tolerance test |
| GU | genitourinary |
| GVHD | graft-versus-host disease |
| Gyn | gynecology |
| **H** | |
| H2RAs | histamine-2-receptor antagonists (or blockers) |
| H/A | headache |
| HAART | highly reactive retroviral therapy |
| HAV | Hepatitis A virus |
| Hb, hgb | hemoglobin |
| $HbA_{1c}$ | glycosylated hemoglobin |
| HBsAg | surface antigen of hepatitis B virus |
| HBV | Hepatitis B virus |
| HCG | human chorionic gonadotropin |
| $HCO_3$ | bicarbonate |
| Hct | hematocrit |
| HCTZ | hydrochlorothiazide |
| HCV | Hepatitis C virus |
| Hcy | homocysteine |
| HD | Hodgkin disease, hemodialysis |
| HDL | high-density lipoprotein |
| HEENT | head, eyes, ears, nose, throat |
| HGH | human growth hormone |

| HH | hiatal hernia |
|---|---|
| Hib | *Haemophilus influenzae* type B |
| HIV | human immunodeficiency virus |
| HJR | hepatojugular reflux |
| HLA | human leukocyte antigen |
| H/O | history of |
| HPA | hypothalamic-pituitary axis |
| hpf, HPF | high-power field |
| HPI | history of present illness |
| HR | heart rate |
| HRT | hormone replacement therapy |
| HS | at bedtime (*hora somni*) |
| HSM | hepatosplenomegaly |
| HSV | Herpes simplex virus |
| HTN | hypertension |
| HT, Ht | height |
| Hx | history |
| **I** | |
| IBD | inflammatory bowel disease |
| IBW | ideal body weight |
| ICP | intracranial pressure |
| ICS | intercostal space |
| ICU | intensive care unit |
| IF | intrinsic factor |
| IFN | interferon |
| IHD | ischemic heart disease |
| IM | intramuscular, infectious mononucleosis |
| INH | isoniazid |
| INR | international normalized ratio |
| Ins | insulin |
| IOP | intra-ocular pressure |
| IP | intraperitoneal |
| ISH | isolated systolic hypertension |
| ITP | idiopathic thrombocytopenic purpura |
| IU | international unit |
| IUD | intrauterine device |
| IV | intravenous |
| IVC | inferior vena cava |
| IVDA | intravenous drug abuse |
| IVDU | intravenous drug use |
| IVF | intravenous fluids |
| IVIG | intravenous immunoglobulin |
| **J** | |
| JVD | jugular venous distension |
| JVP | jugular venous pressure |

| | |
|---|---|
| **K** | |
| KCL | potassium chloride |
| KOH | potassium hydroxide |
| **L** | |
| L | liter |
| LAD | left anterior descending |
| LBP | low back pain |
| LCM | left costal margin |
| LDH | lactic dehydrogenase |
| LDL | low-density lipoprotein |
| LE | lower extremity |
| LES | lower esophageal sphincter |
| LFT | liver function test |
| LH | luteinizing hormone |
| LHRH | luteinizing hormone-releasing hormone |
| LIQ | lower inner quadrant |
| LLE | left lower extremity |
| LLL | left lower lobe |
| LLQ | left lower quadrant |
| LLSB | left lower sternal border |
| LMP | last menstrual period |
| LN | lymph nodes |
| LOC | loss of consciousness |
| LOQ | lower outer quadrant |
| LOS | length of stay |
| LP | lumbar puncture |
| LR | lactated Ringer's |
| LS | lumbosacral |
| LTCF | long-term care facility |
| LUE | left upper extremity |
| LUL | left upper lobe |
| LUQ | left upper quadrant |
| LVH | left ventricular hypertrophy |
| Lymphs | lymphocytes |
| **M** | |
| mcg, μg | microgram |
| MCH | mean corpuscular hemoglobin |
| MCHC | mean corpuscular hemoglobin concentration |
| MCP | metacarpophalangeal |
| MCV | mean corpuscular volume |
| MDI | metered-dose inhaler |
| MEFR | maximum expiratory flow rate |
| mEq, meq | milliequivalent |
| mg | milligram |
| MI | myocardial infarction, mitral insufficiency |
| mL | milliliter |

| MM | multiple myeloma |
|---|---|
| MMA | methylmalonic acid |
| MMR | measles-mumps-rubella |
| MMSE | Mini Mental Status Examination |
| MOM | milk of magnesia |
| Monos | monocyte |
| m/r/g | murmur/rub/gallop |
| MRI | magnetic resonance imaging |
| MS | mental status, mitral stenosis, musculoskeletal, multiple sclerosis |
| MSE | mental status examination |
| MTD | maximum tolerated dose |
| MTP | metatarsophalangeal |
| MTX | methotrexate |
| MUD | matched unrelated donor |
| MVA | motor vehicle accident |
| MVI | multivitamin |
| MVR | mitral valve replacement |
| **N** | |
| N&V, N/V | nausea and vomiting |
| NA | not available |
| NAD | no acute (or apparent) distress |
| NC | normocephalic |
| N/C | non-contributory, nasal cannula |
| NC/AT | normocephalic, atraumatic |
| ND | non-distended |
| Neuro | neurologic |
| Neutros | neutrophils |
| NG | nasogastric |
| NHL | Non-Hodgkin's lymphoma |
| NKA | no known allergies |
| NKDA | no known drug allergies |
| NL | normal |
| NNRTI | non-nucleoside reverse transcriptase inhibitor |
| NOS | not otherwise specified |
| NPH | neutral protamine Hagedorn |
| NRTI | nucleoside reverse transcriptase inhibitor |
| NS | normal saline |
| NSAID | nonsteroidal anti-inflammatory drug |
| NSCLC | non-small cell lung cancer |
| NSR | normal sinus rhythm |
| NT | non-tender |
| NT/ND | non-tender, non-distended |
| NTG | nitroglycerin |
| NVD | nausea/vomiting/diarrhea |
| **O** | |
| OA | osteoarthritis |
| OB | obstetrics |

| OCD | obsessive-compulsive disorder |
|---|---|
| OGT | oral glucose tolerance test |
| OHTx | orthotopic heart transplantation |
| OLTx | orthotopic liver transplantation |
| O/P | oropharynx |
| OSA | obstructive sleep apnea |
| OTC | over-the-counter |
| **P** | |
| P | pulse |
| P & A | percussion and auscultation |
| PaCO$_2$, PCO$_2$ | arterial carbon dioxide tension |
| PaO$_2$, PO$_2$ | arterial oxygen tension |
| PAT | paroxysmal atrial tachycardia |
| PC | after meals (*post cibum*) |
| PCKD | polycystic kidney disease |
| PCN | penicillin |
| PCOS | polycystic ovarian syndrome |
| PCP | *Pneumocystis carinii* pneumonia, primary care provider |
| PCR | polymerase chain reaction |
| PD | Parkinson disease |
| PDA | patent ductus arteriosus |
| PE | physical examination, pulmonary embolism |
| PEFR | peak expiratory flow rate |
| PERLA | pupils equal, reactive to light and accommodation |
| PERRLA | pupils equal, round, and reactive to light and accommodation |
| PET | positron emission tomography |
| PFT | pulmonary function test |
| pH | hydrogen ion concentration |
| Phos | phosphate |
| PID | pelvic inflammatory disease |
| PIP | proximal interphalangeal |
| PKU | phenylketonuria |
| PMH | past medical history |
| PMI | point of maximal impulse |
| PMN | polymorphonuclear leukocyte |
| PMS | premenstrual syndrome |
| PND | paroxysmal nocturnal dyspnea |
| po | by mouth (*per os*) |
| POAG | primary open-angle glaucoma |
| POD | post-operative day |
| POS | polycystic ovarian syndrome |
| PPBG | post-prandial blood glucose |
| ppd | packs per day |
| PPD | purified protein derivative (tuberculin skin test) |
| PPI | proton pump inhibitor |
| pr | per rectum |

| PR | progesterone receptor |
|---|---|
| PRN | when necessary, as needed (*pro re nata*) |
| PSA | prostate-specific antigen |
| PSH | past surgical history |
| PT | prothrombin time |
| PTCA | percutaneous transluminal coronary angioplasty |
| PTH | parathyroid hormone |
| PTT | partial thromboplastin time |
| PTU | propylthiouracil |
| PUD | peptic ulcer disease |
| PVC | premature ventricular contraction |
| PVD | peripheral vascular disease |
| **Q** | |
| Q | every (*quaque*) |
| QD | every day (*quaque die*) |
| QID | four times daily (*quater in die*) |
| QOD | every other day |
| QOL | quality of life |
| **R** | |
| RA | rheumatoid arthritis |
| RAIU | radioactive iodine uptake |
| RBC | red blood cell |
| RCA | right coronary artery |
| RCM | right costal margin |
| Rect | rectum |
| REM | rapid eye movement |
| RF | rheumatoid factor, renal failure, rheumatic fever |
| RHD | rheumatic heart disease |
| R & L | right and left |
| RLE | right lower extremity |
| RLL | right lower lobe |
| RLQ | right lower quadrant |
| RML | right middle lobe |
| RNA | ribonucleic acid |
| R/O | rule out |
| ROM | range of motion |
| ROS | review of systems |
| RPGN | rapidly progressive glomerulonephritis |
| RR | respiratory rate |
| RRR | regular rate and rhythm |
| RSV | respiratory syncytial virus |
| RT | radiation therapy |
| RT-PCR | reverse transcriptase-polymerase chain reaction |
| RUE | right upper extremity |
| RUL | right upper lobe |
| RUQ | right upper quadrant |

| **S** | |
|---|---|
| SA | sinoatrial |
| SAH | subarachnoid hemorrhage |
| SaO$_2$ | arterial oxygen percent saturation |
| SBO | small bowel obstruction |
| SBP | systolic blood pressure |
| SC | subcutaneous, subclavian |
| SCID | severe combined immunodeficiency disease |
| SCLC | small cell lung cancer |
| SEM | systolic ejection murmur |
| SG | specific gravity |
| SH | social history |
| SIADH | syndrome of inappropriate antidiuretic hormone secretion |
| SIDS | sudden infant death syndrome |
| SL | sublingual |
| SLE | systemic lupus erythematosus |
| SOB | shortness of breath |
| S/P | status post |
| SPF | sun protection factor |
| SQ | subcutaneous |
| SRI | serotonin reuptake inhibitor |
| SSRI | selective serotonin reuptake inhibitor |
| STD | sexually transmitted disease |
| SVC | superior vena cava |
| SVT | supraventricular tachycardia |
| SWI | surgical wound infection |
| Sx | symptoms |
| **T** | |
| T | temperature |
| T & A | tonsillectomy and adenoidectomy |
| TAH | total abdominal hysterectomy |
| TB | tuberculosis |
| TCA | tricyclic antidepressant |
| TCN | tetracycline |
| TED | thromboembolic disease |
| TFT | thyroid function test |
| TG | triglyceride |
| THA | total hip arthroplasty |
| THC | tetrahydrocannabinol (cannabis, marijuana) |
| TIA | transient ischemic attack |
| TIBC | total iron-binding capacity |
| TID | three times daily (*ter in die*) |
| TIH | tumor-induced hypercalcemia |
| TLC | total lung capacity |
| TM | tympanic membrane |
| TMJ | temporomandibular joint |

| TMP-SMX | trimethoprim-sulfamethoxazole |
|---------|-------------------------------|
| TNTC | too numerous to count |
| TPR | temperature, pulse, respiration |
| Trig | triglyceride |
| TSH | thyroid-stimulating hormone |
| TTP | thrombotic thrombocytopenic purpura |
| TUIP | transurethral incision of the prostate |
| TURP | transurethral resection of the prostate |
| Tx | treatment |
| **U** | |
| UA | urinalysis, uric acid |
| UC | ulcerative colitis |
| UCD | usual childhood diseases |
| UE | upper extremity |
| UGI | upper gastrointestinal |
| UIQ | upper inner quadrant |
| UOQ | upper outer quadrant |
| URI | upper respiratory infection |
| USP | United States Pharmacopeia |
| UTI | urinary tract infection |
| UV | ultraviolet |
| **V** | |
| VC | vital capacity |
| VDRL | Venereal Disease Research Laboratory |
| VF | ventricular fibrillation |
| VLDL | very low-density lipoprotein |
| VS | vital signs |
| VSS | vital signs stable |
| VT | ventricular tachycardia |
| VTE | venous thromboembolism |
| **W** | |
| WBC | white blood cell |
| W/C | wheelchair |
| WDWN | well-developed, well-nourished |
| WNL | within normal limits |
| w/o | without |
| WT, wt | weight |
| **X** | |
| **Y** | |
| yo | year-old |
| **Z** | |
| Z | zidovudine |

(Source: Medical Abbreviations Dictionary, mediLexicon website, www.medilexicon.com/medicalabbreviations.php)

# APPENDIX F. TABLE OF APGAR SCORING FOR NEWBORNS

## APGAR SCORING FOR NEWBORNS

A score is given for each sign at one minute and five minutes after birth. If there are problems with the newborn, an additional score is given at 10 minutes. A score of 7–10 is considered normal, while a score of 4–7 might require some resuscitative measures. An infant with an APGAR of 3 or less requires immediate resuscitation.

| SIGNS | 0 | 1 | 2 | 1-MINUTE SCORE | 5-MINUTE SCORE |
|---|---|---|---|---|---|
| **Heart rate** | Absent | Below 100 | Above 100 | | |
| **Respiratory effort** | Absent | Slow, irregular | Good, crying | | |
| **Muscle tone** | Limp | Some flexion of extremities | Active motion | | |
| **Reflex irritability Response to catheter in nostril (tested after oropharynx is clear)** | No response | Grimace | Cough, sneeze | | |
| **Color** | Blue, pale | Body pink, extremities blue | Completely pink | | |
| | | | **TOTAL SCORE :** | | |

(Source: Apgar V, A proposal for a new method for evaluation of the newborn infant. Curr Res Anesth Analg 1953;32:260–267.)

**QUALITY OF LIFE IN EPILEPSY:**     **QOLIE-31** (*Version 1.0*)

Today's Date    _____ / _____ / _____ /
                   mm      dd      yy

Name      _____

Age      _____ (years)

## INSTRUCTIONS

The QOLIE-31 is a survey of health-related quality of life for adults (18 years or older) with epilepsy. Adolescents (ages 11-17 years) should complete the QOLIE-AD-48, designed for that age group. This questionnaire should be completed only by the person who has epilepsy (not a relative or friend) because no one else knows how YOU feel.

There are 31 questions about your health and daily activities. Answer every question by circling the appropriate number (1, 2, 3...). If you are unsure about how to answer a question, please give the best answer you can and write a comment or explanation on the side of the page. These notes may be useful if you discuss the QOLIE-31 with your doctor. Completing the QOLIE-31 before and after treatment changes may help you and your doctor understand how the changes have affected your life.

1. Overall, how would you rate your quality of life?

*(Circle one number on the scale below)*

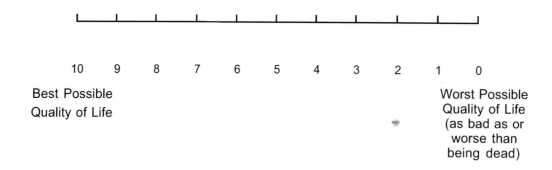

| 10 | 9 | 8 | 7 | 6 | 5 | 4 | 3 | 2 | 1 | 0 |

Best Possible Quality of Life                                    Worst Possible Quality of Life (as bad as or worse than being dead)

These questions are about how you **FEEL** and how things have been for you during the **past 4 weeks**. For each question, please indicate the one answer that comes closest to the way you have been feeling.

How much of the time during the **past 4 weeks...**

*(Circle one number on each line)*

|  |  | All of the time | Most of the time | A good bit of the time | Some of the time | A little of the time | None of the time |
|---|---|---|---|---|---|---|---|
| 2. | Did you feel full of pep? | 1 | 2 | 3 | 4 | 5 | 6 |
| 3. | Have you been a very nervous person? | 1 | 2 | 3 | 4 | 5 | 6 |
| 4. | Have you felt so down in the dumps that nothing could cheer you up? | 1 | 2 | 3 | 4 | 5 | 6 |
| 5. | Have you felt calm and peaceful? | 1 | 2 | 3 | 4 | 5 | 6 |
| 6. | Did you have a lot of energy? | 1 | 2 | 3 | 4 | 5 | 6 |
| 7. | Have you felt downhearted and blue? | 1 | 2 | 3 | 4 | 5 | 6 |
| 8. | Did you feel worn out? | 1 | 2 | 3 | 4 | 5 | 6 |
| 9. | Have you been a happy person? | 1 | 2 | 3 | 4 | 5 | 6 |
| 10. | Did you feel tired? | 1 | 2 | 3 | 4 | 5 | 6 |
| 11. | Have you worried about having another seizure? | 1 | 2 | 3 | 4 | 5 | 6 |
| 12. | Did you have difficulty reasoning and solving problems (such as making plans, making decisions, learning new things)? | 1 | 2 | 3 | 4 | 5 | 6 |
| 13. | Has your health limited your social activities (such as visiting with friends or close relatives)? | 1 | 2 | 3 | 4 | 5 | 6 |

14. How has the **QUALITY OF YOUR LIFE** been during the **past 4 weeks** (that is, how have things been going for you)?

*(Circle one number)*

| Very well: could hardly be better | Pretty good | Good & bad parts about equal | Pretty bad | Very bad: could hardly be worse |
|---|---|---|---|---|
| 1 | 2 | 3 | 4 | 5 |

The following question is about **MEMORY**.

*(Circle one number)*

| | Yes, a great deal | Yes, somewhat | Only a little | No, not at all |
|---|---|---|---|---|
| 15. In the past 4 weeks, have you had any trouble with your memory? | 1 | 2 | 3 | 4 |

Circle one number for **how often** in the **past 4 weeks** you have had trouble *remembering* or **how often** this memory problem has interfered with your normal work or living.

| | All of the time | Most of the time | A good bit of the time | Some of the time | A little of the time | None of the time |
|---|---|---|---|---|---|---|
| 16. Trouble remembering things people tell you | 1 | 2 | 3 | 4 | 5 | 6 |

The following questions are about **CONCENTRATION** problems you may have. Circle one number for **how often** in the **past 4 weeks** you had trouble concentrating or **how often** these problems interfered with your normal work or living.

| | All of the time | Most of the time | A good bit of the time | Some of the time | A little of the time | None of the time |
|---|---|---|---|---|---|---|
| 17. Trouble concentrating on reading | 1 | 2 | 3 | 4 | 5 | 6 |
| 18. Trouble concentrating on doing one thing at a time | 1 | 2 | 3 | 4 | 5 | 6 |

The following questions are about problems you may have with certain **ACTIVITIES**. Circle one number for **how much** during the **past 4 weeks** your epilepsy or antiepileptic medication has caused trouble with...

|  |  | A great deal | A lot | Some-what | Only a little | Not at all |
|---|---|---|---|---|---|---|
| 19. | Leisure time (such as hobbies, going out) | 1 | 2 | 3 | 4 | 5 |
| 20. | Driving | 1 | 2 | 3 | 4 | 5 |

The following questions relate to the way you **FEEL** about your **seizures.**

*(Circle one number on each line)*

|  |  | Very fearful | Somewhat fearful | Not very fearful | Not fearful at all |
|---|---|---|---|---|---|
| 21. | How fearful are you of having a seizure during the next month? | 1 | 2 | 3 | 4 |

|  |  | Worry a lot | Occasionally worry | Don't worry at all |
|---|---|---|---|---|
| 22. | Do you worry about hurting yourself during a seizure? | 1 | 2 | 3 |

|  |  | Very worried | Somewhat worried | Not very worried | Not at all worried |
|---|---|---|---|---|---|
| 23. | How worried are you about embarrassment or other social problems resulting from having a seizure during the next month? | 1 | 2 | 3 | 4 |
| 24. | How worried are you that medications you are taking will be bad for you if taken for a long time? | 1 | 2 | 3 | 4 |

For each of these **PROBLEMS**, circle one number for **how much they bother you** on a scale of 1 to 5 where 1 = Not at all bothersome, and 5 = Extremely bothersome.

|  |  | Not at all bothersome |  |  |  | Extremely bothersome |
|---|---|---|---|---|---|---|
| 25. | Seizures | 1 | 2 | 3 | 4 | 5 |
| 26. | Memory difficulties | 1 | 2 | 3 | 4 | 5 |
| 27. | Work limitations | 1 | 2 | 3 | 4 | 5 |
| 28. | Social limitations | 1 | 2 | 3 | 4 | 5 |
| 29. | Physical effects of antiepileptic medication | 1 | 2 | 3 | 4 | 5 |
| 30. | Mental effects of antiepileptic medication | 1 | 2 | 3 | 4 | 5 |

31. How good or bad do you think your health is? On the thermometer scale below, the best imaginable state of health is 10 and the worst imaginable state is 0. Please indicate how you feel about your health by circling one number on the scale. **Please consider your epilepsy as part of your health when you answer this question.**
    *(Circle one number on the scale below)*

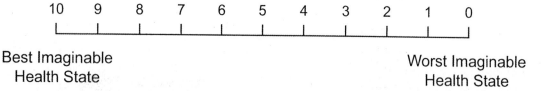

<table>
<tr><td>10</td><td>9</td><td>8</td><td>7</td><td>6</td><td>5</td><td>4</td><td>3</td><td>2</td><td>1</td><td>0</td></tr>
</table>

Best Imaginable
Health State

Worst Imaginable
Health State

(*Source*: Rand Health website, www.rand.org/health/surveys_tools/qolie/. Disclaimer: The authorization of the use of this survey is in no way an endorsement of the commercial product being tested or the trial.)